Hospital Departmental Profiles

Third Edition

Edited by Alan J. Goldberg and Raymond A. Buttaro,
*Applied Management Systems, Inc., for the Healthcare Information
and Management Systems Society of the American Hospital Association*

AHA ®

**American Hospital Publishing, Inc.,
a wholly owned subsidiary
of the American Hospital Association**

The views expressed in this publication are strictly those of the authors and do not necessarily represent official positions of the American Hospital Association.

Library of Congress Cataloging-in-Publication Data

Hospital departmental profiles / edited by Alan J. Goldberg and Raymond
    A. Buttaro for the Healthcare Information and Management Systems Society
    of the American Hospital Association.—3rd ed.
       p.   cm.
    Includes bibliographical references.
    ISBN 1-55648-043-1
    1. Hospitals—Administration.   2. Industrial engineering.   I. Goldberg,
Alan J.   II. Buttaro, Raymond A.   III. Healthcare Information and
Management Systems Society.
    [DNLM: 1. Hospital Departments—organization & administration.
WX   150   H8245]
RA971.H5933   1990
362.1'1'068—dc20
DNLM/DLC   89-18510
for Library of Congress   CIP

Catalog no. 133122

©1990 by American Hospital Publishing, Inc.,
a wholly owned subsidiary of the
American Hospital Association

Printed in the USA

AHA is a service mark of the American Hospital Association used under license by American Hospital Publishing, Inc.

Text set in English Times
5M—03/90—0255

Richard Hill, Project Editor
Sophie Yarborough, Editorial Assistant
Marcia Bottoms, Managing Editor
Peggy DuMais, Production Coordinator
Marcia Vecchione, Designer
Brian Schenk, Books Division Director

Contents

List of Figures

List of Tables

About the Editors

Alan J. Goldberg is the president of Applied Management Systems, Inc., of Burlington, Massachusetts, a major provider of operational management consulting and receivables management support to the health care industry. Mr. Goldberg has been president of the company since 1985 and has been affiliated with it since 1976. He concentrates his activity on the corporate responsibilities of business development, administration, and financial management. Like everyone in the company, he also performs client work. His specialty areas include productivity assessments, operation audits, and physicians' issues.

Mr. Goldberg is a former adjunct professor at Providence College in Providence, Rhode Island, and at the Rensselaer Polytechnic Institute Graduate School of Management in Troy, New York. He is the author of numerous articles in *Hospitals, Medical Laboratory Observers, Health Services Research,* and *Hospital Energy Strategies.* Most recently he coauthored a chapter with Raymond Buttaro in *Productivity and Performance Management in Health Care Institutions* (Chicago: American Hospital Publishing, 1989). Mr. Goldberg served as an editor of both prior editions of *Hospital Departmental Profiles* and in 1984 received the Technical Publication Award of the Hospital Management Systems Society of the American Hospital Association for the book.

Mr. Goldberg's current affiliations include the American Hospital Association, the American College of Healthcare Executives, the Association of Healthcare Enterprises, the Massachusetts Hospital Association, and the New England Healthcare Assembly. In addition, he serves on the board of directors of the Health Care Management Association of Massachusetts, and he is a fellow and past national president and chairman of the board of directors of the Healthcare Information and Management Systems Society.

Raymond A. Buttaro is a manager with Applied Management Systems, Inc. He is a member of the Healthcare Information and Management Systems Society and has written and presented numerous technical papers on health care issues. He coauthored the chapter entitled "Management Systems: A Key Part of the Productivity Strategy" for *Productivity and Performance Management in Health Care Institutions.*

Special Note

The HAS/MONITREND™ System is a comparative, monthly data program providing utilization, financial, and productivity data for all areas of the hospital. The data presented in this book are for an average month within the six-month period ending December 1988. These data may be used as a frame of reference for comparing a hospital's performance with a group of similar hospitals for the same period; however, these data are not intended as standards.

The data presented in this book are medians for national bed size groups. The data are also for a given point in time. If the hospital is a MONITREND II participant, the current MONITREND II monthly report should be examined because data values may change over time. For more information on the HAS/MONITREND II System, contact the Healthcare Administrative Services (HAS) division of the American Hospital Association at 800/621-8096; in Illinois, 312/280-6485.

Preface

The hospital of the 1990s is very different from the hospital of the 1980s. Sophisticated changes in equipment, data technologies, staff skills, patient expectations, service delivery models, and reimbursement methodologies have all contributed to this difference. These changes are most evident in how certain hospital departments operate and what goals and objectives they have.

The objective of this book is to present a brief but current description of how departments or major functions of the hospital are typically organized and what methods and techniques can be used to get the work done. The description is not intended to be an extensive academic review or to present a theoretical discussion of each department. In reality, the actual operation of departments is conducted in different ways in different hospitals. Yet, the overall purpose, goals, and desired outcomes are not different.

The profiles begin with an overview and then lead readers through a discussion of organization and staffing, models and systems, situations and problems, and approaches to departmental analyses. As each area is described, information is also presented on how it relates to the hospital as a whole.

Because this is the third edition of the book, it has a history to it. The book originally evolved from an internal training manual developed by Applied Management Systems, Inc. (AMS), a wholly owned subsidiary of the Massachusetts Hospital Association, in the late 1970s. Believing that the information might be useful to a wide audience in the health care field, AMS released the material to what is now called the Healthcare Information and Management Systems Society for the development of the original manuscript.

The third edition is a significant step forward from our previous work. New chapters profile such departments as clinical engineering, marketing, the medical staff office, public relations, quality assurance, renal dialysis, and risk management. In addition, the book presents extensively revised and rewritten chapters on admissions/registration, ambulatory services, fiscal services, information systems, the laboratory, planning, radiation therapy, respiratory care, the surgical suite, and telecommunications. For the first time, this book includes samples of recent MONITREND data for various functional reporting centers. The book also presents an expanded and updated bibliography. The end result, we hope, is a reference tool that is even more useful in the day-to-day activities of our readership.

Acknowledgments

Since its original publication as a 19-chapter book in 1982, this text has grown in sophistication and nearly doubled in size. To produce a book that now includes 37 profiles has proved to be a monumental task for a group of people volunteering their time and expertise.

This book would not exist today without the significant advice and assistance of Richard P. Covert, Ph.D., of the Healthcare Information and Management Systems Society of the American Hospital Association. Dick was the driving force behind the first edition. We will never forget the joy and mutual satisfaction we shared over the telephone when the first book was released. As this book enters its third edition, Dick continues to offer his guidance to ensure its high quality and usefulness.

Robert A. DeNoble, now of McLean Hospital, Belmont, Massachusetts, brought an increased depth of coverage to the expanded second edition. We know that if Bob were still with us at Applied Management Systems, he too would have been actively involved in this edition. Of course, the third edition could also not exist without the hard work and contributions of the many other individuals gratefully acknowledged in the earlier editions.

The staff of Applied Management Systems labored on this third edition for an entire year, for which we want to express our heartfelt thanks. The following persons were responsible for writing or contributing new or updated information to various profiles of this book: Raymond Buttaro and Kurt Hamke (Introduction); Paul Brzozowski (Administration); Thomas Webb and Thomas Souliotis (Admissions/Registration); Philip Ortolani and Charles Dayhoff (Ambulatory Services); Arthur Lambert (Cardiac Catheterization Laboratory); Eugene McCarthy (Central Services); Charles Dayhoff (Electroencephalography and Electrocardiology); Raymond Buttaro and Michael Foley (Emergency); Alan Goldberg (Energy Management and Maintenance); Charles Dayhoff and Kurt Hamke (Environmental Services); Thomas Souliotis, Thomas Webb, and Doc Fouts (Fiscal Services); Raymond Buttaro and Richard McNeil (Food Services); John O'Brien and Alan Goldberg (Human Resources/Personnel); Patrick Abrami (Information Systems); Donna Watson, RN, and Arthur Lambert (Intensive Care Units); Paul Brzozowski and Michael Foley (Laboratory); Raymond Buttaro and Richard McNeil (Laundry); Richard McNeil and Michael Nix (Maintenance); Michael Nix (Marketing); Patrick Abrami and Michael Nix (Materials Management); Eugene McCarthy (Medical Records, Medical Staff Office); Arthur Lambert and Donna Watson, RN (Nursing Service); Michael Foley and Paul Brzozowski (Pharmacy); Richard McNeil (Physical Therapy); Frances Charles, RN (Quality Assurance); Patrick Abrami and Thomas Webb (Radiation Therapy); Daniel Huntoon and Michael Foley (Radiology); Daniel Huntoon (Renal Dialysis); Daniel Huntoon and Philip Ortolani (Respiratory Care); Michael Nix (Risk Management); Philip Ortolani and Charles Dayhoff (Social Services); Donna Watson, RN, and Eugene McCarthy (Surgical Suite); Daniel Huntoon (Telecommunications); and Patrick Abrami (Transportation). Their work on this book was supported by a dedicated and effective office staff, of whom we'd particularly like to recognize Robin Allaby, Stawn Barber, Marie Murphy, Cynthia Tyndall, and Barbara Wedge. Without their unflagging and enthusiastic participation, this effort would have been less enjoyable.

In addition, a number of professionals at various institutions throughout the country contributed to the writing of many of these chapters. We offer their names here in grateful acknowledgment: Suzanne Lopes, director of materials management, Charlton Memorial Hospital, Fall River, Massachusetts (Central Services); Raymond Zambuto, president, Technology in Medicine, Holliston, Massachusetts (Clinical Engineering); Frank Werbinski, vice-president, Cheshire Medical Center, Keene, New Hampshire, and Edward Cummings, manager of plant engineering and maintenance, Beth Israel Hospital, Boston, Massachusetts (Maintenance); Jo Ellen Mistarz, project director, The Catholic Health Alliance for Metropolitan Chicago, Chicago, Illinois, and Scott Mason, president, National Health Advisors, Vienna, Virginia (Planning); Patricia Powell, nurse manager, outpatient chronic hemodialysis, and Joyce A. Sweet, nurse manager, dialysis home training, The Medical Center of Central Massachusetts-Memorial Hospital, Worcester, Massachusetts (Renal Dialysis); John Pace, director of respiratory care, cardiology, and neurology services, Memorial Hospital of Carbondale, Carbondale, Illinois (Respiratory Care); Murray Edge, director of risk management, University of Tennessee Memorial Hospital, Knoxville, Tennessee (Risk Management); Chris Carpenter, director of social work, Mid Maine Medical Center, Waterville, Maine (Social Services); and Noreen Malloy, director of communications, Charlton Memorial Hospital, Fall River, Massachusetts, and Edward Blythe, owner/operator, CS&M Tele-Systems, Tiverton, Rhode Island (Telecommunications). We would also like to thank the American Medical Technologists and the American Society of Electroencephalographic Technologists for their contributions to the second edition profiles on the Laboratory and the Electroencephalography and Electrocardiology Departments, respectively.

During the writing process we received valuable assistance from a number of other individuals, whose willingness to share their expertise in generous amounts has resulted in a more accurate book. Those individuals are: Kevin Shrake, administrative director of cardiology, Memorial Medical Center, Springfield, Illinois; Sylvia McBeth, director of marketing, Cheshire Medical Center, Keene, New Hampshire; Jeff Cymrot, director of planning, Carney Hospital, Boston, Massachusetts; Sue Foley, director, quality assurance/utilization review systems, South Shore Hospital, Weymouth, Massachusetts; Bea Green, director, quality assurance, St. Luke's Hospital, New Bedford, Massachusetts; Kenneth Trester, director, office of planning and marketing, University of Michigan Medical Center, Ann Arbor, Michigan; Ira Schlesinger, director of planning and marketing, Hillcrest Medical Center, Tulsa, Oklahoma; Michael Sachs, chairman, The Sachs Group, Ltd., Evanston, Illinois; Steven Garlock, senior vice-president, U.S. Health Corporation, Columbus, Ohio; Donald Geller, director of marketing and public affairs, Boston University Medical Center, Boston, Massachusetts; Steven Kukla, regional director of financial services, Sisters of Mercy Health Corporation, West Des Moines, Iowa; Jack Gilbert, principal, Pathfinder Associates, Boyertown, Pennsylvania; and Howard Berman, president and CEO, Blue Cross-Blue Shield, Rochester, New York.

Many organizations reviewed individual chapters of this book and provided us with numerous suggestions for improvements. Those organizations include: the American Academy of Neurology, the National Association of Hospital Admitting Managers, the American Organization for Nursing Executives, the American Society for Healthcare Central Services Personnel, the American Society for Healthcare Human Resources Administration, the American Society for Hospital Food Service Administrators, the American Society for Hospital Materials Management, the Society for Hospital Social Work Directors, the Society for Hospital Marketing and Public Relations, the American Society for Healthcare Environmental Services, the American Society for Healthcare Risk Management, and the Joint Commission on Accreditation of Healthcare Organizations.

We also received assistance from several offices of the American Hospital Association, especially: the AHA Resource Center, the Division of Ambulatory Care and Health Promotion, the Center for Nursing, the Division of Clinical Services and Technology, the Division of Strategic Planning and Marketing, the Division of Health Facilities Management, the Division of Quality Control Management, the Section for Rehabilitation Hospitals and Programs, the Hospital Research and Educational Trust, the Healthcare Information and Management Systems Society, the Division of Medical Affairs, and the Office of Legal and Regulatory Affairs. We are especially grateful to Healthcare Administrative Services and its senior project specialist, Karen McGannon, for providing us with the MONITREND data appearing in selected chapters of this book.

Our list of acknowledgments would not be complete without offering sincere thanks to the staff of American Hospital Publishing, Inc., with whom we worked closely on this project over the past few years. In particular, we want to recognize Richard Hill, project editor; Brian Schenk, books division director; Marcia Bottoms, managing editor; and Sophie Yarborough, editorial assistant, all of whom contributed their editorial and administrative expertise to the work of preparing this new edition. We also want to thank Joseph Kubal and Mark Harju for their keen study of consumer perceptions of the second edition. Their findings helped us immeasurably in planning a new edition that would serve our readers' needs more fully.

Finally, we wish to acknowledge our gratitude to our families, whose support and encouragement were vital to the completion of the third edition. We therefore dedicate this book to our wives, Beverly Goldberg and Sheila Buttaro, and to our children, Jimmy and Marissa Goldberg and Andrew and Katelyn Buttaro.

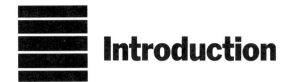

Introduction

A hospital is a large and complex organization. Because each of its many departments performs a different function, each experiences different problems. However, the methods of analyzing and solving such problems may involve similar concepts. This book includes brief profiles of most major departments or areas of the hospital. It explains their organization, functions, and procedures. This book also provides an overview of the systems used in managing personnel, materials, equipment, and information in each department; describes some of the problems that arise in these systems; and suggests topics for management engineering analysis.

A departmental analysis is an assessment of the effectiveness and efficiency of a selected hospital service or area. A combination of managerial and scientific measurement techniques is employed to evaluate, and possibly improve, the department's objectives and operations. The following areas of concern are addressed in a departmental analysis.

Departmental Objectives

The initial step in conducting a departmental analysis is to determine the objectives of the service. Although departmental objectives may be self-evident for surgery and radiology, other departments such as admissions/registration may operate in a multiobjective mode. The identification of all departmental objectives is a prerequisite for progress in the analysis. This initial step should cover such factors as weekend staffing, hours of operation, and special services.

Internal Organization

Once the departmental objectives have been determined, an analysis of the internal organization should be undertaken. The primary purpose of this analysis is to determine whether the department is structured appropriately to meet its objectives. The secondary purpose is to evaluate the span and scope of controls practiced by department members in key positions. Key positions are determined by a review of the department's organizational chart. Excessive or highly limited spans of control should be identified and changes should be proposed.

Policies and Procedures

A review of the department's policies and procedures manual should be made to ensure that all policies and procedures relate to both the hospital's and the department's objectives. The manual should be made available to all department and administrative personnel so that mutual expectations may be developed by department managers and employees. Whenever possible, clearly defined service expectations and requirements should be identified.

Human Resource Utilization

Next, a list of all tasks performed by department members and the time needed to perform those tasks should be compiled. Various methods exist for the determination of task times: supervisors' estimates, time studies, and so forth. A method should be chosen that balances the amount of analysis involved with the depth of detail required. Key tasks should be identified because the department's future labor performance may be tied to these indicative functions.

The task list and associated times are the focal points for determining current staff utilization. Comparing the task times and frequencies with the available staff hours provides the current labor utilization level. When this level consistently exceeds 100 percent, a check of overtime hours and delayed tasks should be made. When tasks are being delayed or overtime hours are being worked, one or more of the following actions should be taken: work (tasks) should be simplified, tasks should be eliminated, or personnel should be added. Should consistently low levels of labor performance be identified, the following actions are recommended: worthwhile functions should be added, or personnel should be reduced.

Related Systems Interactions

In addition to a review of all activities inside the department, an assessment of related systems interactions should be performed. For most departments, any modification of activities affects other departments in the hospital; therefore, a complete departmental analysis should include a review of interactions with other departments. These interactions may occur in the form of communications (both oral and written), products (such as the meal trays provided to patients by the food service department), or services (such as the transportation of patients to the radiology department), among many others. The most effective methods of identifying these interactions entail the departmental activity list and interviews with the department manager.

Because poor performance in one area often has an impact on other areas, systems and productivity should be optimized at the hospital level. It is often possible to improve performance in one area by transferring work or reducing service levels, although this approach may not result in the most cost-effective solution from a hospitalwide perspective.

Management Information Systems

Once an evaluation of a department is complete, the department's managers should be able to evaluate departmental performance on an ongoing basis. To be the most effective tool for managers, the analysis should have led to the implementation of management information systems. These systems are designed to provide feedback to managers by measuring the quality and quantity of work performed by the department. Managers then can translate this information into a measure of efficiency and effectiveness. A procedure should be established to keep these information systems up-to-date.

Work Environment Issues

The environment in which work is performed has a direct relationship to its quality and quantity. An evaluation of the complete work environment (as well as key work stations) should be included in any departmental analysis. Improvements in the work environment generally have a positive effect on work quantity and quality. This step should include a review of the department's layout and the flow through the area assessed (paper, staff, patient, and work).

In addition to a generalized evaluation of the work environment, a review of specific locations may be in order. Specific functions may require access to selected facilities. Easy access to these facilities should be ensured so that the staff can perform its tasks properly.

Safety issues should always be reviewed as well. Hospitals operate under a strict set of safety regulations, and knowledge of these regulations will help ensure a thorough evaluation of any work environment.

Conclusion

A strong departmental analysis should be based on an evaluation of the following factors:

- Departmental objectives
- Internal organization
- Policies and procedures
- Departmental tasks and corresponding times
- Frequency of task completion
- Staffing levels (including minimum staffing)
- Skill levels
- Interaction with other departments
- Service expectations
- Management information
- Work environment

Each departmental analysis will present a new challenge. The inclusion of these 11 areas, as well as the development and execution of a plan to address the uniqueness of the department, will ensure a strong and useful analysis that benefits the entire institution.

Administration

Overview

Hospital administration has become increasingly complex in the past 10 years because of significant changes in the following areas: social forces affecting health care, medical staff relations, medical technology, and federal government initiatives regarding health care reimbursement. As a result, the roles, tasks, and responsibilities of hospital administrators continue to undergo significant changes. In the current hospital environment, the function of a hospital administrator could be described as "shooting at a moving target."

A hospital's administrative staff is made up of a group of individuals who are responsible for continually striving toward and eventually attaining the hospital's objectives through the work of others. No one individual has all the knowledge and know-how needed to manage all the activities of a hospital. Therefore, a group of individuals is assembled, each of whom has some special skill or knowledge of a specific activity, such as finance, planning, or operations. The group collectively provides the necessary management support to the chief executive officer (CEO) or the president of the hospital.

The CEO or president has the ultimate legal authority and overall responsibility for making decisions on behalf of the organization and for placing the hospital in a position of effectiveness and influence in the future. He or she is retained by the hospital's board of trustees and is empowered to carry out the hospital's stated mission. The CEO is usually a member of the board and works under a management contract. In order to manage the day-to-day operations of the hospital, the CEO relies on a staff of hospital administrators who have specialized knowledge in the following areas:

- Ambulatory services
- Financial management
- Information systems
- Medical services (medical staff)
- Nursing administration
- Personnel management
- Professional services (ancillaries)
- Public affairs and community services
- Strategic planning and development
- Support services (purchasing, stores, and so forth)

The major functions of the hospital's administration are to plan and develop an effective health care team of physicians, nurses, and other health care professionals and to provide them adequate equipment and a cost-effective environment in which to provide

1

high-quality health care. This means making decisions about new health care programs, new shared services with other health care facilities, new facilities, and major capital expenditures. It also means keeping a close watch on existing facilities to ensure their efficiency and effectiveness. The administration directs the daily details of hospital operations.

In large health care facilities, the administrator or CEO supervises and coordinates the activities of as many as six to eight highly specialized administrators who manage either administrative, medical, or support services. The administrative staff may also include assistants to whom the administrator delegates certain responsibilities and authority. The staff members have titles such as vice-president, associate administrator, assistant administrator, and administrative assistant, depending on the scope of their responsibilities.

Administrators in progressive health care organizations often do not limit their roles to the management of their own institutions. They may also be active at the local, state, and national levels in professional organizations and thereby may influence national health care policies.

Organization

General administration in a hospital is organized in several different ways, with various titles and various combinations of department responsibilities, depending on the size of the hospital. Figure 1 is an organizational chart for a typical 250-bed hospital. The chart illustrates the staff positions, their functions, and their reporting relationships. Each vice-president or assistant administrator is given the responsibility of managing the day-to-day operations of specific hospital departments. Even though the department heads and supervisors in each department are not included in the chart, they are, in effect, administrators within their departments.

Many administrators use an administrative council type of organization to promote participative management. The council is made up of all vice-presidents or assistant administrators, executive vice-presidents or associate administrators, and the president or administrator. It meets once or twice a week or more often when necessary. All major problems, plans, and budgets are brought to these meetings for discussion and resolution. Each member proposes subjects or issues to be included in the agenda. Although the president or CEO is not bound to accept the advice and suggestions of the council (because the council has no legal authority to act), the council's opinions are highly valued and recognized in any final decisions that are made about hospital operations.

The council members, in turn, consult their own department heads or supervisors for key management information or advice. Thus, communication up and down the lines of organization is greatly enhanced. The president or CEO also has direct contact with personnel in all key phases of the hospital's operations. The sense of participative management and teamwork also helps make the day-to-day administration of the hospital departments smooth and efficient.

In addition to the council's advice, the hospital administrator has access to other information (such as confidential information from assistants, outside consultants, and legal experts) on which to base timely decisions that have a significant impact on the financial viability and effectiveness of the institution.

Models and Systems

Because the administrator makes hospital policy decisions that have a major impact on the future, the systems and models needed for the role are decision support and management information systems such as the following:

- Budget planning and variance system
- Purchase options (such as buy or lease models) for major equipment acquisitions

- Case mix management system (based on different definitions of case mix)
- Decision support system
- Diagnosis-related group (DRG)/case mix (reimbursement) simulation system (a model that illustrates the impact on a particular service when changes in patient population or operational characteristics occur)
- Facility planning (simulation) model
- Facility utilization review system
- Fund development or donor system
- Hospitalwide resource utilization monitoring system
- Management by objectives system (for performance review of key management employees)
- Market or program planning model (market research)
- Medical staff profile analysis system
- Operations monitoring system (management information system)
- Product costing model
- Program profitability analysis model

Figure 1. Organizational Chart for a Typical 250-Bed Hospital

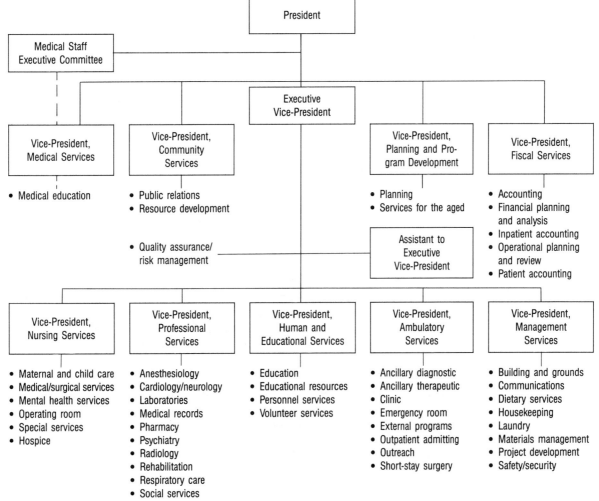

Some of these systems and models may be automated and run on microcomputers or mainframe computers, and others may use a manual system on an ad hoc basis. Most large hospitals use automated systems to provide management information such as occupancy rates, key trends in case mix, budget variances, and productivity. Small hospitals tend to depend on manual systems and their administrative staff to develop management summary reports. However, with the advent of less expensive, more efficient microcomputers, trends suggest that soon all hospitals, small and large, will have microcomputers and use computerized systems and models similar to the ones listed above. Software vendors currently market systems ready for immediate use, which eliminates necessity of laborious and costly system development work for individual hospitals.

Situations and Problems

Recent changes in the reimbursement policies of Medicare and Medicaid and strong competition from neighboring hospitals, freestanding medical centers, and ambulatory care clinics have made it necessary for hospitals to penetrate their local health care markets and increase their market share. As a consequence of the changing climate, hospital administrators have begun to recognize the need for new and additional decision support systems and planning models, which are designed to assist administrators in making rational decisions that will affect the long-term viability of the institution. Such systems and models include procedural level costing systems, expanded interhospital comparative data bases, and feasibility studies for joint ventures and alternative delivery systems (for example, regional laboratories, ambulatory surgery centers, and diagnostic imaging centers). Management engineers can provide assistance in choosing the most useful systems and models.

Departmental Analysis

In addition to the models and systems already listed, typical topics for studies that could be initiated by management engineers include the following:

- Audits of individual department operations to identify major problem areas and solutions
- Analysis of word processing, communications, and administrative systems used by administrative staff
- Strategic planning models, such as facility planning, budget planning, program planning, profitability and venture analysis (surgicenters and so forth), and market planning models
- Analysis of joint ventures with other health care facilities, such as materials management, shared information system services, shared laboratory services, and others
- Evaluation and selection of management information system software for such areas as nursing, DRG case mix, and automated patient care
- Selection of software interfaces to establish an integrated total management information system

These types of studies are ideal for management engineers because they require structural work plans and quantitative analysis. It is often necessary for studies to cross traditional lines of responsibility, and so an objective third party should be used for analysis of the hospital administration.

Admissions/Registration Department

Overview

The admissions/registration department performs reception and registration services for inpatients, outpatients, emergency department patients, same-day surgery patients, ambulatory care patients, and day care patients. In so doing, the department coordinates the patients' arrival, registration, and admissions testing. In many institutions, the department is also responsible for counseling patients about their payment obligations. In addition, the office may be responsible for the hospital's information desk and/or telephone switchboard.

As the patients' point of entry into the hospital, the admissions/registration department plays an important role in establishing the patients' first and perhaps lasting opinion of the institution. The patients' families and the general public may also form their opinions on the basis of the way the department functions.

Admissions and registration affect not only the patients, but also the hospital staff that serves them. The data collected during the admission process are vital to the quality of care provided and to the financial status of the hospital. For example, information gained in the admission interview process is the foundation for the patient's medical record; therefore, because of its effect on the quality of the medical record, the efficiency of the admission process has potential medical and legal ramifications. Data obtained during the admission process are also made available to the nursing units (patient care centers), financial services, the laboratory, utilization management personnel, physicians' offices, the medical record department, social services, respiratory care, radiology, and the food service department. All of these departments need accurate, timely information to function effectively and to provide efficient service.

The effect of the admissions/registration department on patients and on the hospital can be measured by analyzing such factors as the length of time patients must wait during processing, the confidentiality of information, the level of patient satisfaction, and the efficiency of procedures for escorting patients through testing and to their rooms. Measurable financial factors affecting the hospital in general include the accuracy of billing data, the status of accounts receivable, and the amount of lost charges. Still other factors to be measured include the timeliness of information provided to nurses, physicians, and the medical record department as well as the efficiency of admissions/registration staff members.

Admissions/Registration

The admissions/registration department performs the following activities for standard elective admissions. The procedures may be different for patients referred from the emergency department or clinics or for patients registering for ambulatory care or day care.

Reservations/Scheduling

The physician's office contacts the hospital's admissions/registration department, usually by phone, to make a reservation for a patient to be admitted. Such requests are usually made in advance, although referrals of patients may be made directly from the emergency department, the ambulatory care department, or an outpatient clinic. It is important for admissions staff to build good working relationships with physician's office personnel to be sure that they know the hospital's procedures and have the necessary forms or informational brochures to give to patients.

The priority of admissions can be set according to the degree of urgency, which is usually determined by the admitting physician. Three classifications are typically used: emergency, urgent, and elective. Emergency cases require immediate admission, and urgent cases require admission as soon as possible (usually within 72 hours or, at most, within one week). Elective admissions are scheduled in advance according to the policy of the institution. (For example, patients may be admitted in the order in which their reservations were received. Other factors may involve bed availability, patient requests, or physician availability.) Many chronic care or rehabilitation hospitals follow an application and review procedure for admission.

The admissions department checks that a bed will be available and enters the request in the booking list. For elective surgery patients, the admissions department must ensure the availability of both an operating room and a bed. A conference telephone call may be used to coordinate arrangements among the admissions department, the operating room, and the physician's office.

Some admissions/registration departments facilitate surgery and outpatient service scheduling. This is performed in collaboration and direct communication with the hospital's service departments. The function enhances patient flow while improving service to the medical staff by providing a centralized mechanism for patient scheduling.

Preadmission

Once physician's office personnel have made a reservation for the patient, the admissions office mails a preadmission form to the patient for completion or requests the information needed from the patient by telephone. At this time, insurance coverage is verified, and precertification and second opinions are obtained. When appropriate, financial screening is performed. An efficient preadmission process reduces the actual admitting time.

Many hospitals have found preadmission through the mail to be ineffective because of their limited lead time and have opted to use the telephone only. Telephone contact is also viewed by patients as being more personalized and provides a perfect opportunity to answer questions or provide information to patients before their arrival at the hospital. A similar process can be developed for the preregistration of scheduled outpatients and ambulatory care patients.

Inpatient Registration

Elective admissions are generally scheduled in the early morning for same-day surgical patients and in the early afternoon for other elective admissions. This allows sufficient time for the registration and testing procedures and helps ensure a more even flow of patient arrivals, which in turn allows for more effective scheduling of hospital staff. Occasionally, however, congestion may occur, increasing the time patients must wait to be admitted. The arrival patterns of urgent and emergency admissions are less predictable but tend to correspond with physicians' office hours and emergency department activity.

When the patient arrives at the hospital for the actual check-in process, information not obtained during the preadmission process is completed, insurance cards are photocopied, all insurance data are obtained, and release of information and consent forms are signed. Patient identification data include the patient's name, address, telephone number, and birth date.

Billing data include the method of payment, insurance policy numbers, the name of guarantor, and the name of the patient's employer. A bed and room are assigned on the basis of the medical needs of the patient. For previously admitted patients, the medical record is requested from the medical record department, or for new patients, a medical record number is assigned and a new file is established.

As part of the registration process, the patient may also receive instruction and orientation.

Admission Testing

Either before admission or during registration, patients are scheduled for the routine tests required by the hospital and other tests specified by the physician. The admissions/registration department may issue testing requisitions and charge tickets for the tests. Initial tests can be scheduled at the patient's convenience and in compliance with the hospital's guidelines.

In many cases, patients can undergo testing before being admitted to the hospital, which simplifies the admission procedure on the actual day of admission and allows test results to be reviewed before admission. Admission for pretested patients may be scheduled outside the peak admitting periods.

The use of preadmission or admission testing centers is expanding rapidly. In such centers, all testing can be performed in one location, thereby reducing the need to transport the patient to several testing areas throughout the hospital. The centers may also be expanded to include nursing admission assessment, physician history and physical assessment, patient education, and surgical preparation.

Patient Placement

The admissions/registration department coordinates the patient's room and bed assignments and may direct the route the patient takes through testing, therapy, and other types of care and ultimately to his or her room. A staff member or volunteer typically escorts the patient.

The room and bed assignments are based primarily on the medical needs of the patient. Other factors that enter into the assignments include requests from the patient or the patient's physician, the patient's age and sex, the patient's smoking/nonsmoking preference, the hospital's patient census, and other approved restrictions.

In the event that a patient is transferred to another nursing unit, the admissions/registration staff ensures that the patient is moved in a timely manner. In addition, the staff communicates the patient's individual needs to all parties.

Census Management

To maintain the patient census, the admissions/registration department records all admissions, transfers, room and bed assignments, and discharges. Timely and accurate census data are essential and are distributed to the nursing units, financial services, the pharmacy, and other hospital departments that depend on the data to plan their work load.

One system for maintaining the census depends on the use of plastic patient identification plates (similar to credit cards) embossed with the patient's name, room number, and medical record number. The plates are kept in a cardholder that has a slot for each bed number, commonly referred to as the bedboard. The card is used to record the information on charge slips and other forms, and it can be moved when the patient is transferred to another room.

Most information systems offer computerized census-tracking options as part of the admission/discharge/transfer (ADT) system. Such computerized systems typically increase the accuracy of ADT information.

Discharge Notification

When a patient is discharged, the admissions/registration department is usually notified by the nursing unit and adjusts the census status accordingly. In addition, either the admissions/

registration department or the nursing department notifies other departments of the discharge because discharges affect the work schedules of departments such as environmental services, central service, and food service. A growing trend is for the nursing unit to enter discharges into a computerized ADT system, which automatically transmits the information to the other departments.

Having access to timely discharge information is imperative for the admissions/registration staff if it is to have accurate information on available beds for incoming patients. It is also necessary for accurate billing. Problems may arise when discharge notification is slow or when all departments are not informed. For example, the pharmacy may not submit charges for billing until after financial services has submitted the insurance claims or until after the bill has been sent to the patient, which results in lost charges. Therefore, an adequate interdepartmental communication system, either manual or computerized, ensures that charges are captured, or recorded in a central location, on a daily basis or as soon as possible after the patient is discharged.

Organization and Staffing

The location of management responsibility for admissions/registration varies considerably, but it is typically assigned to administrative services or financial services. With recent changes in reimbursement systems, there has been movement toward having admissions/registration report to the chief financial officer (CFO). The department manager is often called the director of registration, the director of admissions, or more recently, the director of patient access services.

Much of the work in the admissions/registration department is performed by personnel with titles such as admissions interviewer, registrar, coordinator, counselor, and registration representative. These personnel should have good general office skills, a working knowledge of medical terminology and medical insurance, and most important, excellent communication and interpersonal skills. They also need to be able to coordinate their duties well. Effective personnel are empathetic to the needs of patients and their families, who are typically uneasy about the prospect of being admitted to the hospital and are often confused. The admissions/registration staff's ability to convey information on hospital policies and procedures at the same time it shows compassion enhances the hospital's image.

Training should include orientation to billing processes, medical terminology and procedures, medical record procedures, nursing services, ancillary services, insurance precertification requirements, and hospital reimbursement policies. Nurses or other professional staff members may also perform the registration function. In such cases, they may have either a full spectrum of responsibilities or such specific duties as patient orientation, test requisitioning, and nursing assessment.

The inpatient admission process is a seven-day-a-week, 24-hour-a-day function. However, coverage during off-shifts varies, depending on the size of the hospital. In many smaller hospitals, after-hours coverage (11 p.m. to 7 a.m.) may be performed by the nursing staff or the emergency department registration staff.

The key to effective personnel utilization is matching staff schedules to patient arrival patterns. This can be accomplished through collecting data on patient arrivals by hour of the day and patient type to determine demand work load. Staff schedules should match this demand pattern.

Alternative Systems

The growing number of patients and the increasing informational requirements for admission, billing, and medical records have resulted in considerable growth in the admissions/registration function. In the past, admissions/registration was a manual operation that used typewriters, card systems, and manual filing. Today, the admissions function has become more and more computerized, with linkage to the hospital's billing and patient care information systems.

Among the options available to hospitals is centralizing or decentralizing the registration process. In a centralized system, all patients are registered at a central registration desk by personnel dedicated to this function. In a decentralized system, each hospital department registers its own patients. When the system is computerized, the patient registers only once and on return visits the information is checked and updated as needed and new consent forms are signed. When the system is not computerized, patients may be required to give information to more than one department, such as the radiology department and the laboratory. Admissions personnel in a decentralized system perform many functions in addition to registration.

Practical considerations can often be the overriding factors in choosing which model is more appropriate. For example, the physical layout and patient flow patterns of the hospital may determine whether it is more practical to centralize or decentralize the registration function. When entrances to the emergency and ambulatory care departments are remote, a centralized registration area is impractical. The advantages and disadvantages of centralized and decentralized systems are listed in figure 2. Hospitals might also consider a combination of the two types of systems.

The level of automation also affects the design of a hospital's registration system. The three basic levels are these:

- *Nonautomated (manual):* Typewriters and manual filing systems are still used in a few registration systems, with each department handling its own registrations. Programmed or automated typewriters may be used.
- *Automated:* In an automated system, admissions staff use an embossed plastic identification card to imprint registration forms. Generally, the system is used for inpatients and centralized outpatient systems. Outpatients usually keep identification cards for

---

Figure 2. Advantages and Disadvantages of Centralized and Decentralized Registration

Centralized Registration	
Advantages	**Disadvantages**
• Consistency in quality of data • Easier supervision • Possible cross-training of staff • Better staff coverage • Reduced staff time • Reduced paperwork • Continuity in patient routing • Easier control of records	• Layout constraints, including size and location of registration area • Schedules of other departments not necessarily known by central desk • Patient not able to go directly to department on the first visit

Decentralized Registration	
Advantages	**Disadvantages**
• Outpatients able to go directly to department • No layout constraints • Departmental control of schedule	• Staff coverage vulnerable to illness and vacation schedules • Continuity lacking for patient orientation and routing • Records control difficult • Increased equipment needs (computer terminals, printers, copiers, embossers) • Increased supply inventory • More staff required to cover station-filled positions • Staff supervision more difficult • Poor-quality demographic information when obtained by ancillary staff rather than registration personnel

subsequent visits. The benefits of the card system include consistency of data, reuse of the card, patient identification with the hospital system, reduced typing time, and accurate and readable charge tickets. Shortcomings, although limited and infrequent, include incorrect or changed data requiring a new identification card, security problems involving imposter patients, the failure of the patients to bring cards back for subsequent visits, and the cost of the card stock and equipment.

- *Computerized:* Computerized systems allow registration data to be entered and retrieved directly. In addition, the computer can handle charge posting and forms printing. The benefits of a computerized system are that it reduces paperwork; captures charges with requisitions; generates requisition slips; centralizes the system without physical centralization; allows entry, maintenance, and retrieval of census data; and uses standard input formats. Shortcomings include the costliness of installation, the amount of training required for staff members, and the system's dependence on automated hardware that may need to be shut down for repairs and thus cause delays and interruptions in record keeping.

The use of computerized systems in the admissions/registration department is now commonplace. Generally, these systems are linked with the hospital's financial services system. A computerized system can allow direct input of admissions information and charge ordering at the point of admission. The manual typing of forms after initial input is eliminated through the use of printers attached to the system. Systems can be expanded hospitalwide, with computer terminals provided at nursing stations and in other departments. Enhanced computerized systems may allow for magnetic striped encoding, laser disk placement in the plastic identification card, and bar coding of forms and arm bands.

Although the level of automation affects the design of the hospital's registration system, it has little or no impact on staffing requirements. However, the greater the degree of automation, the greater the hospital's ability to capture data quickly and accurately and to make information available to other areas of the hospital.

Departmental Analysis

In analyzing the admissions/registration department, the management engineer should consider the following factors and goals:

- *Operational standard:* Identify an acceptable level of patient delay in registration. Acceptable delays typically range from 10 to 20 minutes. Overall staffing is affected by how much delay management is willing to tolerate.
- *Department staff:* Study utilization and determine appropriate staffing levels for day and evening coverage. Demand work load (registering various outpatient types, processing inpatient admissions, and so on) should be measured. In addition, non–demand work load (preadmission phone calls, statistics preparation, staff meetings, and so on) should be measured and used to balance work load during nonpeak periods.
- *Scheduling/preregistration:* Improve procedures to develop an effective system that reduces patient waiting times and levels out work load; evaluate coordination of preadmission testing, credit screening with financial services, and staffing patterns of the department with those of service departments.
- *Systems and forms:* Review the design of forms and the efficiency of record location and retrieval systems.
- *Communication system:* Review admission, discharge, and transfer notice dissemination procedures.
- *Filing and indexing:* Review file contents and recommend an appropriate filing system.
- *Data collection:* Review errors and deficiencies in financial and demographic data collected during registration.

- *Census management:* Design a census management system that includes reservation procedures, patient listing, and bed control.
- *Organizational analysis:* Review organizational responsibility and the feasibility of changes such as the consolidation of the admissions/registration department, emergency admissions, and ambulatory care registration.

Such analyses might result in the following kinds of changes:

- Staff rescheduling to provide staffing adequate for the work load at the least cost
- Development of a productivity measurement system
- Implementation of preregistration and admission procedures that could be coordinated with financial services' billing and collection efforts to reduce bad debt expense
- Improvement of the hospitalwide communication system
- Enhanced systems design for interfacing with a computerized admissions installation
- Design and establishment of a preadmission or admission testing center
- Consolidation, when appropriate, of inpatient, ambulatory care, and emergency department registration
- Implementation of a centralized booking function to coordinate patient flow and improve the use of nursing, operating room, and ancillary department personnel and resources
- Development of a clinical screening function to determine the appropriateness of each admission, potential disallowment of payment by third-party payers, and requirements for discharge planning. Such a system requires increased lead time for an admission as well as coordination of personnel from the medical staff office, the medical record department, financial services, and utilization management.

Ambulatory Services

Overview

Historically, hospital ambulatory services were established to provide essential health care to the economically indigent population. Because of the high concentration of such people in urban areas, outpatient clinics were primarily located in, or affiliated with, large public teaching hospitals. Using medical interns and residents to provide the professional care, clinics were able to keep operating costs at a minimum while creating a practical training ground for physicians. Usually, operating revenues were subsidized by tax revenues from the local, city, or county government and sometimes from grants by private or governmental organizations.

In recent years, the increasingly widespread movement toward the delivery of health care in ambulatory settings has resulted in the expansion of outpatient clinics. This shift toward outpatient activity has been further encouraged by the impact of prospective payment systems. Originally designed with a limited scope, outpatient clinics are diversifying their services, establishing more accessible locations, and in some cases, broadening their population base. Because such clinics are not necessarily located within the hospital complex, they need to be considered separately from emergency departments, which may act as outpatient clinics for hospitals where there is no other source of outpatient care.

The types of services offered by ambulatory services departments are as varied as the hospitals that provide these services. For example, a large teaching institution typically offers an extensive array of services, for example:

- Allergy
- Dental
- Dermatology
- Diabetes
- Endocrinology
- Eye and ear
- Gastroenterology
- Gynecology and women's health
- Hand
- Hypertension
- Infectious disease
- Internal medicine
- Language disorders
- Learning disorders
- Medical walk-in

- Neuromedical
- Neurosurgery
- Nutrition
- Obstetrics
- Occupational health
- Oral and maxillofacial surgery
- Orthopedics
- Pediatrics
- Psychiatry
- Pulmonary
- Renal
- Social service
- Sports medicine
- Substance abuse

Some hospitals even offer subspecialization within various categories.

Although small hospitals or nonteaching institutions may not have the medical staff to support all the clinics a large hospital may provide, small hospitals often have arrangements with other hospitals and/or physicians to offer clinics on a periodic basis. For example, a group of physicians and nurses may visit a hospital once a week or once a month to conduct a special ambulatory care clinic.

The hours of operation for ambulatory services depend on a number of factors. The hours of operation often follow what may be considered a standard nine-to-five schedule, or they may be open odd hours to attract clients or to serve the unusual needs of the local population. The hospital needs to assess the cost of operating a service at off-hours compared to the potential benefit to patients who might use the service. In some cases, staff availability as well as cost restrictions may limit the hours of operation.

Freestanding outpatient clinics are primarily a marketing tool inasmuch as patients who need hospitalization or more sophisticated diagnostic testing are referred to the parent hospital. In fact, some hospitals have established satellite primary ambulatory care facilities that are strictly targeted at private-pay clientele. Moreover, some private enterprises (investor-owned firms, physician groups, and others) have also taken advantage of the changing health care environment to set up similar clinic operations.

Organization

Typically, there are four major organizational components of the outpatient clinic: physician staff, clinical staff, ancillary staff, and clerical staff. In teaching hospital settings, the physician staff consists of a medical director, who usually holds teaching privileges at an affiliated medical school, and house staff physicians (interns and residents), who provide professional consultation and care. Sometimes private physicians may augment the core staff to provide specialty coverage.

The primary clinical support staff is made up of nurses, including registered nurses, licensed practical nurses, and nurses' aides. Ancillary staff, such as radiology, laboratory, and ECG technologists, is usually provided as needed by the respective hospital departments when the clinic is located within the hospital complex. In satellite clinics, such ancillary staff may be dedicated to the clinics. Finally, the clinic must have the clerical staff necessary to carry out the registration, patient accounting, secretarial, and medical record functions.

Staffing levels for the physician, clinical, ancillary, and clerical staffs depend on the number of patients and the hours of operation. The size of the hospital has very little impact on ambulatory services staffing levels in that ambulatory volumes do not necessarily relate to inpatient volumes. This is especially true in today's reimbursement climate. In assessing ambulatory services staffing levels, the hospital should consider patient volume by hour of the day and day of the week. When possible, smaller services should look into sharing some staff functions, such as receptionist, clerical, and medical records. It is also common to have the nursing staff serve a number of clinics.

The management structure of the outpatient clinic may vary considerably among hospitals. Quite often, the medical director also functions in the department manager's role, with direct responsibility for all personnel (physicians, nurses, ancillary staff, and clerks) and all operations, both clinical and business related. However, many hospitals are moving toward a structure in which the medical director is responsible for clinical activities and an outpatient clinic manager is responsible for all administrative and personnel functions, excluding physicians. This arrangement allows the medical director to concentrate on the provision of health care while taking advantage of the clinic manager's managerial and financial skills. The clinic manager may have been trained in business or health care administration or may be a clinician who has been promoted from within. The use of the clinic manager is particularly common where there are several different clinics operating in one hospital. Depending on the size of the clinics, the manager should be able to direct several clinics by using head nurses to provide daily supervision in each individual clinic.

Outpatient clinic managers always report to the administrative level of the hospital. In hospitals in which outpatient clinics constitute a substantial part of the hospital's operation, the clinic manager may actually function at the administrative level. However, it is most common for the clinic manager and medical director to report to an assistant administrator.

Models and Systems

The key to operational efficiency in outpatient clinics is efficient patient flow. All systems related to the clinics affect the flow of patients. An efficiently run clinic must develop sound policies and procedures to ensure that patients are promptly registered and treated.

The first step toward establishing efficient patient flow is the development of an effective patient scheduling system. Traditionally, patients have been scheduled for clinic visits in block appointments. In this system, many patients are given appointments at the same time, usually at the beginning of the morning or afternoon hours. Inherent in this system are long waits for patients and high productivity for physicians and staff. A specific appointment system in which each patient is given an individual appointment time is more convenient for patients and will generally improve patient flow, but it may lower physician productivity. Some hospitals have adopted compromise systems that schedule patients in small blocks of time to better balance patient arrivals with staff resources.

Although it is desirable to limit patient waiting time to less than 20 minutes, it is not always possible to do so. Scheduling of patients and staff obviously has an impact on patient waiting time and on staff productivity. Average waiting times depend on the type of clinic and the economic circumstances under which the clinic functions. In cases where a clinic is offered to patients who can choose from a wide variety of providers, the ambulatory services department may choose to run the clinic so that appointment times are kept and/or waiting time for walk-ins is very short. Conversely, when a clinic is offered once a month in a rural area and a high percentage of care is provided free of charge on a walk-in basis, it may be very hard to avoid long waiting times for patients.

Closely related to the patient appointments process is the process of registering patients once they arrive at the clinic. This process includes gathering pertinent demographic and payer information. The registration process sets in action the rest of the service provision by acknowledging the patient's arrival, notifying the patient care staff, and initiating medical record retrieval.

The system for filing, retrieving, and making available the medical records of outpatients for clinic visits is extremely important. Because of the fragmented, episodic nature of the care given through outpatient clinics, managing record keeping can be difficult. Historically, outpatient records were located and handled within the hospital's medical record department.

More recently, as outpatient volume has increased dramatically, the trend is toward keeping separate records for outpatient visits located in areas more convenient to the clinics.

As a general rule, utilization of clinic facilities has been quite poor. Significant planning is needed to ensure that the medical resources (physicians, nurses, equipment, and supplies) are available in the right amounts and at the right times to treat the patients who need them. Full utilization of the examination rooms and staff is a result of properly managing these resources.

To maximize available resources, the ambulatory services department needs to coordinate patient and staff schedules and, as mentioned earlier, cross-utilize staff from clinic to clinic. The most effective way to manage resources would be to control the patient schedule so as to distribute patient volumes evenly throughout the day. However, shifts in demand and unforeseen circumstances are common and often mean that there are highs and lows in patient activity throughout the day. This shift in demand causes occasional overstaffing or understaffing.

Another important system in outpatient clinic functions is charge collection. Beginning with patient registration and continuing through charge identification and gathering and fee collection, the financial viability of the clinic operation depends on properly designed charge collection procedures.

All of the systems discussed earlier can be significantly improved through automation. The patient volumes in most large outpatient clinics can justify on-line computerization to make appointments, process registrations, identify records to be retrieved, produce staff work or patient assignments, capture charges, and bill patients. The episodic nature of the patient's relationship with the clinic presents problems for manual systems and creates an excellent environment for computerized systems.

Situations and Problems

Perhaps more than any other hospital department, ambulatory care services pivot on physician involvement and commitment because the physician is central to the delivery of care. Owing to the complicated organizational relationships among physicians and other hospital staff, numerous problems in developing common goals and daily work objectives can occur. All changes in outpatient clinic operations require close communication and involvement with the clinic's medical staff.

The issue of financial interdependence among hospital departments requires that the efficacy of sharing resources between inpatient and outpatient departments is practically and objectively considered. In other words, when is it better to use an ancillary department's services (for example, laboratory or electroencephalography) as opposed to taking advantage of the convenience and potentially improved effectiveness of having the same resource dedicated to the outpatient clinic?

A variable that can significantly affect patient flow is the centralization or decentralization of the registration and appointment systems. The centralization/decentralization issue involves both the organizational structure and the physical location of ambulatory services. Numerous studies have been conducted that demonstrate the advantages of both centralization and decentralization. Many factors can influence this decision, including the peculiarity of the patients' illnesses, the level of clinical knowledge required of clerical personnel, the physical proximity of the registration area to the reception area, and the physician and support staff organizational relationships.

The advantages of centralization are these:

- Multiple examinations can be coordinated and the hospital's ancillary services can be used.
- The location and retrieval of medical records are simplified.
- Registration personnel are used more efficiently.

The advantages of decentralization are these:

- The patient deals directly with the staff at the clinic where services are being provided.
- There is less confusion at registration.
- Reactions to changes in patient scheduling and arrival are faster.

A computer-based appointment and registration system allows the ambulatory services department to take advantage of both centralized and decentralized scheduling, provided that there is access to the system at central registration and in individual departments. Such a system allows patients to register at a central registration point when they first come to ambulatory services. When they are repeat patients, they can go directly to a specific department and register for repeat visits at that department. The location of the clinics has an impact on the system, and for small ambulatory departments, it may be just as convenient to have all patients register at a central location.

The physical location of the outpatient clinic facility in relation to the main hospital can also influence operational decisions. This is particularly true for satellite clinics that are not located on the hospital campus. Generally, the more remote the clinic's location, the more self-sufficient the operation must become. However, as the clinic needs to become more self-sufficient, it may not be able to utilize staff effectively. Cross-utilization may not be possible, and downtime during nonpeak hours may be unavoidable. Actual patient volumes and hours of operation affect utilization levels for remote clinics as well as hospital-based clinics.

Perhaps the biggest problem that clinic managers must cope with is walk-in and no-show patients. A walk-in patient is defined as a patient who is seen by a physician in an outpatient clinic but who did not have an appointment. A no-show patient is simply a patient who has an appointment but does not keep it. The number of walk-ins and no-shows in outpatient clinic environments is much greater than in a typical private physician's practice. Walk-in patients are difficult to serve because of their unpredictable arrival rates, and no-show patients create inefficiencies because the staff and other resources reserved for them are not utilized. Several hospitals have implemented measures to remedy this problem, but most have achieved only limited success. The main point to understand is that no-shows and walk-ins are a reality in ambulatory care and must be factored in to any operational planning.

Departmental Analysis

Outpatient clinics hold many challenges for the management engineer or analyst. The unique blend of multidisciplinary staff, episodic ambulatory patient care, dependence on information flow, and oftentimes complex fiscal issues makes outpatient clinics an ideal setting for systems analysis and improvements. Some of the principal areas for study include the following:

- *Staffing requirements:* Determining staff requirements and skill level mix and analyzing the use of incremental inpatient department resources
- *Examination room usage:* Determining how well rooms are used during available hours and identifying the resources and reasons that limit the usage
- *Patient scheduling systems:* Evaluating the advantages and disadvantages of various scheduling methods, determining the method most appropriate, and developing a system that is reasonable for the specific situation
- *Records handling:* Analyzing the filing, transfer, and use of medical records
- *Patient waiting:* Determining average patient waiting times and finding ways to shorten them when necessary
- *Patient flow:* Using flowcharting techniques to analyze the movement of patients through clinic facilities in order to maximize resource utilization and minimize patient waiting times

- *Information systems:* Assessing information needs and designing appropriate systems to meet the needs, possibly including the evaluation and implementation of a computerized information system
- *Management information:* Determining the type and availability of information that clinic managers need to manage effectively
- *Financial management:* Evaluating the fiscal viability of the clinics in areas such as cost inputs, microcosting, revenue sources, and mix of services
- *Quality assurance:* Developing an objective measurement tool for evaluating the quality of operations

As the preceding list indicates, there is no one simple study that can be done to measure productivity or determine the effectiveness of overall systems. Rather, the many interactive and interdependent systems of ambulatory services often need to be reviewed at the same time. For example, to measure productivity accurately, the analysis should include assessments of staff requirements by patient visit. In some cases, an average time can be determined, and in more complex cases, the staff may need a mechanism to indicate their involvement on a case-by-case basis. In analyzing staff utilization, it is also necessary to take into consideration room utilization and scheduling practices.

Cardiac Catheterization Laboratory

Overview

Cardiac catheterization is the insertion of a catheter (a long, narrow, flexible tube) through a blood vessel into the heart. This procedure makes it possible for the cardiologist to explore within the heart to find out precisely how well the patient's heart and coronary arteries are working and, in some cases, to treat heart disease. Although cardiac catheterization is a highly specialized diagnostic technique performed only in a specially equipped hospital laboratory, it is a common procedure in many hospitals.

The procedures performed in the cardiac catheterization laboratory can be classified as either diagnostic or therapeutic. The procedures can be further grouped as valvular heart disease procedures, electrophysiological studies, congenital heart studies, cardiomyopathy studies, or coronary artery disease studies. These procedures are often performed in combination. Therapeutic procedures cannot be performed unless the hospital has an open-heart surgery program as a backup and the surgeons are on standby during each procedure. Examples of therapeutic procedures are angioplasty (balloon catheterization), thrombolysis (injection of clot-dissolving agents), and installation of pacemakers. Examples of diagnostic procedures are right and left heart catheterizations, ventriculography, and coronary angiograms (the injection of a substance through the tube that allows the coronary arteries to show up on X rays).

Hospitals without an open-heart surgery program primarily perform angiograms; patients are then referred to another hospital for surgery. Another major difference between cardiac catheterization programs is whether pediatric patients are treated. Different equipment specifically sized for infants and small children is needed for pediatric patients.

Organization

The organizational structure of the cardiac catheterization laboratory is partially determined by the relationship between the cardiologists and the hospital. Physician staffing may be arranged through a contractual relationship whereby physicians directly bill patients for any procedures performed. In teaching hospitals, the hospital may do the billing for the physicians. Regardless of the billing arrangements, the laboratory is usually organized under the medical director of cardiology.

The department usually has a supervisor or manager who reports to the hospital's administration or to the department's medical director. In some hospitals, the supervisor reports to the manager of radiology and diagnostic imaging or to the assistant administrator of ancillary services. The cardiac catheterization department manager may also supervise other areas of the hospital in addition to the cardiac catheterization laboratory.

Cardiologists are required to be board certified in cardiology and internal medicine. The qualifications for the nonphysician staff vary from hospital to hospital; however, most personnel receive extensive on-the-job training. The following positions are commonly found in the laboratory:

- *Physiology technician, also called cardiovascular technician, cardiopulmonary technician, or cardiac catheterization technician:* The employee occupying this position usually has a baccalaureate degree in science, biology, or physiology and may be registered by the National Society for Cardiopulmonary Technology. Frequently, the physiology technician also acts as the laboratory supervisor.
- *Registered nurse or sometimes licensed practical nurse:* The employee occupying this position has had experience in the cardiac care unit or the intensive care unit and usually is able to interpret electrocardiograms. The employee may be associated with the American Association of Critical Care Nurses.
- *Radiology technician or technologist:* The employee occupying this position is usually registered by the American Association of Radiology Technology and has experience in performing special procedures.

Other positions such as darkroom technician, clerk, and aide are not common. These employees usually receive on-the-job training.

Models and Systems

The typical cardiac catheterization laboratory has the following physical layout:

- Catheterization laboratory, a clean procedure room similar to a radiology special procedures room (there is a sterile field consisting of the patient, the back table with supplies, the angiographer, and the assistant; many departments have only one laboratory, which may also be used for special procedures)
- Darkroom for 35-millimeter film processing and sometimes large spot film processing
- Clerical area with filing space for films and records
- Film viewing area for the cardiologists
- Small chemistry support section for blood-gas analysis and quality assurance for film processing
- Patient holding area, a separate area, frequently located away from the catheterization laboratory (this area is most common in laboratories that were converted from radiology special procedure rooms)

The following staff specialists are needed during the cardiac catheterization procedure:

- *Angiographer:* The cardiologist who inserts the catheter, oversees the medical aspects of the procedure, and reads and interprets the film afterward
- *Scrub or assistant angiographer:* The physician or technologist who assists the primary physician in the sterile field
- *Float or circulating nurse:* The nurse who administers medications, gets supplies, and helps the angiographer
- *Monitoring or recording technician:* The technician who monitors the electrocardiogram, hemodynamics, and blood gases of the patient throughout the procedure
- *Darkroom technician:* The technician who reruns the videotape for the cardiologist to determine whether the views are adequate before the procedure is terminated and who develops the film

Some of these positions are frequently combined, particularly the float, monitoring, and darkroom positions. The number of laboratory personnel required for these duties depends on the type of procedure, the condition of the patient, the preferences of the cardiologists, or the policies of the hospital. In addition, the laboratory staff is responsible for preparing the room, supplies, and patient before and after the procedure and for monitoring the patient's recovery.

In addition to assisting with the actual procedure, the laboratory staff must also perform or arrange for the following activities:

- *Scheduling:* The method used may be block scheduling, which allows one day for each cardiologist group, or conventional scheduling, which operates on a first-come, first-served basis except in emergencies.
- *Preparation of case carts:* The laboratory may use a case cart system similar to that used in an operating room. Under this system, the setup for the procedure is done by the cardiac catheterization staff; the preparation and autoclaving of the procedure tray is done by central service.
- *Patient transportation:* The type of personnel assigned to transporting the patient to and from the catheterization laboratory depends on the condition of the patient. For diagnostic procedures, a nontechnical escort can be used. For therapeutic procedures, a technician or a nurse is needed.
- *Transcription:* A medical transcriber or secretary types the cardiologist's report. The work may be performed by centralized transcription, by radiology transcription, or by a secretary in the laboratory who also performs other duties.
- *Records management:* The films are usually archived in the laboratory. The laboratory may keep a file card on each patient and a patient folder with the hemodynamic data, the physician's order, computer reports, and raw data on blood pressure and blood gases. Some laboratories keep the transcribed report and electrocardiograms, although copies of these materials are also part of the patient's medical record.
- *Clerical functions:* In addition to filing records and scheduling procedures, clerical or technical staff may answer the telephones, process charging or billing data, order supplies, perform quality control, and provide clerical support for the supervisor and the medical director.
- *Patient education:* Prior to the procedure, a member of the technical staff may review with the patient the steps, preparation, follow-up, expectations, and other details associated with the procedure.

In nonteaching hospitals, the laboratory staff is often involved in procedures usually performed by physicians in teaching hospitals. Technicians may inject the coronary dye, read pressure strips, and calculate additional patient data.

Departmental Analysis

The cardiac catheterization laboratory is similar to the operating room and to the special procedures area of the radiology department. The laboratory may have many of the same management problems and may be analyzed with many of the same methods. Potential areas of study include the following:

- The department's staffing patterns, including staff scheduling and productivity standards
- The department's physical layout, particularly the patient holding area
- The type of equipment used
- Certificate-of-need (CON) studies for new cardiac catheterization laboratories or for expanding or replacing facilities

Productivity statistics can be based on the number of cases, the number of procedures, or the number of actual hours spent performing the procedures. For hospitals with teaching programs and fellowships, the amount of time needed to perform the procedures may increase significantly. Samples of recent MONITREND data for the catheterization laboratory functional reporting center are provided in table 1.

In a typical cardiac catheterization laboratory with one procedure room, the staff size is small, and the patient load fluctuates on a day-to-day basis. Therefore, one of the largest areas for potential improvement is cross-training. Although it can be time-consuming, cross-training within the cardiac catheterization laboratory and with other departments provides coverage when key personnel are absent or the patient load temporarily increases. Surgery, cardiac care unit, intensive care unit, and open-heart surgery nurses or radiology special procedure technicians are the best sources of shared staffing. Similarly, cardiac catheterization personnel can be used in other hospital departments when the laboratory's work load is low.

In addition, the cardiac catheterization laboratory can be staffed more effectively by sharing personnel from other departments rather than employing underused nontechnical staff within the department. However, the efficiency of interdepartmental staffing depends on the proximity of other departments to the cardiac catheterization laboratory. Examples of such usage are escorts from X ray, surgery, or recovery; nurses from the intensive care unit, the cardiac care unit, or recovery; and clerical or secretarial assistance from another department, which is helpful when the technical staff is too busy to answer the telephones.

A holding room for the patients also increases the efficiency of the laboratory. When the holding room is equipped with electrocardiogram monitors, the patient can be monitored while the staff is in the procedure room. In addition, a patient can be prepped in the holding room while a case is being finished in the laboratory.

Table 1. HAS/MONITREND Data for Catheterization Laboratory: Six-Month Medians for Period Ending December 1988

Indicator	National Bed Size Groups							
	Under 50	50–74	75–99	100–149	150–199	200–299	300–399	400 and Over
Procedures per calendar day[a]	0.0	0.0	1.73	0.91	1.30	2.22	3.98	7.30
Paid hours per procedure[b]	0.0	0.0	8.60	19.50	10.65	12.59	11.30	9.93

[a]Procedures per calendar day = catheterization laboratory procedures/days in period.

[b]Paid hours per procedure = catheterization laboratory paid hours/catheterization laboratory procedures.

Source: HAS/MONITREND, 1988. Please refer to page x for more information about the data presented in this table.

Central Service Department

Overview

The central service department operates in a number of different functional models ranging from one that offers very limited support services to one that offers broad-based support services. Under one common configuration, central service furnishes most nondrug supplies for the nursing units and surgery, the emergency department, the laboratory, the radiology department, and ambulatory services. The activities of the central service department include supplying, reclaiming, sterilizing, and stocking supplies such as glassware, gloves, needles, syringes, linens, surgical packs and kits, intravenous solutions, trays, and instrument sets. When the department has a broad-based support service function, the department may also price the items and charge them to the appropriate accounts. The department is also some-times called the central sterile supply department, the central processing department, the central supply department, or the central medical supply department.

Sterilization is generally considered the main function of the central service department. Sterilization of instruments, surgical packs, trays, and similar materials is performed by heating them with pressurized steam exceeding 122°C (250°F) or by sterilizing them with special gases such as ethylene oxide. Steam sterilization, also called autoclaving, is performed in stainless steel pressure tanks. Certain items such as delicate instruments and plastic materials are usually sterilized by using ethylene oxide or similar gases. Gas sterilization requires more safety precau-tions (such as aeration of the sterilized materials for 12 hours prior to use and special exhaust ventilation) than does autoclaving.

The use of disposable sterile supplies has had a significant impact on central service. Many items that traditionally were reusable are now disposable and need only be stored and dispensed through central service. However, the use of disposables tends to vary with the cost of supplies and the attitudes of medical staff members. With increased concern for infec-tion control issues, the use of disposables has now proliferated in spite of some significant increases in costs.

Organization

Traditionally, central service was part of the nursing department. However, with increased emphasis on efficient materials management, there are a significant number of hospitals in which the central services function reports to a materials manager. The department may be located next to the surgical suite for ease of transporting sterile packs. However, the physical location of the sterilization function is becoming more diverse as hospitals undergo substan-tial renovations and remodeling. The increased emphasis on ethylene oxide safety has resulted in the location of this department in areas of the hospital with better ventilation access. More stringent personal safety standards for the transportation of contaminated supplies has also affected the choice of location for this function in many hospitals. Some surgical departments perform their own sterilization procedures and have limited interaction with the central service department.

Today, the central service department is usually a centralized service for the entire hospital rather than a support function for the surgical and nursing units only. The department often functions under different models or levels of service. The most common current trend is to place central service under the direction of a materials manager, a purchasing agent, or a general services administrator.

Alternatively, the central service department might be structured primarily as an instrument-reprocessing service that performs the cleaning, wrapping, sterilization, and assembly of surgical packs, kits, and trays. Under this structure, a separate function or department may handle the restocking and issuance of medical supplies.

Traditionally, central service has been supervised by a nurse or a person with paramedical training, although this nurse-supervisor model is changing. The supervisor usually participates in the activities of the hospital's infection control, product evaluation, and standards committees. Central service personnel are usually not formally trained in instrument processing and are most often trained on the job. However, professional training and certification within the area of central services have become more formal in recent years, and central services activities now represent a recognized discipline. Although limited numbers of formal educational programs provide structured training in most areas of the country, some changes within vocational educational systems are becoming noticeable. To meet the more exacting contemporary skill and training environments, many hospitals are developing formal in-house training programs that are affiliated with educational institutions.

Depending on the extent of services provided, it is common to find central service providing coverage seven days a week on both day and evening shifts. Evening and weekend staffing is usually reduced. Some hospitals provide around-the-clock coverage.

Models and Systems

Central service models and systems follow a functional model similar to the one characteristic of materials management. The basic functions that central service performs are equipment–instrument management, materials acquisition (or purchasing), storage (or warehousing), and distribution and charging.

Equipment–Instrument Management

Equipment–instrument management includes sterilization, cleaning, instrument processing, kit assembly, inspection of surgical linen, and preparation of sterile water and saline solutions. In recent years, the operation of the hospital's portable medical equipment program has also commonly become a responsibility of the central service department. Portable medical equipment includes intravenous control equipment, suction machines, orthopedic equipment, and other portable equipment routinely used in many areas throughout the hospital. The responsibilities of central service include cleaning, calibration, safety testing, periodic maintenance, and delivery/pickup.

Instrument processing includes assembling appropriate instruments and supplies into kits and wrapping the kits with linen. Examples of kits and trays include various surgical instrument kits, suture kits for nursing units and emergency departments, cut-down trays for nursing units (used to find accessible patient veins for intravenous therapy), and special procedure trays for radiology. Central service may also be responsible for the maintenance and repair of medical instruments. Most departments have specific procedures for processing instruments.

Instrument processing may be handled either by assembling regularly used instruments to make prewrapped kits or by processing kits as needed or ordered. The prewrapped method provides a stock to meet after-hours requirements; however, this method requires a large inventory of instruments. The use of a combination of the two methods is common. Also common in many hospitals is the use of exchange carts for various supplies and linens. These exchange carts can double as backup for disaster or unplanned usage, thus reducing the amount of after-hours coverage necessary.

Sterilization, as mentioned previously, is performed by using either autoclaving or gas sterilization. Under both systems, sterilization is performed on cleaned instruments that are wrapped in special linen. The wraps may be either single- or double-thickness surgical-quality linen. The acceptable or preferred thickness and composition varies from institution to institution.

The sterilization is performed in batches, which include several packages in a single sterilization load. For infection control purposes, these packages must be marked and logged with test indicators that are reviewed periodically. Thus, any bad batches can be identified and the packages can be removed from the shelves. Once a wrapped kit is sterilized, it is considered sterile only for a designated length of time, after which it must be resterilized.

Flash sterilization, or the autoclaving of an unwrapped instrument, is usually not performed in the central service area. Rather, it is more likely to be performed by a user department (such as the surgical suite) to resterilize something that is needed immediately or that has been dropped.

The cleaning and washing of instruments, trays, and other equipment must be performed prior to reassembling and wrapping instrument kits. Washing and cleaning can be performed either by hand or by using automatic washers. Tubing is washed and rinsed by using the type of nippled water connectors typically used in laboratories for water and gases. One form of automated cleaning can be compared to a kitchen dishwasher. Also available are ultrasonic cleaners, which are considered the most effective method for cleaning because they clean all hinges, joints, and similar hard-to-reach areas. A shortcoming of ultrasonic cleaning, however, is the ongoing erosion of the instrument's surface, which shortens the useful life of the instrument. The introduction of silicon-based soluble solutions to protect instruments from damage by ultrasonic cleaning has increased the acceptance of this method.

Surgical linen is inspected before it is used for wrapping instruments or linen packs. The linen is passed over a light table (a frosted glass table with underlighting) to identify rips, tears, and holes that would reduce its effectiveness in retaining sterile conditions. Delinting the linen is usually performed in conjunction with the inspection of linens. The purpose of delinting is to reduce any materials that could potentially enter the sterile field during a procedure and remain as a foreign body inside the patient's body. The use of disposable linen for wrapping instrument packs, kits, and trays has increased dramatically in recent years.

Linen packs of sheets, drapes, towels, and wraps are assembled for sterile areas, mainly the surgical, labor, and delivery areas. Custom linen packs are made for such procedures as orthopedic hip surgery, laparoscopy, and mastectomy. Packs may also include minor disposable items as well as reusable linens.

The preparation of sterile water and saline solutions is sometimes performed by the central service department. Basically, the process involves the distillation, bottling, and sterilization of intravenous solutions. The bottle size is usually 1 liter. However, because the required quantity of sterile water or saline solution is often smaller than 1 liter, considerable waste may occur. The trend is to purchase sterile water and saline solutions in plastic pouch containers, which reduce breakage and are convenient for handling. The containers are available in various sizes and thus reduce the amount of waste.

The other factor encouraging hospitals to purchase sterile water and saline solutions from outside the institution is the consistency and quality control of the products. In some settings, the level of saline is critical because it is the absolute level of foreign particles in the sterile water. Commercial products adhere to closer quality control standards than are practical in some hospitals without substantial investment in, and upgrading of, preparation equipment.

Materials Acquisition or Purchasing

As the use of disposable products increases, the central service staff may become involved with the actual purchasing and procurement of supplies. Some central service managers may issue purchase orders directly to hospital vendors. Others may requisition new or replacement supplies from the purchasing department. In either case, central service may spend considerable time on materials acquisition.

Storage or Warehousing

The central service department typically stores both disposable and reusable goods. Substantial amounts of medical and surgical supplies for the nursing units and user departments may be stored. Special consideration must be given to sterile instrument and linen packs. Because their sterility can become outdated, stock must be dated and rotated.

The extent of the central service department's involvement in warehousing is generally related to the service level available from the hospital's main materials management function. When the service level is high, the need for central service to warehouse supplies may be significantly diminished. When the hospital does not have a comprehensive materials management capability, the central service function may effectively duplicate many activities and functions in the areas of purchasing, warehousing, and receiving.

Distribution and Charging

Many central service departments deliver goods and supplies to nursing units and user departments. Typical methods include delivery in response to requisitions, replenishing stock at specific locations to a predetermined par level, and utilization of exchange carts. In addition, some items may be dispensed by the central service department through a requisition system.

Central service's responsibility in the distribution process may include issuing, transporting, and pricing all patient-chargeable supplies. The hospital's computer system can be used for inventory management of routinely used items. A common procedure is to attach charge tickets or stickers to individual items. Central service may price items manually or use prepriced patient charge stickers. Other methods of charging include the use of computer-coded patient charge checklists and direct patient charge entry into the hospital's automated order-entry system. Central service may spend a considerable amount of time on the patient charging and pricing process.

Many central service or central processing departments have implemented case cart distribution systems for surgical procedures. A case cart system requires that an individual cart of supplies be prepared for each surgical procedure. This cart usually includes surgical drapes, instruments, sponges, suction equipment, a variety of medical–surgical supplies required for the case, and often implantables (pacemakers, hip replacements, intraocular lenses, vascular grafts, and so on).

Hospitals that use the case cart system usually have one individual (a case cart coordinator) who serves as a liaison between the surgical suite and the central service department. The coordinator is responsible for selecting appropriate supplies and implantables and following the physician's preferences for each case. He or she ensures that the carts are prepared and delivered as scheduled.

The case cart coordinator is also responsible for updating and maintaining physician preference files. Some hospitals have physician preference files computerized in conjunction with the surgery scheduling management system.

Case cart systems will probably become more common as hospitals enter the 1990s. In fact, many hospitals have already taken implants, internal stapling sutures, and several specialty supplies out of the surgical suite and put them into the central service department, where more appropriate levels of supplies can be maintained.

The case cart system extends the useful lives of instruments because central service technicians are experts in the reprocessing function. They ensure that instruments are properly cleaned, that all joints and crevices are inspected, and that specialty items are lubricated as required and wrapped very carefully to protect tips and edges.

Potential Problems

Traditionally, central service has been part of the nursing department. Because the interaction among personnel in nursing units and support service departments is critical to effective materials flow and patient care, attempts at reorganizing central service may meet resistance. Nevertheless, the duties and responsibilities assigned to the central service function should be consistent with the organizational model used throughout the hospital.

As a support service to the patient care areas of the hospital, the central service department is often criticized for providing inadequate supplies and equipment, offering poor accessibility to supplies after hours, and being too stringent in identifying and reducing lost charges (supplies for which no patient charges have been submitted). Conflict may result between central service and user departments, especially when departments attempt to hoard supplies.

Conflicts may often arise regarding the use of disposable versus reusable supplies. Various staff members may have preferences for one or the other. For example, the use of disposable versus reusable thermometers is usually a controversial issue. Such problems should be resolved by hospital clinicians in consultation with the central service department.

Departmental Analysis

An analysis of the central service department might include the following areas:

- Staffing and staff scheduling
- Purchasing and stocking procedures
- Charging system
- Quality control program
- Materials delivery systems and schedules
- Interface with materials management program
- Cost determination for alternative methods of assembling and stocking instrument kits
- Department layout and location (for example, proximity to the surgical suite)
- Make-or-buy analyses for disposables, reusables, sterile water, and saline solutions

Recent MONITREND data for the central services functional reporting center are provided in table 2.

Table 2. HAS/MONITREND Data for Central Services: Six-Month Medians for Period Ending December 1988

Indicator	National Bed Size Groups							
	Under 50	50–74	75–99	100–149	150–199	200–299	300–399	400 and Over
Paid hours per adjusted patient day[a]	0.38	0.33	0.32	0.43	0.41	0.45	0.47	0.50

[a]Paid hours per adjusted patient day = central service paid hours/(total patient days/central services RCC). The central services RCC (ratio of charges to charges) is an adjustment factor that is computed as follows: Central services RCC = central services inpatient revenue/(central services inpatient revenue + central services outpatient revenue).

Source: HAS/MONITREND, 1988. Please refer to page x for more information about the data presented in this table.

Clinical Engineering Department

Overview

The maintenance of medical equipment in the United States is a billion-dollar industry. According to unpublished data compiled over a five-year period and completed in the mid-1980s by Hospital Maintenance Consultants (Lebanon, Wisconsin) for the Committee on Shared Clinical Engineering Services, equipment maintenance costs for a 100-bed hospital should average between $400 and $800 per bed per year. A university medical center should expect to spend up to $1,600 per bed per year. Not surprisingly, the public pressure to contain costs has led many hospitals to form their own medical equipment maintenance departments in the expectation that services could be provided more economically in-house than by profit-making vendors. Although this is often true, all hospitals still use outside suppliers to provide maintenance services on at least some of their medical equipment because the variety of technologies used in the various clinical areas cannot be cost-effectively supported in-house in any but the largest institutions.

The typical clinical engineering department of just one or two technicians cannot maintain its proficiency on all types of complex medical equipment. In addition, the cost to maintain spare parts for some high-technology equipment can become prohibitive to the institution. Most often, X-ray and clinical laboratory equipment is maintained by the manufacturer or by independent vendor(s). Anesthesia, respiratory therapy, nuclear medicine, ultrasound, laser, and other highly specialized instrumentation may also be supported from outside. Table 3 illustrates the approximate breakdown of maintenance dollars spent by hospitals on the various technologies.

An in-house clinical engineering department's core responsibility is the "all other" category of equipment. The 22 percent of maintenance dollars spent in this category includes the equipment used in the intensive care unit, the surgical suite, the obstetrics department, emergency

---

Table 3. Percentages of Maintenance Dollars Spent on Hospital Technology

Technology	Percentage
X ray, imaging	55
Clinical laboratory	17
Nuclear medicine/ultrasound	3
Respiratory therapy	3
All other	22

Source: Hospital Maintenance Consultants, Lebanon, Wisconsin. Unpublished data from five-year study completed in 1986 for the Committee on Shared Clinical Engineering Services.

services, central supply, step-down units, intravenous therapy, clinics, and physical therapy, as well as all other general equipment in patient areas. The clinical engineering department may also branch out into handling low-technology laboratory equipment such as centrifuges and microscopes and is often called on to provide support in related areas of technology ranging from the evaluation of equipment prior to purchase to the investigation of hazard bulletins, recalls, and incidents involving equipment. In many hospitals, the clinical engineering department is represented on the equipment and/or safety committees.

Because much of the work entailed in maintaining a hospital's technical equipment falls outside the capacity of a hands-on clinical engineering department, efforts to manage the hospital's overall technology in terms of cost and effectiveness can become fragmented. The early direction of the clinical engineering discipline was toward the development of departments that could not only maintain the full range of technology in the hospital, but also function as a clearinghouse for equipment assessment, planning, utilization, and disposal.

Fiscal realities aside, this technology management function is not carried on at most hospitals. Most of the current development in areas outside of maintenance and repair remains the province of outside suppliers and shared services, although some of the major medical centers have developed unique programs.

Organization

The maintenance of medical equipment, when it exists as a separate staffed department, may be called clinical, biomedical, or medical engineering. When clinical engineering is not an in-house function, the work is contracted out to individual manufacturers, independent service firms, or shared service organizations. The approaches used by these outside firms vary from full-service contracts to time and materials arrangements and from field-service support to part-time or full-time in-residence technicians.

Those hospitals that do staff this function most often set up clinical engineering as a part of the maintenance department. It has also been placed under nursing, respiratory therapy, and purchasing. In large teaching hospitals, it may be set up as a freestanding department reporting directly to the hospital's administration.

Regardless of the reporting structure, there are several consistent features in the operation of the clinical engineering department. The first is that the hospital's clinical staff expects clinical engineering to be able to respond 24 hours a day to equipment problems. Although the department is called on infrequently to provide service in the off-hours, 24-hour coverage requires the availability of off-site paging for the technician on call. A one-person department cannot be placed on call constantly. Therefore, some means of alternate call as well as sick leave and vacation backup must be provided. Contingency plans must be in place to cover the hospital in the event of personnel turnover, and on-call pay and overtime pay must be included in the department's budget.

The second feature found in most clinical engineering departments is that they require a minimum of 200 square feet per person of clean shop space to accommodate a bench, desk, stock, records, and a repair area for large equipment. This area should be directly accessible to major concentrations of equipment so that the technician does not need to travel outside the facility or between levels over stairs.

Third, in addition to the usual utilities, the shop should be provided with outlets on the medical gas and suction systems, a sink with hot and cold water, and telephone call forwarding capability or an answering machine to cover the telephone when the shop is left unattended. To maintain the records required, a personal computer terminal with communications capabilities should be provided.

Whenever possible, the scope of work allocated to clinical engineering should be limited to responsibilities involving medical equipment. This limitation eliminates potential confusion when more traditional maintenance functions are included in the department's work load. Although clinical engineering reports in the chain of command to the hospital engineer or another manager, the work is performed on equipment allocated to many different departments throughout the hospital. This reporting relationship requires that a system for prioritizing work be in place. Because the clinical engineering department staff usually has no technical peers available within the hospital, care must also be exercised to ensure that the routine work required is not overlooked in favor of performing more interesting tasks and that the clinical engineering staff does not become enmeshed in work that is inappropriate to its job descriptions and skills.

With the increasing need for cost accountability, many hospitals are adopting internal charge systems for their support departments. The activities of the clinical engineering department are appropriate for such a charge-back system, which also helps management maintain control of the work product by providing an audit trail on productivity. A charge-back system should reflect actual costs, including factors for productivity, overhead, fixed costs, and benefits as well as salaries. The realistic cost of maintaining a clinical engineering department is in excess of $40 per staff hour.

Operations

The clinical engineering department's goal is to maintain the medical equipment in a safe and efficacious operating condition. This goal falls within the hospital's broader objective of managing its technology. Clinical engineering provides repair services when the equipment fails in addition to such services as ongoing maintenance, operator instruction, record keeping, and cost management.

There are several overlapping systems of state, federal, and voluntary codes and standards that must be met in maintaining medical equipment. The Joint Commission on Accreditation of Healthcare Organizations (JCAHO) devotes one-quarter of its plant, technology, and safety management standards to medical equipment and greatly emphasizes the management of risk from improper maintenance, improper use, and intrinsic hazards. In order to meet the requirements of the JCAHO, the clinical engineering department must maintain a unique inventory of medical equipment, maintenance histories of that equipment, descriptions of the clinical risks associated with the equipment, and other pertinent data such as special uses or risks, recalls, and incidents.

According to JCAHO standards, clinical engineering must analyze the causes of equipment failures and take steps to preclude recurrences of the problems. The results of these efforts must be monitored to ensure their effectiveness. These procedures apply to operational problems as well as to equipment failures.

To meet the growing needs of the hospital for fiscal integrity, the clinical engineering department should have cost-to-maintain data on all of the hospital's medical equipment and the ability to analyze both these data and the equipment's downtime statistics. Clinical engineering is expected to make informed capital replacement recommendations to administration on the basis of such data.

The clinical engineering department needs specific test equipment to carry out the operations involved in testing and repairing medical equipment. In addition to the typical electronic test instruments, meters, and displays found in all electronics shops, the clinical engineering department must have specialized equipment for testing leakage current, defibrillator outputs, electrosurgical unit outputs, and ultrasound equipment as well as temperature, pressure, and flow levels. Simulators of the various physiological signals measured by medical equipment are also needed. These include electrocardiograms, blood pressure readings, temperature readings, and cardiac output. Departments that service specialized areas such as respiratory therapy, dialysis, and anesthesia must have appropriate equipment.

The stocking of spare parts presents particular problems owing to the need for rapid turnaround of items to be repaired. The department maintains such a wide variety of equipment that it can be very difficult to manage the cost of spare parts. Much of the newer electronics equipment is most quickly repaired by replacing circuit boards that cost hundreds of dollars each. The rate at which technology changes creates a high risk that large spare parts inventories might become obsolete before they can be used.

Staffing and Productivity

The staffing of the clinical engineering department depends on the size of the hospital and the amount of equipment in the inventory. The productivity of a clinical engineering department may vary from 40 percent to 80 percent. This productive time includes the time required to provide the system and management functions required by the JCAHO.

Measures of productivity in a clinical engineering department tend to be somewhat subjective. Most individuals lose between 160 and 400 hours from the basic 2,080-hour work year for vacation, illness, holidays, and other unavailable time. Therefore, the base of available time on which to compare productivity among departments is highly variable. To define productivity as productive time divided by available time, it is necessary to determine the tasks to be included as productive time.

Although preventive maintenance and repairs clearly constitute productive time, there is significant disagreement over the inclusion of other tasks such as writing reports, ordering parts, maintaining records, evaluating equipment, conducting in-service education, and similar tasks. Excluding these tasks can lead to artificially low levels of productivity, as low as 50 percent or less. Conversely, overly generous consideration of this indirect productive work may inflate productivity to unreasonable levels, as high as 80 percent or more.

In light of the emphasis on cost containment and cost effectiveness, a more appropriate measure of productivity is the effective cost per hour. Because clinical engineering services are available from equipment manufacturers and other outside organizations on a quantifiable dollars-per-hour basis, the calculation of an effective charge rate for the clinical engineering department provides a basis for measuring productivity that can be compared to the performance of the private sector.

The effective charge rate is the total cost of operating the department divided by the total number of billable hours. The total cost of operating the department includes budget-line items such as salaries, benefits, rent and utilities, depreciation, and so on, and it must include *all* costs associated with supervision, clerical support, and other indirect functions. A factor reflecting the hospital's overhead should also be considered in the calculation.

Billable hours literally include all hours that are (or could be) billed out to the other departments of the hospital. The actual use of a charge-back system by clinical engineering allows the department to determine what types of work can be billed out to the users.

Under the charge-back system, the department's effective rate should be between $40 and $65 per hour. A rate lower than that level indicates that all costs are not being considered; a rate above that range suggests that the department's productivity indicators and expenses should be seriously analyzed to identify inefficiencies and/or inappropriate expenditures.

The work of the department is accomplished by biomedical equipment technicians (BMETs). A full-time BMET whose time is devoted solely to the maintenance of medical equipment and who is not called on for other types of work or supervision should be able to maintain up to 1,000 pieces of equipment. (A typical 250- to 275-bed community hospital would have about 1,000 pieces of equipment.) However, in a one-person department, this level of productivity cannot be achieved because the BMET is responsible for maintaining all the hospital's operating systems and performing overhead functions, typically without secretarial support.

An entry-level BMET working in a hospital should have a minimum of two years of experience maintaining medical equipment. More experience is required if the BMET is to work without direct supervision. In large hospitals, the supervising BMET should have at least five years of experience.

Many BMETs are trained in the U.S. military services. Other experienced BMETs come to hospitals after working for equipment manufacturers, shared services, independent service organizations, and schools. Many technical schools offer a two-year associate's degree in engineering with an emphasis on biomedical technology.

Although there is an international certification program for BMETs, only a small fraction of people working in the field are certified as bioengineering technicians (CBETs). There are no national licensing standards for BMETs; however, the JCAHO now requires that individuals who maintain medical equipment provide proof of ongoing education. Under any circumstances, the hospital's potential liability for mistakes made by improperly trained maintenance personnel should be reason enough to ensure that the staff charged with maintaining the hospital's medical equipment is properly trained.

In large teaching hospitals, the clinical engineering department may employ a clinical engineer. The clinical engineer holds a bachelor's or master's degree in science and may also be a certified clinical engineer (CCE). The scope of work requiring the presence of a clinical engineer on staff includes problem solving, fiscal management of the program, environmental testing, and general technology management functions. Those hospitals that do not have a sufficient volume of such activities to justify staffing a position typically use outside consultants or shared services staff to perform these functions.

Situations and Problems

Although clinical engineering departments often are strong in technical areas, many are weak in management capabilities. Individuals trained in a highly technical skill are asked not only to provide that skill, but also to manage the budget, the record keeping, and the productivity of the department.

The department's mission may be so weakly defined that the staff finds itself providing services that stray from the original departmental objectives. When this situation occurs, the natural response of the staff is to accept the added responsibilities and expand the scope of the department's services and then to request additional personnel to perform the work required under the original mission. A more appropriate response to such situations is to first evaluate the new services, however interesting they may seem to the staff, in terms of their relation to the specific mission of the department.

The most successful clinical engineering departments are those that operate in large institutions. In such settings, the work load is sufficient to support a functional department with a manager trained in clinical engineering who can directly represent the needs and opinions of the department at the professional levels of the hospital. Unfortunately, many management engineering studies attempt to superimpose this model on small hospitals. The result is often ineffectual and expensive changes. Management studies must concentrate on the needs of the individual institution for clinical engineering services and then evaluate the various methods available to meet those needs and the comparative costs of each approach.

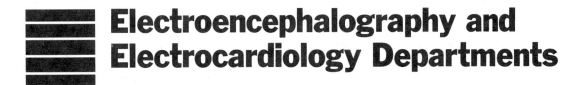

Electroencephalography and Electrocardiology Departments

Overview

The departments of electroencephalography (EEG) and electrocardiology (ECG is the preferred abbreviation, but EKG is also used) provide diagnostic support services. Electroencephalography equipment records the brain-wave patterns produced by the electrical impulses of the brain. This procedure aids in diagnosing various injuries and diseases of the brain. Electrocardiography equipment records the activities of the heart and helps to determine the existence and/or extent of heart disease. Inpatients, outpatients, and emergency department patients may receive both EEGs and ECGs to diagnose a variety of conditions, but inpatient care usually represents at least 80 percent of the departments' work load. This proportion is changing, however, due to the overall growth in outpatient activity brought on by contemporary prospective pricing systems.

Electroencephalography is routinely used to assess neurological and psychiatric disorders. It is one of the few noninvasive tests available to aid physicians in the diagnosis of disease processes that may alter brain functions. Epilepsy is one area in which EEG is particularly useful. Studies can reveal the type of abnormal electrocortical activity, thus enabling physicians to classify seizures and choose appropriate therapy. Studies of electrocerebral inactivity play a major role in determining brain death in patients who have suffered severe brain injury. In addition, laboratories increasingly are performing EEG recordings to assess sleep disorders such as sleep apnea and narcolepsy.

Organization

The EEG and ECG departments in most hospitals are organized as one department and typically are included in the cardiopulmonary department. In many institutions, this department reports to a clinical services vice-president. Historically, the EEG and ECG departments were organized under the direction of the clinical laboratory. Some institutions still have this reporting structure. The services may also be provided under a contract arrangement. Most EEG and ECG departments are centralized, although large hospitals may take a decentralized approach in specialty areas.

Typically, the departments consist of a manager who provides technical direction, technologists and technicians, and clerical support staff. Depending on the size and patient mix of the institution, supervisory responsibility may be delegated for functional areas and operational shifts. Clinical direction is provided through the appointment of a physician as the medical director of the department.

35

Administratively and medically, EEG and ECG department managers may report to a physician who seldom is actually present in the department. When these managers have obtained their authority on the basis of their technical rather than administrative skills (which is a common occurrence), the department may lack the necessary managerial direction and support. This situation can create a difficult working environment and low productivity levels.

Licensing is not required for the technical staff for either the EEG or ECG department, although voluntary certification is available through national associations. The educational background and preparation of the technical staff vary widely. A general qualification guideline is that a technical staff member be a high school graduate who has taken courses in the physical sciences. The technical staff is often prepared through three to six months of on-the-job training programs in hospital settings. Formal educational programs are also available at many hospitals, community colleges, universities, and technical institutes. Such programs are generally one to two years long.

The generally recognized credentials for EEG and ECG technologists are as follows:

- *Registered EEG technologist:* Voluntary certification is available through the American Board of Registration of Electroencephalographic Technologists and requires successful completion of a one-year training program, a one-year internship, and an examination.
- *Registered cardiology technologist:* Voluntary certification is available through the American Cardiology Technologists Association and requires two years of ECG experience and successful completion of an examination.

Technical personnel without certification are usually referred to as technicians. However, terminology is not standardized, and in some institutions they may also be designated as technologists.

The hours of operation of the ECG department vary according to the size of the hospital, its work load, and its patient mix. Staffing patterns generally conform to the department's work load, with most staff members on duty during the day shift. In most large hospitals, ECG departments function seven days a week, varying the number of staff on duty only on weekends. When the ECG department does have limited operating hours, provisions are often made for other clinical staff, such as nursing, laboratory, or respiratory therapy staff, to provide ECG coverage. In contrast, EEG departments are usually staffed five days a week, from 8 a.m. to 5 p.m.

Cross-training of staff can often be used advantageously in these departments. For example, in small hospitals, EEG and ECG staffs may be cross-trained and combined with respiratory therapy or laboratory staff. This system allows the staffing flexibility needed to cover seasonal variations in demand caused by seasonal outbreaks of respiratory diseases such as influenza and asthma. Although cross-training is useful for this reason, a hospital must be careful not to allow untrained personnel to perform tests outside their fields. As the technology associated with these departments becomes increasingly complex, it becomes more difficult to cross-train staff effectively. Because of the critical nature of determining such issues as brain death, only skilled EEG technologists should conduct such examinations.

Required clerical functions include activities such as patient scheduling, telephone answering, transcription of physicians' interpretations, billing, and filing. Both the EEG and ECG departments usually maintain records and may also send tracings and interpretations to the medical record department. The technical staff often performs many clerical functions, particularly in small departments or when assigned to evening or night shifts.

Because of the varied needs for electrocardiograms, ECG units can be found throughout the hospital, and they are used in many different ways. Mobile units are often kept in or near the emergency department, surgical suite, cardiac care unit, laboratory, respiratory therapy area, and other locations where they may be needed immediately. Other ECG equipment may be permanently installed in the stress test laboratory and as part of an intensive care unit's monitoring systems.

Systems have been developed that allow electrocardiograms to be transmitted via radio or telephone to a centralized computer network for interpretation. Such systems are especially useful in isolated rural areas. Some ambulances are also capable of transmitting electrocardiograms to hospital emergency departments from accident scenes or while en route to the hospital. This capability can allow for physician-directed treatment prior to the patient's arrival at the hospital.

Operating Systems and Problems

Most routine ECG work is performed at the patient's bedside or in an ambulatory care setting. Procedures are also performed in the ECG department when specialized instrumentation is required. Special procedures include stress or exercise testing; Holter monitoring; vectorcardiograms, which produce a "stereo" version of the ECG; phonocardiograms, which record heart sounds; echocardiograms, which use ultrasound waves; and cardiac scans, which require the injection of a radioactive substance.

Electrocardiograms must be interpreted by a physician. This interpretation may be provided by the department, by qualified medical staff members on a fee-for-service basis, or by the patient's personal physician.

Electroencephalograms are performed by an EEG technologist in either an inpatient or outpatient setting. After the diagnostic testing is completed, the results of the EEG must be interpreted by a physician. Medical interpretation may be provided as a professional service by the department or by the patient's personal physician. Physicians who interpret EEGs should have the necessary qualifications to do so, such as board certification in EEG or neurology.

Patient charges for EEG and ECG procedures usually include the following components: labor, supplies and services, depreciation, professional fees, and an estimated amount to cover overhead, supervision, hospital administration, and allowance for bad debt. Clerical staff may be assigned to assist with billing functions. The increasing use of computer applications helps to ensure that requisitions and charges are captured correctly.

The charge system may be an area of concern when the departments use manual transcription of technical staff data for billing purposes. Cash flow can be affected adversely when the posting of charges is not timely. This problem can be significantly reduced by using computerized billing procedures.

Financial issues may also be an area of concern. A conflict of interest may arise when the medical director orders many of the services rendered by the department because remuneration incentives may outweigh cost-containment objectives. In teaching hospitals, services may be provided by medical students, interns, and residents who do not properly document the patient information required to ensure proper billing of a diagnostic test. This can have an unfavorable impact on departmental revenue.

Both the ECG and EEG departments are usually responsible for maintaining clinical files. The filing system is a crucial component in providing a satisfactory level of service because a record of previous diagnostic tests is important in making current diagnoses. The organization and management of the filing function can often be improved by implementing color coding and using microfiche for storing older files.

Advances in technology have stimulated changes in the direction and operation of the departments. Labor requirements for routine procedures have been reduced by the development of equipment that eliminates such tasks as cutting and mounting diagnostic tracings. Computerized order and charge-capture systems have decreased clerical requirements. At the same time, the availability of increasingly sophisticated equipment has increased the demand for staff who have the appropriate level of technical skills. As technical specialization becomes more common, such as for echocardiography, staffing the department becomes more difficult.

Staffing and Productivity

Basic staffing requirements can be determined through the use of detailed labor standards. In many institutions, the primary staffing determination is based on adequate coverage. The volume of testing may vary significantly on the basis of the ordering practices of a few physicians.

Issues to consider when reviewing staffing requirements include the characteristics of the patient population, the variability of service demand by hour of day and by day of week, the types of testing offered, the amount of travel time, the amount of clerical time, and the amount of delay or downtime. Recent MONITREND data for the ECG and EEG functional reporting center are provided in table 4.

The fact that much ECG work is performed away from the department may result in control problems for the manager. Staff utilization may be difficult to monitor because the staff is not observed directly. This supervision problem may be compounded when the staff is cross-trained for different functions or among different departments. Equipment use and maintenance may be difficult to monitor because of the need for equipment mobility. These facets of departmental operations suggest the need to establish appropriate evaluation and control mechanisms such as shift reports and monthly statistics reports.

Departmental Analysis

Departmental analyses generally focus on the departments' staffing, filing, charging, and clerical systems and on work-load reporting. Other topics of analysis can include the merging of departments to gain the advantages of cross-training, the separation of departments because of the increased technological skills required of staff, the evaluation of equipment purchases, and the analysis of the cost of contract services.

Table 4. HAS/MONITREND Data for ECG and EEG: Six-Month Medians for Period Ending December 1988

Indicator	National Bed Size Groups							
	Under 50	50–74	75–99	100–149	150–199	200–299	300–399	400 and Over
Work-load units per adjusted patient day[a]	2.88	3.76	3.12	4.26	3.72	4.04	4.24	4.08
Paid hours per adjusted patient day[b]	0.06	0.10	0.10	0.14	0.14	0.17	0.19	0.18

[a]Work-load units per adjusted patient day = ECG and EEG work-load units/(total patient days/ECG and EEG RCC). The ECG and EEG RCC (ratio of charges to charges) is an adjustment factor that is computed as follows: ECG & EEG RCC = ECG & EEG inpatient revenue/(ECG & EEG inpatient revenue + ECG & EEG outpatient revenue).

[b]Paid hours per adjusted patient day = ECG and EEG paid hours/(total patient days/ECG and EEG RCC).

Source: HAS/MONITREND, 1988. Please refer to page x for more information about the data presented in this table.

Emergency Department

Overview

The emergency department provides a central facility for the treatment of the following types of patients:

- Emergency cases that require immediate examination and treatment such as injuries or illnesses of a traumatic nature
- Nonemergency cases that may not require immediate attention, such as headaches, respiratory infections, dressing changes, and suture removals
- Hospital employees and/or private patients of physicians on the staff (in some hospitals)

It should be noted that people who use emergency services are seeking immediate medical assistance and are likely to believe that theirs is a case needing immediate attention regardless of their actual condition. The emergency department is responsible for evaluating the medical needs of patients and determining the appropriate place and method of treatment. Many institutions have established walk-in care areas designed to provide treatment to nonemergency patients. Thus, a patient may be referred to an outpatient clinic, a walk-in care service, or some other hospital service to relieve the patient load in the emergency department.

The importance of the emergency department in the delivery of primary health care is undisputed. More and more people are looking to the emergency department to provide all their medical care. Several factors have been suggested as causes of this increased demand, including the following:

- The public awareness of, and confidence in, the hospital as the most appropriate place to obtain around-the-clock care for unexpected injuries or illnesses
- The acceptance of the hospital by the medical community as the preferred location for treatment of trauma and other life-threatening episodes
- The trend toward specialization in medical practice with a consequent decline in the proportion of practitioners serving as primary family doctors
- The reluctance of physicians to make house calls and the unavailability of physicians at night, on weekends, and on holidays
- The rise in accident rates and in chronic diseases
- The increasing inability of many persons to afford private medical care
- The availability of around-the-clock hospital-based emergency physicians through salaried emergency physician and resident programs

The emergency department is a source of many patients who utilize ancillary hospital services such as laboratory and radiology diagnostic services. Although the use of ancillary services is a source of hospital revenue, the emergency department is a costly area to maintain because of its high fixed costs and periods of low utilization. A utilization rate of 50 to 60 percent is not unusual.

Organization

The emergency department staff consists of physicians, physician assistants, nurses, nursing aides, department managers, orderlies, technicians, receptionists, and clerks. In order to free physicians for the actual treatment of patients, the nursing staff performs the initial assessment of the patient and with appropriate guidelines may order routine diagnostic procedures prior to the physician's examination of the patient. In small-volume departments, night-shift coverage may be provided by the night-shift nursing supervisor. Physician assistants are often used to reduce delays caused by the unavailability of a physician. Physician assistants are typically found in high-volume departments, where they treat routine, nonurgent cases under the direction of a physician.

Generally, the nursing staff reports to the head nurse of the department, and physicians report to the hospital's administration. However, several alternative organizational models are possible. For example:

- All emergency department staff (physician, nursing, clerical) may report to the administration (clinical services, ambulatory services, or patient care services).
- All emergency department staff may report to a physician director, who in turn reports to the administration.
- The emergency department staff may report to the administration while the nursing department supervises the nursing staff indirectly (that is, recruiting, credentialing, and in-service education). In some instances, this model has been formalized to include contractual agreements between the nursing and emergency department administrations.

The members of the ancillary staff (that is, laboratory, radiology, electrocardiology, and so on) usually report to (and are scheduled by) their respective departments. Staff coverage (hours and staff levels) is determined by ancillary administration in consultation with the emergency department.

Volunteer workers may be assigned to the emergency department on a part-time basis to perform routine clerical tasks during peak periods. In some states, the law stipulates that at least one physician and one nurse must be on duty around the clock.

The emergency department may be designated as a base station as part of an areawide emergency medical system. As such, the department includes a radio communication center for providing clinical advice to paramedical units or remote treatment centers.

Hospital-based emergency physician staffing may be arranged through a contractual relationship with an outside service or practice, or the physicians may be paid directly by the hospital. Salaried physicians are often compensated at an hourly rate for on-duty periods of 8, 10, 12, or 24 hours. Private physicians may also attend patients in the emergency department.

Board certification for physicians who treat emergency patients is a growing dimension of medicine. Nurses working in the emergency department must also have appropriate credentials.

Models and Systems

Models and systems commonly found in emergency departments are designed to set priorities for patient treatment and to ensure efficient charging, registration, and record keeping.

Setting Priorities for Treatment

The emergency department system must accommodate patients who need treatment in several areas. The emergency department is the primary area of treatment, but it also requires additional diagnostic services such as radiology, laboratory, and electrocardiography. Thus, a key to the effective delivery of treatment is the policy that sets priorities for the treatment of patients.

The emergency staff is trained to recognize the nature and relative severity of a patient's condition. In order to avoid civil liability suits against the physician and/or the hospital, the staff must also know the legal requirements pertaining to the treatment of patients who present themselves in the emergency department. In large hospitals that experience a heavy influx of emergency patients, a triage sorting system establishes priorities for treatment of critical or emergency patients. The priority for treatment is determined by the degree to which the patient's life is threatened.

Typically, patients are classified as follows:

- *Emergency:* The patient requires immediate medical attention; life, limb, or sight is threatened.
- *Urgent:* The patient requires medical attention within a few hours and will be in danger if left unattended; medical follow-up is required.
- *Nonemergency:* The patient's disorder is minor and not acute (such as removal of a cast); the visit might have been scheduled by a physician.

Patients are also described according to the type of medical problem involved (surgical, medical, obstetrical, pediatric, or orthopedic) and according to the type of physician who will provide treatment (private physician or physician service).

Contingency plans are established in hospitals to cover those situations in which several emergency visits occur simultaneously (for example, a car crash, a fire, or another type of disaster). Personnel outside the emergency department are instructed to respond to certain codes, such as "Code Blue" or "Code 99," so that timely and proper patient care may be provided in these situations.

The established policies and procedures of the hospital, the personal preferences of the emergency physician, the specialized equipment available for examination and treatment, and the size of the staff with respect to the rate of patient arrival affect the length of time required to treat emergency patients. For example, all emergency departments have the capacity for typical ancillary services (laboratory, radiology, electrocardiology, and so on). However, emergency departments designated as trauma centers have 24-hour coverage of anesthesiology and trauma surgery. Depending on patient mix and services, emergency departments may have facilities for dental, psychiatric, and pediatric patients as well.

One area of conflict that may arise in the emergency department involves the relationship between the patient and his or her private physician. A patient may visit the emergency department in response to the family doctor's instruction or in the hope of finding the doctor there. Some hospitals, by policy or tradition, require a house physician to provide care for all emergency patients. Others may allow the house physician to assess the severity of the emergency and take action only when necessary or after it becomes evident that the family physician is delayed or unavailable. The conflict involves the patient's preferences and the question of which physician collects the fees.

Emergency department policies and procedures are influenced by guidelines established by the Joint Commission on Accreditation of Healthcare Organizations (JCAHO) and by the applicable statutes contained in the general laws of the state in which the hospital is located.

Charging, Registration, and Record Keeping

Hospitals use various charging systems. Two typical models for charging are the following:

- *Flat rate:* Patients are charged an established fee for the visit and for each treatment in the emergency department.
- *Sliding scale:* Patients are classified according to the level of treatment provided and are charged corresponding rates.

Hospital-based physicians' charges are generally issued by the hospital. Private physicians' charges are often billed separately by the physician.

Manual registration and charge systems may be replaced with computerized systems that include order-entry systems. Large emergency departments may have substantial computerization. The registration staff may not be part of the emergency department staff but may instead be part of the central registration or admitting staff.

All documentation of diagnosis, treatment, and so forth is made on the emergency record. The medical record department is usually responsible for retaining the record. In addition, a log of all individuals who seek treatment in the emergency department must be maintained.

Departmental Analysis

Analysis of the emergency department should focus on the following topics:

- *Staff:* Measure staff utilization and productivity; identify the clinical and nonclinical skills needed for each shift; determine the appropriate number of part-time and full-time staff members needed. Examples of productivity measures are hours per patient encounter and hours per patient type. (Recent MONITREND data for the emergency service functional reporting center are provided in table 5.) Because of the standby nature of the emergency department's activities, staff utilization is typically not very high. Representative utilization ranges are 40 to 60 percent for the night shift, 50 to 75 percent for the evening shift, and 60 to 80 percent for the day shift.
- *Treatment room:* Develop a profile of utilization by hour, day, physician, and treatment room; study the adequacy of the department's facilities.
- *Patients:* Study the number of patients requiring treatment by day of the week and time of the day. Review procedures for patient examination and routing, and recommend improvements.
- *Minor surgery:* Analyze the adequacy of present surgical facilities; consider alternatives and improvements.
- *Materials management:* Review procedures for acquisition, stocking, control, distribution, and transportation of supplies; check for pilferage problems.
- *Management reporting:* Develop a reporting system for managers to monitor utilization and productivity regularly.
- *Ambulance service:* Assess the adequacy of ambulance service.

Table 5. HAS/MONITREND Data for Emergency Service: Six-Month Medians for Period Ending December 1988

Indicator	National Bed Size Groups							
	Under 50	50–74	75–99	100–149	150–199	200–299	300–399	400 and Over
Visits per calendar day[a]	9.85	21.81	28.37	42.29	55.10	72.81	83.63	100.93
Paid hours per visit[b]	1.56	1.89	2.00	2.02	2.13	2.20	2.29	2.66

[a]Visits per calendar day = emergency visits/days in period.

[b]Paid hours per visit = emergency paid hours/emergency visits.

Source: HAS/MONITREND, 1988. Please refer to page x for more information about the data presented in this table.

- *Staff education:* Through surveys and interviews, measure staff skills and recommend special training as appropriate.
- *Housekeeping:* Study staffing, scheduling, and quality control.
- *Management:* Study the management structure and policies for meeting JCAHO standards; examine issues related to the billing and collection of physicians' fees.
- *Ancillary support:* Determine the effectiveness of the support services provided by ancillary departments to assess the impact of patient delays on the effectiveness of the emergency department staff.
- *Patient registration and transportation:* Study the factors relating to emergency patient registration; study transportation patterns for the emergency department and for the hospital; analyze patient needs and staffing requirements.
- *Charging procedures:* Review procedures for charging for visits and evaluate alternative charge systems; review cost and revenue data.
- *Clerical staff:* Review clerical procedures, task assignments, and the design and use of forms.
- *Logs and record books:* Review records to determine whether statistics are maintained as required by the hospital's bylaws and accreditation regulations.

A thorough analysis of the emergency department should encompass all areas of the hospital. It is often true that problems elsewhere in the hospital have a significant effect on emergency services. For example, if abnormal lengths of inpatient stays have led to high hospitalwide occupancy levels, an inpatient bed may not be available for a patient being admitted from the emergency department. Delays and extra staffing demands in the department may be reduced by giving careful attention to problems in seemingly unrelated areas of the hospital.

Energy Management and Maintenance

Overview

Public awareness of energy costs and the need for conservation have increased in recent years largely because of sharply increasing energy prices, scarcity of energy resources, and legislative activity on energy issues. A twofold message seems to have evolved that stresses the importance not only of conservation of present resources, but also of the development and use of alternative sources. Hospitals, whose energy costs may represent as much as 5 to 7 percent of the operations budget, are well aware of this message.

The energy management and maintenance function may be treated as a separate hospital department in large hospitals. In small facilities, it is often a subsection of the maintenance department or a function assigned to one individual. The size and complexity of the institution are definite factors in the department's organization.

In essence, the hospital's use of energy is similar in purpose to that of residential homes and other facilities, but some special applications exist. The basic hospital functions that consume energy and resources are the following:

- Environmental control, including heating, ventilating, and air-conditioning (HVAC)
- Heating and cooling water
- Lighting
- Cooking, refrigerating, and freezing food
- Operating medical, sterilization, incineration, laundry, and other types of equipment

Over the years, as hospitals have been built, the types of power plants installed have been determined by the geographic location of the facilities and by the environmental and economic conditions of the time. Currently, environmental impact is of great concern in determining the type of power plant to install in a new or remodeled facility.

Major Types of Energy

Typically, natural gas, fuel oil, coal, steam, electricity, or a combination of these is the hospital's primary source of energy for heating. In addition, solar power might be used in conjunction with other power sources.

Natural Gas

Natural gas is a very clean and efficient fuel that has a positive effect on boiler and chimney maintenance. Storage is also relatively easy because gas can be either piped in or bottled.

The availability and the use of gas are influenced by the geographic area and by whether the location is urban or rural. However, natural gas is the most commonly used fuel in hospitals.

Gas consumption is usually measured in units of 1,000 cubic feet. For piped-in gas, meters are used to measure monthly consumption. For bottled gas, delivery records or installed meters may be used. The price of gas may be a function of the amount consumed and/or the rate of consumption. A hospital may have several gas accounts, depending on various uses, such as main heating, kitchen, and residential use. Some hospitals use interruptible gas service, which is cut off at a predetermined temperature. Such hospitals maintain a secondary fuel, usually oil, as a backup.

Fuel Oil

Fuel oil, usually used to fire boilers, is available in various grades, with number 2 and number 6 oil the most commonly used. Although less costly than number 2 oil, number 6 oil is a cruder form of oil and therefore requires additional processing to make it burnable. For instance, number 6 oil must be reheated before burning to maintain an appropriate level of viscosity. In addition, number 6 oil does not provide as much thermal energy per gallon as number 2 oil.

The consumption of fuel oil is measured in gallons. Billing records usually indicate both the number of gallons and the dollar value of the fuel oil consumed. Because oil deliveries vary with the weather, billing periods are sporadic and the exact monthly consumption may be difficult to measure. However, some hospitals obtain accurate readings by installing a meter at the boiler or by measuring tank level at least once a month.

Coal

The use of coal as a heating fuel has fluctuated in recent years, largely in response to changes in its availability and price. Environmental restrictions have also affected the use of coal. Measuring and comparing British thermal units (Btus) of coal is difficult because the heating value of different types of coal varies considerably.

Coal consumption is measured in tons. The measurement of consumption depends on the type and size of boiler in use. For example, a small, hand-fed boiler may contain no gauge with which to record daily consumption, but a large installation may weigh the coal as it is fed into the furnace.

Steam

Most hospitals use fuel oil, gas, or coal to produce steam in a boiler plant, but some hospitals purchase steam from a central facility or utility. The steam is transported via underground steam pressure lines or pipes. Steam is used for heating, air-conditioning, heating water, sterilizing medical instruments (autoclaving), and drying laundry and linen. Whether the steam is purchased or produced by the hospital's boiler, the measuring unit of consumption or production is expressed as the heat energy in 1,000 pounds of steam. The rate of consumption is expressed in pounds per hour.

Electricity

Electric energy has many applications, among them lighting, equipment operation, air-conditioning, ventilation, and sometimes heating. Electricity differs from other energy sources in that it is directly consumable, whereas other sources must be converted in a central power plant to produce power. The measuring unit of consumption for electricity is the kilowatt-hour, and the unit of demand, or rate of consumption, is the kilowatt.

The cost of electricity is usually based on both consumption and demand. The billing procedure reflects the utility's total cost of producing electricity. Typically, about two-thirds of an electric utility's revenues are used to pay for installed equipment, which must be sized to meet peak demands. The cost of electricity can vary widely by utility, even within the same state, depending on the age of the power plants, whether nuclear plants are used, and what rate increases for abandoned projects or power plants have been authorized to be charged to consumers by the rate payers. Generally, the cost is lower when the nuclear power plant is operating at full capacity. Consequently, the cost rises when existing power plants are not operating and alternative fuels such as imported oil must be used.

The cost of capital equipment is recovered in part through a demand charge based on peak demand, and the cost of fuel to generate electricity is based on the amount consumed. In other words, a hospital's electric bill consists of two parts: a demand charge and a consumption charge. Peak demand usually occurs during the summer months to meet air-conditioning needs. This yearly peak is often the basis for demand charges during the winter months as well, when the actual, registered demand is low. Thus, in effect, the hospital must pay year-round for high summer demand, a billing procedure referred to as "summer ratchet." To compute the bill each month, the utility assigns a billed demand equal to or greater than the actual demand. Billed demand depends on a number of factors, the most important one being the summer ratchet.

The hospital may have several electricity accounts for various uses and with varying rates. Monthly electric bills provide good consumption and cost data. Traditionally, electricity used as the major heating source has been the most expensive of the options.

Organization

The director of engineering and maintenance is responsible for energy management in most hospitals. Another common title for this position is administrative engineer. A developing trend is to give the administrative director responsibility for environmental services (housekeeping), food service, and maintenance. The department has 24-hour coverage or on-call access and responsibility, especially with regard to the operations of the power plant.

Traditionally, energy conservation was practiced informally, primarily from a power or physical plant orientation. In most cases, the utility bills (fuel oil, gas, and electricity) were reviewed by the director of engineering and then forwarded to accounts payable. The basic shortcoming of this traditional assignment of responsibility is that it does not involve all personnel within the hospital who can affect energy usage. For instance, many people have an effect on thermostat settings and electricity and hot water usage.

The present concern over energy conservation has prompted many hospitals to form energy committees or energy management committees. The organizational structure of these committees may include a core group of representatives from the administrative, engineering and maintenance, nursing, and medical staffs. Additional members might include the department heads and supervisors, depending on the specific topics of study. The purpose of the committees is to gain support and commitment from top-level management for energy conservation and eventually to involve all hospital personnel. The energy committee may be a subcommittee of the hospital's cost-containment committee.

Models and Systems

Analyzing and evaluating energy consumption and conservation requires both engineering and economic analysis skills. Because the largest energy-consuming function is usually heating, ventilating, and air-conditioning, theoretical knowledge of thermodynamic principles as well as a practical understanding of boiler plants and air-conditioning are essential. Engineering skills in relation to electromechanical devices (motors and generators), circuits, and lighting systems are also required. Cost analyses employ such classic engineering and economic principles as payback period, return on investment, and ranking of alternatives. The engineering terms and indicators can be translated into economic terms for costing purposes.

Energy Consumption Indicators

Two basic engineering measurements used for analysis are the degree-day and the British thermal unit. A degree-day represents one degree of difference between 65°F (degrees Fahrenheit) and the mean daily outdoor temperature. For example, if the mean daily temperature is 40°F, the number of heating degree-days is 65 minus 40, or 25. Cooling degree-days are measured in a similar manner when outside temperatures are higher than 65°F. Degree-days can be tallied daily to obtain a monthly total, and degree-day statistics can also be obtained monthly from the local U.S. Weather Service. Such statistics are the best available measurement of heating and cooling requirements.

The British thermal unit is considered the common base for calculating energy use. It is defined as the quantity of heat required to raise the temperature of 1 pound of water 1°F at or near a temperature of 39.2°F. For example, the energy given off by a large wooden match is about equal to 1 Btu. The various sources of energy (fuel oil, gas, electricity, or other) are measured in different types of units, but each measurement can also be expressed as a British thermal unit equivalent. For example, 1 cubic foot of gas contains approximately 1,000 Btu (equivalent to 1 MBtu). By converting from British thermal units to a measurable volume, a cost can be assigned. Approximate equivalents for common energy sources are listed in table 6.

Energy indicators and their economic impact are usually expressed in terms of calculated values; five such factors are as follows:

- Total energy costs in dollars (may be compared on an annual, monthly, or seasonal basis)
- Energy costs as a percentage of the operating budget
- Total energy costs per gross square foot (may be calculated as a universal indicator for comparing hospitals located within the same climatic area)
- Total energy consumed per gross square foot (may be expressed in British thermal units)
- Cost per unit of energy in dollars per million British thermal units (may be calculated for various energy sources, allowing comparison among hospitals; such measurements may be separated by energy source)

Rule-of-Thumb Data

Rule-of-thumb data are helpful in determining which cost reduction efforts would be worthwhile to pursue. For instance, a potential 10 percent reduction in heating fuel consumption would save far more than a 10 percent reduction in lighting costs. Because the sizes of hospitals and their environments and systems vary, simple indicators do not provide an accurate guideline. However, the sample allocation of energy usage in table 7 may be informative.

Table 6. Approximate MBtu Equivalents for Common Energy Sources

Energy Source	Unit of Measurement	MBtu Equivalent
Electricity	Kilowatt-hour	3.41
Steam	Pound	1,000.00
Natural gas	Cubic foot	1,000.00
Fuel oil (no. 2 burner)	Gallon	139.00
Coal (bituminous)	Ton	28,000.00

Table 7. Sample Allocation of Energy Usage

Energy Application	Percentage of Total Energy Consumption
Environmental control	40–65
Lighting and electrical outlets	10–20
Food service	5–10
Medical equipment	3–5
Sterilization and incineration	2

Other Considerations

The political issues concerning energy conservation are evident on the local, state, and national levels. Legislation regulates energy usage. The uncertainty of fuel prices makes energy planning difficult. In the first half of 1989, the energy component of the consumer price index rose dramatically. However, funds for energy-saving programs and construction have become available from the government. Private sector companies and foundations, especially energy and fuel companies, have also distributed funds for energy conservation studies, energy audits, technical assistance, and other projects.

In terms of hospital employee involvement, energy conservation in the hospital might tend to receive more lip service than action. For example, individuals may lack the incentive to turn off the lights when they do not pay the electricity bill personally. Building support for a conservation program requires the commitment of top-level management, the involvement of all personnel, and possibly an incentive or reward system.

Hospitals may have internal financial competition for funds allocated to conservation. That is, most hospitals have limited capital available, and requests for clinical technology often take precedence over plant equipment, even though such equipment may save energy dollars over the long term. In addition, capital expenditures may require certificates of need from the state government. The result is that large-scale investments for energy conservation that should occur as part of new building programs may not be included because of their initial costs.

Departmental Analysis

Three types of energy studies can be undertaken: an energy audit, specific studies, and an energy program. The procedures for analyzing energy use are discussed in the following paragraphs.

Energy Audit

An audit is usually the first step in analyzing a hospital's use of energy. The audit should include a fact-finding study of the types and amount of energy used, as well as a survey of the building and all equipment.

The fact-finding study answers the question, "What energy sources are we using for what purposes?" by quantifying and summarizing energy usage. The hospital's consumption of energy is tabulated and analyzed by checking existing records and invoices. Both usage and cost may be plotted on graphs to reveal trends and patterns. The fact-finding data are useful for identifying problem areas, forecasting future consumption, and analyzing the cost of improvements.

A survey of the building and the equipment, an analysis of systems and their effectiveness, and a quality control check are necessary before planning cost reductions. Survey checklists can be used for all major factors in energy use, including heating, ventilation, and air-conditioning; laundry; windows and doors; and insulation. Sample survey questions include: "What is the maximum temperature measured in the hot water system(s)? Do regulations require it to be so high?" The information from the fact-finding study and from the building and equipment survey can be used to identify problem areas and to determine the nature and extent of specific in-depth studies to be undertaken.

Specific Studies

Specific analyses can range from simply measuring the effect of reducing lighting to planning technical changes in the boiler plant equipment. The analytical process is much the same, however. Basic engineering and cost analysis techniques should be used. In each study, energy costs and expected savings from alternative systems or equipment can be predicted. The technical expertise required varies. For example, changes in HVAC systems may require evaluation by both hospital engineering personnel and professional engineering consultants. Energy providers, such as electric companies and oil distributors, can provide valuable information, particularly in regard to their pricing structure.

Specific studies may include the following topics: cost benefits of insulation, electric power factor improvement, piping insulation, window and door insulation, lighting reductions and compliance with regulated lighting standards, hot water temperature reduction, steam pressure reduction, boiler conversion to alternative fuel, cleaning and maintenance of HVAC vents and filters, descaling of boilers, scheduled air-conditioning, and the feasibility of a computer-monitored and computer-controlled environmental system.

Energy Program

The process of establishing an energy management program parallels that of a cost-containment program, and the principles of cost containment are useful in conducting studies. In fact, a hospital's energy committee may be a subcommittee of the hospital's cost-containment committee.

The basic issues that should be assessed and addressed regarding an energy management program include the following:

- The policy of top-level management regarding conservation and energy management programs
- Such specific goals, objectives, and considerations as reducing energy costs and planning for a new building
- The organization and involvement of personnel, the responsibility of individuals, and the formation of committees
- The documentation of study findings
- The availability of funds to be invested in saving energy
- Plans to encourage the cooperation of all personnel, including incentives, bonuses, and recognition programs

Sources

The following agencies and organizations may be helpful:

- Department of Energy (DOE), on the state as well as the federal levels
- Public utilities that provide electricity and gas
- State department of public utilities, rates and research division
- Environmental Protection Agency (EPA)
- Local societies of engineering personnel
- State hospital associations
- Political action groups that provide up-to-date information on legislation and regulation issues, such as public interest research groups
- State energy policy offices

Environmental Services

Overview

Environmental services, also called the housekeeping department, is primarily responsible for maintaining a clean, safe, and functional environment in the hospital. The department has an effect on patient care and on the morale and performance of the entire hospital staff. The department performs a wide variety of tasks, which include:

- *Daily cleaning:* Mopping floors, dusting furniture, cleaning rest rooms, and so forth in patient rooms as well as offices, corridors, waiting rooms, and other areas
- *Scheduled project work:* Washing windows, stripping and waxing floors, shampooing carpets, washing walls, cleaning vents, and replacing curtains and draperies
- *Trash removal:* Moving trash from various points within the hospital to an incinerator, compactor, or dumpster
- *Furniture moving:* Rearranging or moving furniture as needed
- *Discharge cleaning:* Cleaning the room for a newly admitted patient after the discharge or transfer of another patient
- *Infection control:* Ensuring conditions for good patient care by using proven techniques and procedures to minimize the chance of spreading infections

The department's responsibilities may also extend to interior decorating, laundry, the disposition of hazardous materials, the purchase of furniture, and contract negotiation and management.

Organization

The staff of the environmental services department is often one of the largest in the hospital and typically consists of a director, shift supervisors, line personnel, and clerical workers. Depending on the size of the facility, the department may also have an assistant director.

The director generally reports to the vice-president for support services or to an assistant administrator. The director is responsible for many administrative duties, including budget preparation and monitoring, requisitioning, purchasing, scheduling, and report preparation. The director must be a problem solver, supervisor, trainer, scheduler, coordinator, morale builder, and disciplinarian.

The director should be knowledgeable about labor relations, systems development, chemicals, infection and inventory control, and right-to-know and waste-handling regulations, as well as regulations from the Occupational Safety and Health Administration. He or she must be familiar with medical terminology as applied to housekeeping procedures and must have the ability to communicate with staff and other department directors. In addition, the director should be able to delegate authority; be able to plan, develop, and administer all phases of a comprehensive housekeeping program; use cost analysis methods and manpower utilization studies; and understand sanitation standards. Currently, it is reasonable to expect an environmental services director to hold a bachelor's degree in a subject related to hospital environmental services or basic management.

The assistant director and/or the shift supervisors schedule the work of line personnel and manage and monitor the work activities of the department, including the training, discipline, and motivation of the staff. They act as liaisons between environmental services workers and other workers in the hospital and make arrangements to carry out special tasks. They must be completely familiar with housekeeping procedures and must be able to communicate with all hospital staff effectively.

Line personnel (often called housekeepers, service workers, environmental assistants, or environmental technicians) must receive on-the-job training because they often come to the department with little or no experience. Most institutions today require that line personnel be able to read and write English. Furthermore, institutions may require that line personnel hold a high school diploma or its equivalent. At the minimum, line personnel must be able to read labels, prepare chemicals at the proper dilution ratio, and identify an isolation sign.

Clerical workers perform routine functions such as answering telephones, relaying messages, and communicating with the admissions/registration department and the nursing service.

Staffing and Supervision

There are no strict guidelines for environmental services staffing because staffing levels depend on many variables, including:

- *Scope of environmental services:* What administrative and/or union expectations govern the scope and frequency of required activities? (For example, is the department responsible for delivering clean linen and removing soiled linen from nursing units? Does the department clean food service areas? Does it change light bulbs and clean vents? Are office wastebaskets emptied twice per day or three times per week?) In addition, what are the expectations regarding desired levels of environmental appearance?
- *Facility:* Is the hospital in new or aging facilities? What is the location of the hospital? How many beds does the hospital have? What is the square footage of cleanable space? Are the facilities centralized or decentralized? What are the hospital's interior surfaces (carpeted or hard-surface floors, painted or vinyl-covered walls)?
- *Specialty units:* What are the number and types of specialty units requiring special care in the hospital? To what extent is the department responsible for providing services to these units? Such units might include lithotripsy, operating and recovery rooms, intensive care units, maintenance areas, and the labor and delivery suite.
- *Federal, state, and local regulations:* What standards or criteria have regulating bodies imposed on the operation of the department?

Work Schedule and Work Assignment

The work schedule of the environmental services department should be established for staffing on all three shifts. A large part of the cleaning, particularly on the nursing units, is done during the day shift. Staff on the evening and night shifts handle high-priority cleaning on the nursing units and in the emergency department. In addition, the administrative and clinical areas are cleaned mostly after scheduled business hours to avoid interfering with peak activity periods during the workday.

Of highest priority for the department is ensuring that patient rooms are available after patients have been discharged or transferred. During periods of high patient census, other scheduled housekeeping activities should be rearranged to facilitate readying patient rooms.

Supervision

Due to the assignment of environmental services staff to all areas of the hospital during all shifts, supervision is difficult. In many hospitals, shift supervisors oversee the cleaning functions, providing hands-on supervision to ensure that duties are performed adequately. Inadequate supervision can result in poor performance, inefficiency, and low employee morale. Similar problems may result when the supervisor cannot gain the cooperation of fellow workers.

Interdepartmental Communications

One of the environmental services department's keys to efficiency and effectiveness is good communications with the admissions/registration department and the nursing units. The three areas should cooperate closely in setting priorities and in communicating their needs in order to reduce potential conflict among departments.

Communication between environmental services and the admissions/registration department is especially important when the hospital has a high occupancy rate. When rooms are not cleaned quickly after patients are discharged, newly admitted patients may have to wait for their rooms. With prompt notification of new admissions, transfers, and discharges, the shift supervisors can streamline and organize the work load so that rooms are cleaned and readied for new patients as quickly as possible. The supervisors should then notify the admissions/registration department and the nursing units that the rooms are ready.

Environmental services personnel should also work very closely with nursing personnel in the patient care areas, and good communications among them is essential. Nevertheless, conflicts sometimes arise regarding the following issues:

- The time of day that major cleaning is performed
- The environmental services staff's responsiveness to requests from nursing personnel
- Clarification of the specific duties and responsibilities of the nursing units and environmental services with respect to housekeeping functions
- Notification of admissions, transfers, and discharges
- Attitudes of other personnel toward housekeepers

Open and consistent communication, and respect for fellow workers, can help minimize potential conflicts.

One particularly vital subject for interdepartmental communications is infection control, which has become an important aspect of environmental services activities. In most hospitals, an infection control committee is responsible for ensuring that all reasonable steps are taken to prevent nosocomial, or hospital-acquired, infections. The environmental services director is usually an important member of the committee, which may assess the appropriateness of housekeeping techniques with respect to infection control as well as determine the sources of patient infections.

Departmental Analysis

Analysis of the environmental services department can identify opportunities for improving staffing, quality of service, communications, and coverage. The following topics are typical areas for management engineering studies in the department:

- *Staffing requirements:* Rudimentary staffing requirements could be calculated by reviewing MONITREND and other data. Recent MONITREND data for the housekeeping functional reporting center are provided in table 8. Particular attention should be given to staffing for areas where cleaning activities are required.
- *Quality of service:* Quality standards should be established and monitored in an ongoing manner. Simple checklists can be used to tally acceptable and unacceptable standards for each day. These can then be monitored over time to help focus attention on quality. Quality standards might include whether the task was completed correctly and on time, whether complaints were received concerning the task, and whether appropriate safety guidelines were followed, such as the use of caution signs on wet floors.
- *Supervision problems and labor relations:* The effectiveness of supervision should be studied to determine whether improvements in staff morale and productivity can be made. As with quality standards, one effective way for supervisors to monitor staff productivity is through the use of checklists. A checklist can detail tasks to be performed and can indicate whether and when the work was actually completed. This enables the supervisor to review and document the activities of several housekeepers who may be performing tasks throughout the hospital.
- *Communications systems:* A study evaluating manual and automated systems could be carried out to select the most appropriate system or to improve communications among environmental services, admissions/registration, and the nursing service.
- *In-service education:* A study could be done to evaluate the skills possessed by environmental services personnel and to identify the skills that they need to acquire. The results of such a study would indicate what type of training should be provided.
- *Work-load scheduling:* An evaluation of the routine cleaning required in relation to patient discharges and admissions might improve the utilization of personnel.
- *Environmental services logistics:* An analysis of the methods of distributing housekeeping supplies and equipment might identify ways to save labor and improve the use of equipment.
- *Materials management:* An evaluation of the use of supplies might identify potential savings through appropriate use or substitution of products. Examples might include the substitution of less costly but equally effective cleaning solutions or the substitution of more costly but much more durable cleaning equipment.

The keys to the effective operation of an environmental services department are good supervision, careful selection and training of employees, and consistently followed housekeeping procedures. A contract-managed arrangement could be made if the hospital did not have the internal resources necessary to provide comparable services. However, the cost of a contract service should be carefully compared to its potential benefits.

Table 8. HAS/MONITREND Data for Housekeeping: Six-Month Medians for Period Ending December 1988

Indicator	National Bed Size Groups							
	Under 50	50–74	75–99	100–149	150–199	200–299	300–399	400 and Over
Square feet per bed[a]	870.17	946.09	925.93	965.26	1074.11	1030.30	1116.03	1036.71
Paid hours per 1,000 square feet[b]	26.42	28.96	28.20	29.71	28.80	30.14	29.18	29.29

[a]Square feet per bed = housekeeping serviced square feet/total beds.

[b]Paid hours per 1,000 square feet = housekeeping paid hours/(housekeeping serviced square feet/1,000).

Source: HAS/MONITREND, 1988. Please refer to page x for more information about the data presented in this table.

▤ Fiscal Services

Overview

In most not-for-profit as well as for-profit hospitals, the fiscal services division is responsible for the long-term oversight as well as the day-to-day operational management of its institution's fiscal resources. The division's overall goal is to ensure and optimize the financial viability of the hospital so that it can continue to provide the high-quality health care services its community needs, at an acceptable level of cost. Under the leadership of the chief financial officer (CFO) or controller, the division performs the following general financial management activities as part of the day-to-day operations of the hospital:

- General accounting
- Payroll distribution
- Internal control
- Budget preparation

In addition, hospital fiscal services perform two operations not required in other types of organizations:

- Patient accounting
- Third-party reimbursement processing

Hospitals are unlike commercial organizations in that a significant portion of their total revenues are generated by services provided to patients but paid for by third parties other than the direct consumers of the services; that is, third-party payers (including governmental programs such as Medicare and Medicaid, Blue Cross/Blue Shield plans, and commercial insurance companies) are responsible for reimbursing hospitals for the services provided to most patients. This factor presents unique administrative, operational, and information management challenges to fiscal services divisions in hospitals.

In the past, the role of the CFO or controller and the functions of the fiscal services division in hospitals primarily focused on such short-term, day-to-day operations as bookkeeping and business office activities rather than on long-term planning activities aimed at ensuring the future financial viability of the hospital. Today, however, ongoing changes in the health care industry and growing pressure from government, business, and third-party payers to reduce the cost of health care and make hospitals and other health care institutions more efficient have made it clear that strong financial management is as crucial to health care organizations as it is to commercial organizations and U.S. industry in general. The role of the CFO as an executive officer of the hospital at the policy-making level will continue to gain importance in the foreseeable future.

Organization and Functions

The administrative leader of the fiscal services division is usually referred to as the CFO or the vice-president of finance. In some smaller hospitals, however, the head of fiscal services is still called the controller. No matter what title this manager holds, the CFO most likely reports directly to the hospital's chief executive officer (CEO) and is responsible for all of the financial functions of the hospital.

Many of the specific functions of a hospital's fiscal services division may be delegated to subordinate managers, although the specific organizational structure varies widely among various sizes and kinds of hospitals. In the organizational structure for a large institution suggested by Russell A. Caruana [*Organizing a Healthcare Financial Services Division,* 3rd ed. (Westchester, IL: Healthcare Financial Management Association, 1989), p. 3] and shown in figure 3, the various departments within the fiscal services division are headed by managers who report to three associate vice-presidents, who in turn report to the vice-president of finance. These associate vice-presidents oversee the operations of the following areas:

- Financial services (general accounting, budget and reimbursement, and financial planning)
- Patient administration (patient accounting, medical records, and admissions/registration)
- Information services (computer operations and services support and development)

Smaller institutions may consolidate these responsibilities rather than assigning them to separate departments (see figure 4). In addition, the presence of the medical record, admissions/registration, and information systems departments under the umbrella of fiscal services depends on the organizational structure of the hospital as determined by the governing board and the CEO as well as the degree to which the hospital has developed its own information systems.

The functions of the fiscal services division can be summarized in three broad categories:

- Keeping records of financial transactions and conducting internal control procedures
- Planning, budgeting, and rate setting
- Measuring and reporting on organizational performance

Keeping Financial Records

The principal—and traditional—function of hospital fiscal services is to keep records of all the financial transactions of the hospital. In most hospitals today, this record-keeping function includes the areas of general accounting, patient accounting, and reimbursement. Accounts payable, cash application, and payroll administration are generally subsumed under general accounting, although they are handled separately. Also related to financial record keeping is the hospital's system for planning and coordinating its internal control process.

General Accounting

General accounting can be defined as the appropriate recording, allocation, and monitoring of all financial transactions in the hospital's general ledger. The general accounting staff can be held responsible for ensuring that sound accounting practices are implemented within the institution. General accounting data are the basis for a variety of analyses and reports central to effective financial management.

Accounts Payable

Accounts payable involves the accounting and disbursement of funds (payments) owed to vendors for goods or services provided to the hospital. An authorization form, generally

Figure 3. Consolidated Fiscal Services Division

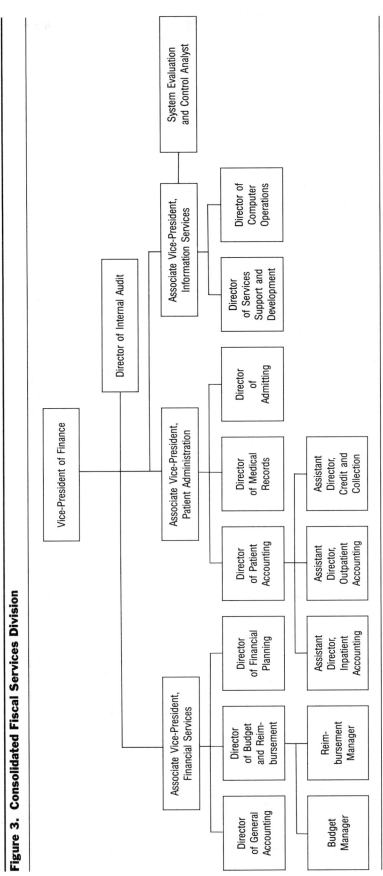

Adapted from Russell A. Caruana, *Organizing a Healthcare Financial Services Division*, 3rd ed. (Westchester, IL: Healthcare Financial Management Association, 1989), p. 3.

Figure 4. Organizational Structure of Fiscal Services for a Small- to Medium-Size Acute Care Community Healthcare Organization

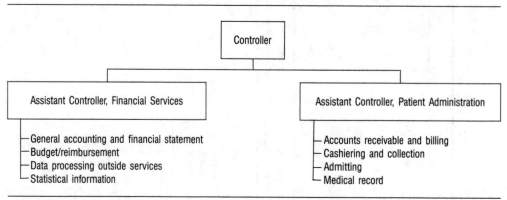

Adapted from Russell A. Caruana, *Organizing a Healthcare Financial Services Division,* 3rd ed. (Westchester, IL: Healthcare Financial Management Association, 1989), p. 144.

referred to as a purchase order, acts as the vehicle for generating the payment. This authorization is usually a multipart document that allows for various review and/or authorization points established within the originating departments' administrative channels and accounts payable protocol. This protocol usually includes dollar limits, budgeted versus unbudgeted evaluations, and other criteria. Furthermore, the authorization form acts as an auditable verification vehicle to ensure that the original contract or agreement has been received and fulfilled.

The authorization form is reviewed by accounts payable staff and processed through an information system accounts payable application to generate a check payable to a vendor. The accounts payable staff works with the general accounting and internal control staff to ensure that the proper checks and balances are in place and enforced so that hospital funds cannot be misallocated.

Cash Application

Cash application entails the receipt, posting, depositing, accounting, and reconciliation of all payments to the hospital. The majority of payments to the hospital are for clinical services provided to patients and billed through patient accounts. Other payments may be generated from nonclinical services such as the hospital's cafeteria, gift shop, and parking garage.

An extension of cash application is the cashier function. Most if not all hospitals provide cashier services in convenient locations easily accessible to patients. Optimally, the hospital's information system would support payment at the time of service via generation of an accurate bill; this is referred to as point-of-service billing.

In general, at the end of each day, the cashier assembles all payments (cash, checks, and credit card slips) and prepares the necessary paperwork to deposit the daily receipts at the bank. Simultaneously, the detailed documentation that identifies the proper allocation of the payments is assembled and delivered to the cash application staff. The cash application staff initiates and controls the transactions necessary to adjust the appropriate patient account through the hospital information system patient accounting application.

Payroll Administration

The payroll administration staff of the fiscal services division generates, issues, and accounts for payments of salaries and wages to employees. In addition, the payroll staff is responsible for maintaining and reporting all the employment information required by government and regulatory agencies.

Payroll receives an authorization form (such as a time card or a sign-in/sign-out log sheet) for each employee that identifies the employee's work hours and other authorized paid hours for a specific pay period. This form is reviewed and processed through an information system payroll application that generates paychecks. In addition, the payroll application may update each individual employee's record regarding benefit time (sick days, holidays, vacation days, personal days) accrued or expended during the pay period. In some hospitals, records of benefit time may instead be maintained by the human resources/personnel department.

The payroll application should interface with the general accounting general ledger application to properly account for salaries, wages, taxes, and fringe benefits on the general ledger by appropriate expense code. The payroll system should be able to monitor actual payroll expenses compared to budgeted expenses to ensure effective financial management. In addition, payroll information is an integral part of the work of the human resources/personnel department.

Patient Accounting

The patient accounting area (business office) of the fiscal services division is responsible for ensuring the accurate, timely billing of patients and third-party payers for services rendered to patients by the hospital. Effective patient accounting depends on the degree to which a number of internal and external activities are handled well. The internal activities include:

- Capturing accurate data at the point of registration or preregistration
- Verifying insurance information, preferably before the patient is discharged
- Responding effectively to patient queries
- Gathering all charges on the patient's bill as quickly as possible to facilitate timely billing after discharge
- Maintaining effective billing cycles (for example, 15, 30, 45, 60, and 90 days)
- Managing payments so that copayments (that is, payments by a second insurer or deductibles paid by patients) are made and posted accurately
- Tracking accounts effectively, preferably by making only one individual responsible for monitoring a given patient's account
- Working with utilization review and quality assurance personnel to identify unnecessary costs in the care of patients, such as inappropriate length of stay or inappropriate use of services

The external activities include:

- Maintaining good relations with third-party payers and understanding their rules and procedures to maximize the possibility for prompt payment
- Maintaining on-line linkages with third-party payers when possible to speed payment
- Maintaining an effective process for resolving disputes
- Following up regularly on delinquent accounts and utilizing collection agencies when necessary
- Monitoring the effectiveness of collection agencies

The formal billing process begins when a patient arrives at the hospital and is registered, a situation similar to a guest arriving at a hotel. (The chapter on the admissions/registration department provides a more comprehensive explanation of the detailed information obtained during the registration process.) Inherent to the billing process is the assignment of a unique series of numbers to establish an individual account, referred to as the patient account. The patient is then assigned a room or bed number. During his or her hospital stay, the patient receives hospital services (such as meals and supplies), which are charged to the patient's account number. All these charges are posted to the patient's account. The backup documentation of care provided and related services is referred to as charting and takes place continuously during the patient's stay in the hospital. The charting function is performed by the department responsible for providing the service (the nursing service, the laboratory, respiratory care, and so on). When the patient is discharged, this information is forwarded to the medical record department, where it is abstracted, assembled, coded, and filed.

When the patient is discharged from a hospital, the situation is similar to a guest checking out of a hotel room. However, the hotel receives payment (generally via a credit card signature) at check-out time. Payment for television and telephone services is usually made on a patient's discharge from the hospital, but the hospital typically must bill a third-party payer (Medicare, Blue Cross/Blue Shield, or a commercial insurer) to secure reimbursement for the other services provided.

If the patient is not insured, attempts should have been made before discharge to receive payment from the patient directly. If the patient does not have the financial resources to pay the hospital or has inadequate insurance coverage, attempts should have been made to arrange payment before discharge so that the hospital would receive at least partial payment from local or state public assistance programs. Such programs are also considered third-party payers. The growing number of uninsured and underinsured individuals, sometimes referred to as the medically indigent, has broadened the extent of free or charity care provided by many hospitals. Information on this phenomenon as it applies to an individual hospital must be carefully monitored and fed into the planning and budgeting process; depending on the nature and extent of uncompensated care, some hospitals may seek creative solutions such as creating a position that assists patients in seeking public assistance.

Most patients do have insurance coverage through a third party, a fact established at the time of admission. Therefore, the hospital must bill the third party. To accomplish this, several days may elapse from the time of discharge to the time of billing to ensure that all charges are posted to the patient's account before the bill is generated. Any charges posted after billing are referred to as late charges.

Billing information is transmitted to the responsible party by the following methods:

- A paper bill may be mailed directly to the responsible party. If the responsible party is an individual, it is referred to as a bill. If the responsible party is a third-party payer, it is referred to as a claim.
- The institution may generate a computer tape that is mailed to a third-party payer.
- The institution's central processing unit (CPU) may be linked to a third-party payer's CPU for direct transmission of claims information.
- The institution may manually enter the necessary billing information into a personal computer terminal from which diskettes containing the information are generated for transmission to the third-party payer. It is appropriate to note that recent advances in computer technology and increased utilization of personal computers have expanded the use of diskettes as a method for transmitting claims information.

In 1986, Medicare implemented a uniform billing format requirement referred to as a UB82. This format was designed to standardize the information submission process, and it requires submitted claims to contain 96 specifically defined data elements in specific locations for payment. These data elements can be submitted via paper, tape, or diskette in accordance with the Medicare intermediary's requirements and capabilities. The Medicare intermediary is generally an insurance company contracted to act as an agent of the Health Care Financing Administration (HCFA), which is the government agency responsible for administering federally funded health care programs such as Medicare. Its offices are located in Baltimore, Maryland.

The uniform billing form format (UB82) is accepted by most third-party payers. However, individual payers may define some of the 96 fields differently than HCFA does. This situation produces unique data requirements even though the format is the same.

Many times, the patient has more than one type of third-party insurance coverage, in which case patient accounting must bill each third-party payer separately. Such billing activities may delay the receipt of payment for services and thereby adversely affect cash flow. The health care industry measures the success of a hospital's patient accounting system by the number of patient days of revenue that are outstanding [accounts receivable (AR) days].

The calculation of the number of AR days outstanding is carried out as follows:

$$\text{AR Days Outstanding} = \frac{\text{Total Accounts Receivable}}{\text{Average Daily Revenue}}$$

This calculation can be expressed in two forms, either as net AR days outstanding or as gross AR days outstanding. Net AR days outstanding are used to identify the true number of days of collectible cash outstanding. This calculation requires the removal of those dollars included in total accounts receivable (numerator) that are not expected to be collected, such as payments for charity or free care, bad debts, and contractual allowances. In general, contractual allowances are discounts third-party payers and health care institutions have negotiated or discounts mandated by state or federal law; therefore, the difference between actual charges for services and contractual allowances is considered uncollectible. Because the gross AR days outstanding figure does not take any of these factors into consideration, it is less meaningful than the net figure.

The total accounts receivable dollar amount typically includes both inpatient and outpatient revenues. This figure is identified through the hospital information system patient accounting management application, which is integrated with the general ledger application.

Reimbursement

The reimbursement staff of the fiscal services division is responsible for the optimization of payments from public programs (Medicare and Medicaid) and other contract payers (Blue Cross/Blue Shield and health maintenance organizations, for example). In addition, the reimbursement staff may be responsible for monitoring third-party contracts.

The reimbursement staff assembles supportive statistical and financial information in a format specific to each third-party payer. This is referred to as a cost report. The cost report is reviewed by the third-party auditors to determine the appropriateness of payments to the hospital for the services provided to patients in accordance with the contract. These data can be very valuable to the institution's management, particularly in carrying out its planning process.

The reimbursement staff works with the patient accounting and cash application staff to properly control contractual allowances. The staff ensures that the difference between the total charges incurred by the patient and the amount paid to the hospital is in accordance with its contract with the third-party payer. The amount paid is referred to as the reimbursement amount.

In general, third-party payers generate a reimbursement check and a remittance advice or remittance schedule periodically, usually weekly, for processed claims. The check is deposited by the cashier, while the remittance advice is processed by cash applications. The term *remittance advice* refers to the document that identifies the patient, the total billed amount, the total reimbursement amount, and the related contractual allowance. The remittance advice also identifies the deductible dollar amount due from the patient as defined by the contract. In addition, the remittance advice may indicate the amount due from any other secondary insurance (or coinsurance) company.

It is important to understand that Medicare reimburses inpatient claims on the basis of diagnosis-related groups (DRGs), which in turn are the basis for a prospective pricing system. Under prospective pricing, the rates of payment to the hospital for its services are established in advance on the basis of an extensive data base developed over many years and updated annually. The hospital is paid a predetermined amount that depends on the discharge diagnosis of the Medicare patient and not on the actual costs incurred by the hospital in providing services.

The prospective pricing system requires the hospital to assign an appropriate DRG on the basis of the discharge diagnosis and the procedure codes assigned by medical record personnel and accompanied by a physician's authorization. The physician's authorization is called an attestation. Therefore, to submit a claim to Medicare, the medical record department must have assigned an appropriate DRG. The prospective pricing methodology has also been adopted by other third-party payers, further linking reimbursement to the nature of the services provided rather than to the hospital's charges or to the costs incurred in providing those services. (The chapter on the medical record department provides a more comprehensive explanation of this process.)

Internal Control

The internal control (or internal audit) staff is responsible for the periodic review of hospital functions to ensure the proper fulfillment of hospital policies, procedures, and established accounting practices. The internal control staff monitors ongoing activities and participates in the establishment of new, enhanced operational practices. This function generally has a direct reporting relationship to executive management to maximize the independence and objectivity required for successful internal control.

The American Institute of Certified Public Accountants defines *internal control* as "the plan of organization and all of the coordinate methods and measures adopted within a business to safeguard its assets, check the accuracy and reliability of its accounting data, promote operational efficiency, and encourage adherence to prescribed managerial policies." An additional function of the internal control staff in a hospital is to verify the extent to which the institution is complying with government regulations and to which it is observing its contractual obligations. Many hospitals designate an internal auditor to handle internal control procedures and to coordinate the internal audit with the activities of independent auditors. The internal auditor is an accountant who may report to the CFO, the CEO, or the hospital's governing board.

Planning, Budgeting, and Rate Setting

The second major function of the fiscal services division is to help hospital managers to make informed decisions in their various planning activities, to allocate resources appropriately for achieving the hospital's goals, and to set reasonable rates for the provision of services to patients.

Planning

As a member of the executive management team, the CFO plays an integral part in the hospital's various planning processes. These processes are undertaken to put into place financial, strategic, and business plans for guiding and monitoring the hospital's future activities.

Financial planning is the establishment of both long- and short-term plans that are compatible with the hospital's objectives and that ensure its financial viability. When engaging in financial planning, the management and governing board of the institution set policies for controlling the receipt of its revenue, the expenditure of its funds, and the conservation of its various assets. The CFO and his or her staff contribute to the financial planning process by performing such tasks as:

- Preparing and evaluating financial data on existing programs
- Preparing financial feasibility studies
- Evaluating managed care contracts for profitability
- Searching for alternatives when financing capital improvements

When participating in strategic and business planning, the CFO ensures that the hospital's strategies and implementation plans are financially sound and enhance rather than endanger the hospital's financial health. (For definitions of strategic and business planning, see the chapter on planning later in this book.) According to Edward Kazemek and Daniel

Grauman ["The CFO's Role in Strategic Planning," *Healthcare Financial Management,* vol. 41, no. 2 (February 1987), pp. 94, 99], four issues must be evaluated when the hospital is considering its strategies and plans of action:

- *Cost and pricing:* How the hospital's cost per discharge has changed over a certain period of time and how the hospital's cost structure compares with that of its competitors
- *Third-party payments:* How the mix of third-party payers has changed and how this mix compares with that of the hospital's competitors
- *Financial position:* How the hospital's financial position has changed and how this position compares with that of the hospital's competitors
- *Financial analysis of strategies:* The profitability and risk of each strategy, the size and type of investment needed (whether capital or otherwise), the effect of the strategy on the hospital's long-term financial health, and the fit between the strategy and the hospital's financial plans

Public accounting firms are often utilized to assist the hospital with its planning processes. Among the services they provide are financial forecasts and feasibility studies, profitability studies, and analyses of new ventures, new products, and product pricing.

Budgeting

The hospital's budget is a tool for managers to allocate resources on the basis of planning decisions and to monitor the results of those decisions. A well-crafted budget establishes the proper relationship between expenses and revenues at a projected volume of services that will generate an acceptable patient margin. According to Charles M. Bley and Cynthia T. Shimko [*A Guide to the Board's Role in Hospital Finance* (Chicago: American Hospital Publishing, 1987), p. 17], the budget process has five outcomes:

- Establishes operating objectives and management policies that enable the hospital to achieve its goals
- Provides a systematic way to develop, evaluate, and set priorities for changes in programs and capital expenditures
- Plans the flow of hospital funds so that financing decisions can be made effectively and necessary financing arrangements can be anticipated
- Coordinates the various levels of responsibility within the hospital and sets measurable departmental performance standards
- Facilitates early recognition of changes in the hospital's circumstances so that timely operating adjustments can be made when necessary

Figure 5 illustrates the essential features of the budget process, which include gathering historical data, evaluating rates for hospital services, and projecting service volumes, expenses, revenues, and deductions (such as for charity care). The master budget is a product of three types of budgets—the operating budget, the capital budget, and the cash budget.

The *operating budget* is built from the detailed budgets submitted by individual departments before the beginning of each fiscal year. Departmental budgets are based on information provided by the hospital's budget manager. This information includes past, current, and future forecasts of service volumes (numbers of patient days, numbers of laboratory tests, numbers of radiological examinations, and so on) and case mix intensity (the differences in resource use among patients with regard to their diagnosis and resulting health care needs), information on salaries and other expenses, revenue projections, and capital equipment information. Once prepared, the individual departmental budgets are then submitted through the proper administrative channels for final administrative authorizations. The fiscal services division supports the administrative authorization process and incorporates the departmental budgets into the master budget.

The *capital budget* provides the institution with guidelines for acquiring new buildings and equipment and for replacing or refurbishing present assets. Whereas the operating budget covers one fiscal year, the capital budget covers at least three years.

The *cash flow budget* anticipates the levels of receipts and disbursements that the hospital can expect at various times throughout the fiscal year. As such, this budget ensures that the hospital has enough working capital on hand to meet its short-term financial obligations.

The master budget establishes final forecasts of revenues and expenses that generate the next fiscal year's projected bottom line. After the fiscal year's budget has been agreed on at the administrative level, it is reviewed and/or accepted by the finance committee of the hospital's board of directors.

The authorized master budget for the forthcoming year is sometimes submitted to various third parties for acceptance and/or used to justify any necessary contract cost adjustments with third parties responsible for payments. This practice, however, is becoming increasingly less common.

Figure 5. The Budget Process

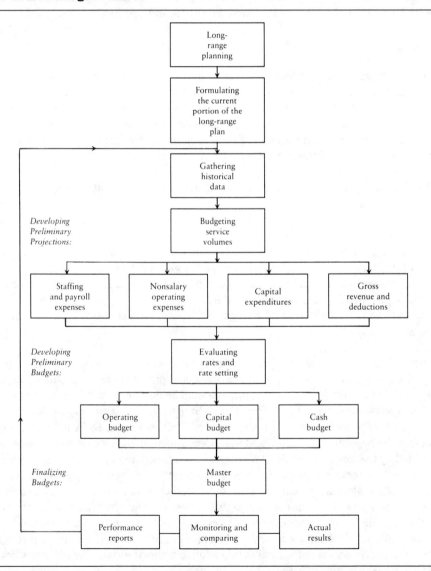

From Charles M. Bley and Cynthia T. Shimko, *A Guide to the Board's Role in Hospital Finance* (Chicago: American Hospital Publishing, 1987), p. 18.

Management engineers should be aware that the budget process varies widely from institution to institution. Hence, it is important for an engineer to understand how budgeting works in the particular hospital being studied. As managers in a hospital are given more responsibility for meeting their budgets, they become more involved in the give-and-take of the budget process.

Rate Setting

The evaluation and setting of rates during the budget process must take into account the costs of providing those services as well as such external factors as competitors' rates and the prospective pricing system. The rate that is set for a service must be high enough to enable the hospital to recover its direct costs in providing the service (such as labor and materials), to help defray the indirect costs that the hospital incurs as overhead (such as administrative staff salaries and heating and lighting), and to yield a certain amount of profit. The desired profit margin is computed by estimating the hospital's projected costs for maintaining and enhancing its services to the community, whether by buying new equipment, building new facilities, replacing existing assets, financing indigent care, or meeting other financial obligations.

The final decision on rates is a function of direct costs, indirect costs, the desired profit margin, the external factors mentioned earlier, and other modifications, such as the hospital's ability to operate a needed community service at a loss or for a low return on investment. Rate setting is always performed with the full knowledge of the CFO as part of the overall financial planning process.

Measuring and Reporting on Organizational Performance

The third major function of the fiscal services division is to collect and report information on the performance of the hospital as a whole as well as the performance of each unit, department, or line of service. This information enables managers to make informed decisions in planning, budgeting, and rate setting and facilitates the monitoring of the hospital's financial performance. The primary source of financial information is the hospital's cost accounting system.

According to Steven Kukla [*Cost Accounting and Financial Analysis for the Hospital Administrator* (Chicago: American Hospital Publishing, 1986), p. 1], the initial function of cost accounting is to "assemble revenues, costs, and standard performance criteria by individual product in order that management can plan and control the subelements of the organization's lines of operations." Once this information is assembled, it is analyzed and interpreted for incorporation into various reports to managers and board members.

Cost accounting utilizes three general methodologies for determining the actual costs of providing a hospital service (see Kukla, pp. 5–22, for a full discussion):

- *Responsibility costing, or the assignment of operating costs to individual organizational units or departments (such as medical records, nursing, or environmental services):* The cost accounting system records the costs each unit incurred over a certain period of time; this in turn allows for a measurement of the unit's performance and any deviations from its budget. Top-level management can therefore determine from its cost accounting system whether the unit is being managed efficiently as well as what its net contribution is to the hospital's overall revenues.
- *Full costing, or the sum of the direct costs of producing a particular line of service plus a portion of the indirect costs that the hospital incurs as overhead:* Given that the costs for a particular line of service can generally be attributed to more than one hospital department or unit, full costing involves the collection of data from many sources such as medical records, patient bills, service cost allocation sheets, the hospital's general ledger, and the payroll system.

- *Differential costing, or the estimation of how costs and revenues might be different for different courses of action within a given line of service:* Data are collected from the same sources used for full costing.

Separate cost accounting systems are generally maintained for each of the three methodologies, but the systems should all share a common data base.

Reports are generated from the hospital fiscal services division periodically and take the form of budget performance reports, financial statements, and financial ratio analyses. *Budget performance reports* show the variances between the actual revenues and costs of a hospital unit, department, or line of service and the budgeted revenues and costs. These reports also show statistics that are meaningful to the particular reporting area, such as the number of procedures performed, the cost per procedure, the cost of supplies per procedure, and the like. Data for the current period as well as for the year to date are generally included. Budget performance reports give managers at various levels of the organization a basis for analyzing variances and taking corrective action when warranted. The level of detail in budget performance reports becomes more and more unit or department specific as one moves down the chain of command. In other words, persons at higher levels of authority receive budget performance reports in which data for the units or departments under their command are aggregated into meaningful categories. The CFO should always take part in executive-level discussions of variance analyses.

Financial statements are reports that are prepared not only for hospital managers, but also for members of the board of directors. These statements, as described by Charles K. Bradford and John F. Tiscornia [*Monitoring the Hospital's Financial Health* (Chicago: American Hospital Publishing, 1987), pp. 3, 9–19], include the following:

- Balance sheets reveal the financial condition of the hospital on a designated date in terms of its assets (cash, accounts receivable, inventory, investments, property, and so on) as opposed to its liabilities (long-term debts, accounts payable, interest payable, payroll and fringe benefits, and so on) and its fund balances or equity (that which has been invested in the institution by the community).
- The statement of operations (or statement of revenue and expenses) shows whether the hospital is currently achieving its expected operating margin. Although the categories comprising this statement vary widely from institution to institution, the most common categories are gross patient revenues, deductions from those revenues (such as deductions for bad debts, charity care, and contractual allowances for Medicare and Medicaid, health maintenance organizations, preferred provider organizations, and the like), other operating revenues, operating expenses (such as salaries and wages, supplies, services, depreciation, and interest), profit (or loss) from operations, unrestricted contributions and investment income, and net profit (or loss).
- The statement of changes in fund balances (or equity statement) generally displays beginning and ending fund balances for a particular period of time along with the intervening additions (net profit, restricted contributions) and/or deductions (such as the amounts of restricted contributions used for purchasing equipment).
- The statement of changes in financial position (or cash flow statement) generally displays beginning and ending cash balances for a particular period of time along with the intervening sources of cash (net profit, depreciation of assets, new borrowings, funds transferred from restricted contributions for the purpose of buying equipment, and so on) and applications (or spending) of cash (such as equipment purchases, repayment of debt, and new investments).

Financial statements are used for many purposes, among which are the following:

- To study trends in the hospital's financial condition, such as whether the working capital of the institution is growing or declining

- To evaluate actual financial performance against budgetary expectations and financial goals
- To determine the current financial needs of the institution and to predict future needs
- To evaluate the organization's rate structure
- To help managers determine how to use financial resources to best advantage, such as how to invest the hospital's new resources (profits)

The general accounting staff generates financial statements for a predetermined fiscal period, usually a calendar month. If desired, the monthly data can be rolled together to provide management with cumulative information by quarter, half-year, or year. General accounting also prepares financial statements for each fiscal year, which can span any 12-month period. Financial statements are generally presented for review to a committee of the hospital's board of directors, often called the finance committee. The fiscal year-end financial statement is usually audited by an independent, outside auditing firm to ensure its validity.

In addition to generating financial statements, the fiscal services division may provide or arrange for *financial ratio analyses,* which aid managers and board members in understanding the institution's financial solvency and profitability. Bley and Shimko place financial ratio analyses into four major categories (*A Guide to the Board's Role in Hospital Finance,* pp. 30–31):

- Liquidity ratios, which measure the hospital's ability to meet short-term obligations, that is, the hospital's bills
- Leverage (or capital structure) ratios, which measure the hospital's ability to meet long-term debts
- Profitability ratios, which reveal how well the hospital is managing its assets in order to make a profit
- Turnover (or activity) ratios, which measure the hospital's ability to generate operating revenue from its capital investments and investments in cash and marketable securities

By supplementing financial statements with financial ratio analyses, managers can readily see key trends in the hospital's performance and its movement toward or away from predetermined goals. As with variance analyses, the CFO should always take part in executive-level discussions of financial ratio analyses.

Management engineers should ensure that hospital executives and managers outside the fiscal services division find all financial reports and analyses complete, timely, and easy to understand and interpret. Narratives should accompany reports whenever possible to assist managers and board members in their deliberations.

Staffing

The functions of the fiscal services division are generally completed and/or overseen by accounting professionals, who are supported by various supervisors and technicians. The number of accounting professionals employed by the hospital depends on the size, type, and organization of the institution. Individual backgrounds vary according to subspecialty, managerial responsibilities, and the department's level of sophistication.

Chief Financial Officer

The CFO, or vice-president of finance, holds at least a bachelor's degree in accounting and has often completed graduate study in either accounting or business administration. In addition, he or she is usually certified by the State Board of Certified Public Accountants. In most cases, accounting and management experience for this position has been gained either directly or indirectly in the health care field.

Staffing for General Accounting

The general accounting department is administered by the director of general accounting. Staff members include accountants, some of whom may serve as fund managers; supervisors of such functions as accounts payable, payroll, and inventory control; and knowledgeable technical staff. Most routine fiscal services are relatively predictable, with tasks occurring daily, weekly, monthly, or annually. Therefore, staffing requirements typically are not linked to an activity indicator as staffing in other hospital departments is.

Comparative statistics for various fiscal services do exist, for example, the American Hospital Association's MONITREND statistics and statistics published by the journal *Healthcare Financial Management*. Such comparative statistics are grouped by hospital size to increase their sensitivity. However, staffing requirements also depend on factors other than bed size, such as:

- Type of hospital
  - Community versus teaching
  - Not-for-profit versus for-profit
- Information systems support
- Financial management philosophy
- State and local reimbursement philosophy

Staffing for Budgeting and Reimbursement

Larger hospitals may have a director of budget and reimbursement as well as a budget manager and a reimbursement manager. The director coordinates the hospital's budgeting activities and oversees reimbursement from third-party payers. He or she holds at least a bachelor's degree in accounting and may have completed a master's degree in either accounting or business administration. The budget and reimbursement managers usually hold bachelor's degrees in accounting as well. All three positions require accounting experience in the health care field and some supervisory experience.

Budgeting and reimbursement involve tasks that are generally predictable and do not vary in relation to any indicator such as tests or procedures. Both activities may be supported by a staff of technicians, whose number and level of expertise depend on the size of the hospital and the organization of its fiscal services.

For its reimbursement staff, today's hospital is increasingly looking for college graduates with two to five years of experience working for third-party payers. Such experience gives candidates a basis for anticipating reimbursement patterns, understanding the multiple regulations for each third party, and thereby helping the hospital to maximize reimbursement.

Staffing for Financial Planning

Financial planning in a large institution is undertaken in part by a director of financial planning, who supports the planning activities of the CFO and the associate vice-president of financial services. This director maintains regular communication with the directors of general accounting and budget and reimbursement to share information on financial feasibility studies, managed care contracts, accounting records for facility construction projects, and the like. A minimum of a bachelor's degree in accounting is required, although many institutions also require a master's degree in business administration and significant health care accounting and supervisory experience.

Staffing for Patient Accounting

The hospital's patient accounting staff requirements are related to the number of inpatient discharges and outpatient visits. However, with the ever-increasing regulatory environment, claims submission criteria vary by third-party payer and by type of patient (inpatient, outpatient, rehabilitation patient, psychiatric patient, and so on). In addition, follow-up on delinquent accounts with either the third-party payers or individual patients affects the department's work load. As a result, quantification of staffing requirements in this department can be very complicated. Staffing decisions may ultimately depend on the level of accounts receivable and the corresponding need to maintain or reduce accounts receivable, thereby improving cash flow.

The director of patient accounting usually holds a bachelor's degree in business administration and has experience in health care accounts receivable and credit and collection. Other managers in this department also have significant accounts receivable experience but may or may not hold bachelor's degrees. Patient accounting staff generally have one to two years experience in health care and some experience in accounts receivable. Staff members are organized into one of three common staffing models: the alphabetical staffing model, the financial class staffing model, and the combination model.

Alphabetical Staffing Model

The staffing model that places all responsibilities related to the timely billing and payment of a particular patient's account with one individual in the patient accounting area is called the alphabetical staffing model. This individual, or patient account representative, begins his or her responsibilities with the routine activities usually conducted through the admissions/registration department (preregistration, registration, insurance verification, and so on). The account management responsibilities continue through the inpatient stay, discharge, medical records/utilization review, bill generation, bill submission, and follow-up processes. Thus, one patient accounting staff member continuously communicates with his or her assigned patients to coordinate and ensure timely total payment. In addition, all subsequent patient visits continue to build on this beneficial interaction between the patient and the patient account representative.

In general, patient account representatives are assigned segments of the alphabet. For example, in a hospital with four patient representatives, one may be assigned patients whose last names begin with the letters A through E, another may be assigned F through M, another N through S, and another T through Z. In assignments of segments of the alphabet, the distribution of accounts should be balanced among staff. Different sets of staff may exist for inpatient and outpatient accounts.

The alphabetical staffing model requires each patient account representative to be knowledgeable about all third-party payers' claims requirements. Development of this expertise requires extensive training (approximately six months). The hospital's facility design should support this staffing model through centralized registration features that allow patient account representatives to be in close proximity to service areas where they can interact with patients.

The positive features of the alphabetical staffing model include the following:

- Positive patient interaction for public relations as well as accurate first-time billing
- Simplified supervision and performance monitoring
- Comprehensive integration of the processes affecting patient accounts:
  - Registration
  - Charge posting
  - Discharge
  - Medical records completion
  - Bill generation
- Cross-trained staff for sick day, holiday, and vacation coverage

Negative features of this model include:

- Extensive learning curve
- Need for long-term staff retention

- Unique support features:
  - Long-term staff
  - Centralized registration facility design
  - Information system support

Financial Class Staffing Model

The organization and allocation of staff resources according to third-party payer is referred to as staffing by financial class or product line. This staffing model assigns a team of staff to handle claims for specific third-party payers such as Medicare, Medicaid, Blue Cross/Blue Shield, and individual commercial insurance providers. Of the three staffing models described in this section, the financial class staffing model is the most popular.

Under certain conditions, inpatient and outpatient responsibilities may be combined. In some operations, Medicare and Medicaid claims processing may be combined. All follow-up is generally the responsibility of a team of staff members.

The foundation of this model is the development of a specialized knowledge of each specific third-party payer because senior patient accounting staff members support the growth and development of junior patient accounting staff members. The major benefit of this pyramid effect is that the specialized expertise is in a dynamic state of growth. In addition, this model is less sensitive to staff turnover than is the alphabetical staffing model. This becomes significant when patient accounting has a history of high staff turnover.

The positive features of the financial class staffing model include:

- Junior and senior staff relationship creating a pyramid effect or a dynamic state of staff growth
- Less investment in training

The negative features include:

- Minimal patient contact
- Minimal involvement with patient account until bill generation
- Minimal cross-training in other third-party payer billing characteristics

Combination Staffing Model

A third model for allocating staff resources is a combination of the alphabetical staffing model and the financial class model. The positive features of each model may be merged to create the optimal situation for that specific hospital. The wide variety of combinations available does not allow for any specific organizational structure. Factors affecting this type of model include the following:

- *Inpatient patient mix and volume:* A concentration of any third-party payer (such as Medicare) would necessitate a patient accounting staffing model that focuses on developing billing and follow-up expertise for working with that payer.
- *Outpatient services and volume:* A hospital with extensive outpatient services would organize a patient accounting staffing model to deal with high-volume billing activities. Outpatient services, with the exception of emergency room services, generally can be scheduled in advance, thereby providing opportunities to collect payments at the time of service.

Choosing the Best Model

When choosing one of these three models for organizing the patient account staff, the hospital must look for the best way to maintain an aggressive patient accounting philosophy. Account resolution can be expedited through policies and procedures that are adhered to throughout the admissions/registration and billing processes and that have the proper allocation of staff and managerial support. Conversely, a staff organized and working under a less aggressive philosophy probably would not have adequate resources and support, thereby allowing for greater account delinquency.

The choice of a model may be influenced by the configuration and sophistication of the information systems serving the patient accounting area. A hospitalwide, integrated information system supports timely and accurate information flow, which directly affects the billing process and allows for more flexibility in assigning staff responsibilities.

Departmental Analysis

Management engineers should focus on three key areas for improving the organization and functioning of a fiscal services division: reducing accounts receivable days, serving the needs of hospital executives fully, and ensuring that there are no deficiencies in audits by third-party payers.

The factors involved in reducing accounts receivable days include the following:

- Organizing the work load properly
- Hiring qualified staff and offering them thorough training
- Ensuring that all necessary systems are in place, whether automated or not
- Using efficient billing, dunning, and collection processes
- Maximizing reimbursement

In order to serve the needs of executives fully, hospital fiscal services must:

- Ensure that all data reported to managers, executives, and board members are appropriate and timely
- Minimize redundant, missing, or confusing data
- Submit financial reports with accompanying narratives to help managers analyze the information they are given

Possible approaches for the management engineer in studying the fiscal services division include interviews, work-flow analyses, work-load analyses, data-flow analyses, and quality checks on the accuracy, completeness, and usefulness of data.

Food Service Department

Overview

The general purpose of the food service department is to prepare and serve food for patients and employees at the hospital. In various institutions, the department is called the food service department, the dietary department, or the nutrition service department. Shortened lengths of stay, profit incentives, computerization, and increased emphasis on good nutrition continue to affect the operation of the department.

Food service uses approximately 6 to 10 percent of the hospital's work force. The department's size depends directly on the types of services the hospital offers, the size of the hospital, and the type of equipment used for food preparation and delivery.

Beyond basic food and nutrition responsibilities, the department may be involved in other services, including catering functions outside the hospital and providing services for special functions within the hospital (for example, meetings, luncheons, and board meetings). Such services range from offering coffee and cookies to serving full meals that require extensive preparation. The department may also operate a coffee shop (in addition to a cafeteria), prepare infant formulas and gourmet meals (on request), provide outpatient nutrition counseling, train students, offer educational programs to community groups, operate a meals-on-wheels program, and consult with medical staff in preparing experimental or special therapeutic diets or tube feedings. In addition, many departments are actively marketing their catering, therapeutic, and consulting services through nursing homes, physicians' offices, community groups, and other agencies.

Organization

A functional organization chart for a typical food service department is illustrated in figure 6. In some hospitals, food service and nutrition service may be organized as two separate departments. In other hospitals, these two functions may be established within one department, emphasizing the growing awareness of both the clinical and production aspects of the food service department's services.

A food service director is usually responsible for the work of the department and may also be called director of dietetics, director of nutrition service, dietary director, or food and nutrition service administrator. The director usually reports to an administrator, assistant administrator, or vice-president for general support services.

Other types of workers in the food service department include the following:

- *Managers:* Depending on the size of the department, individual managers may be responsible for such functions as nutrition care and tray assembly, food procurement and production, and nonpatient services (for example, cafeteria services and catering).

73

Figure 6. Functional Organizational Chart for a Typical Hospital Food Service Department

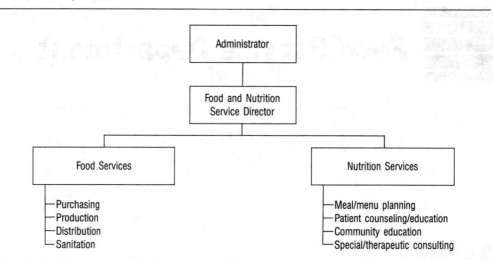

- *Dietitians and dietetic technicians:* Dietitians have usually completed a bachelor's degree program in dietetics, nutrition, or food systems management; in addition, they may have earned the designation registered dietitian (RD) by successfully completing a national registration examination. Dietetic technicians have usually completed an associate's degree program and most often work under the supervision of a registered dietitian. In small hospitals, a dietitian may serve a dual role as both dietetic supervisor and food service department director.
- *Other workers:* Other workers commonly employed in the food service department include cooks, tray assemblers, sanitation workers, and various clerks and aides.

The food service director may or may not be a registered dietitian. In fact, professional food service managers are becoming more acceptable in hospitals. The educational backgrounds of such managers vary, but degrees such as master's degrees in business or hospital administration and/or specialty degrees in dietetics, food service, or hotel management are common. Some hospitals may utilize professional contract management firms for managing their food service departments.

Operating Systems

Because the food service department's primary mission is inpatient nutrition, the discussion of models and systems in this profile focuses largely on patient services. Patient services traditionally include providing three meals, plus snacks or nourishments, each day. An alternative model, which has become less acceptable, is a five-meal plan. Under this plan, patients receive two main meals (early lunch and early supper) and three snacks or minimeals (early morning, midday, and early evening). The five-meal plan was designed primarily to reduce labor costs by eliminating the need for a full staff to prepare and clean up after serving a traditional full evening meal.

Virtually all hospitals operate under a centralized model in view of the advantages in cost, control, efficiency, and sanitation. Food service functions for inpatients can be grouped into five categories:

- Meal planning, including therapeutic nutritional evaluation and patient education
- Supply management

- Food production
- Food service and delivery
- Cleaning and sanitation

These basic functions are discussed in the following paragraphs.

Meal Planning

Meal planning involves the systematic selection of the foods to be served to patients and patrons. The meals, and the menus used to describe these meals, are established by a dietitian or dietary consultant. Patients are usually allowed to select their meals from menus that are often tailored to their specific dietary needs (for example, low calorie, low sodium, bland, and so on). Menus are usually distributed only once per day by dietary supervisors and/or aides, who may assist patients in the ordering process. When all meal selections have been made, the tallied amounts become a cook order.

Two basic types of menus can be used, cycle and restaurant. With a cycle menu, a patient's choice of entrees and other items is somewhat limited. The menu changes daily over a cycle of several weeks. Reduced cost and economies of scale can be realized with this type of menu, but patient satisfaction may suffer.

Restaurant menus are becoming more common than cycle menus, especially as advances are made in food preparation techniques. A restaurant menu has a much larger variety than a cycle menu, but it does not change from day to day.

For patients with special dietary needs, a registered dietitian assists in patient therapy. Based on a physician's orders, nutritional therapy may require modification of the content, consistency, and/or method of preparation of a normal diet. In most cases, the master menu is modified, but a specially prepared diet usually must be written for the individual patient. Therapeutic menus and meals are clearly marked as such. The ordering procedure is similar to regular diet selection, with additional assistance from a dietitian or dietetic technician. The dietitian performs therapeutic management of patients (including education of the patient, family, and medical staff), nutritional diagnosis and diet recommendation, and overall nutritional monitoring of the patient population.

Trends in the meal-planning function include:

- Interactive menu selection on a closed-circuit television system, with an automated tally of the cook order
- Outpatient dietary counseling
- Provision of educational films for the patient population
- Gourmet meal preparation (for items not on the menu) on request
- Increased interfacing with other departments (laboratory, pharmacy, nursing)

Supply Management

Food supplies and other materials for food service are required in substantial amounts. Hence, the food service department is involved in most materials management functions, including inventory, purchasing, storage, processing, and distribution. The choice of menu can have a significant effect on the quantity, frequency, and types of foodstuffs that must be ordered and stored.

The constraints created by the storage requirements of perishable foods and the seasonal availability of some foods often demand decentralized purchasing and storage procedures. A useful technique for purchasing perishable (as well as nonperishable) foods is a system of bids and standing orders. This process eliminates the need for numerous purchase orders and reduces the amount of paperwork. Goods may also be purchased through group purchasing arrangements to reduce costs. Increasingly, purchasing is computerized so that the manager can place orders by using a terminal linked to a vendor or a group purchasing program.

Food storage systems should be designed to facilitate stock rotation and allow for proper cleaning and pest control procedures. Stock control and accountability, however, are often very difficult to achieve in food service departments. The usual approach to pilferage reduction is to keep storage areas locked, which can be a time-consuming system for the management staff responsible for locking and unlocking the areas to provide access to the materials needed. Some hospitals have installed surveillance systems to address this problem.

Food Production

The five basic food groups are milk and milk products; meat, fish, poultry, and eggs; fruits and vegetables; breads, cereals, and other starches; and fats. Food production consists of all the activities required to bring these foods from purchase to serving condition as prescribed by the cook order and appropriate recipes. Activities can involve peeling, slicing, mixing, heating, steaming, cooking, broiling, frying, baking, refrigerating, and freezing.

Significant changes in this function continue to evolve in order to improve food quality, reduce preparation time and expense, and achieve economies of scale. Increasingly, food vendors are able to provide a broader range of preprepared, prepackaged, and preportioned convenience foods. "Scratch" kitchens are rare in today's hospitals. Scratch preparation is now more a matter of institutional tradition, equipment capability, and individual skills availability.

Computerization has helped to keep costs down. Recipes typically written in increments of 20 or 50 portions can now be produced in much smaller increments that correspond to actual census and make use of historical consumption patterns. On-line access to nursing and automated data transmission systems can reduce the volume of late trays and meals delivered to the wrong nursing unit. Meals for relatives and friends are more readily available.

But even with the added benefits of computerization, food service departments must ensure that adequate procedures for ordering and delivering these meals are in place. Food is usually prepared in batches, which may be limited in size by equipment capacity. As much as possible, food is prepared in advance to meet expected demands. For some foods (for example, soft-boiled eggs and ice cream), consideration must be given to plating times, delivery times, and methods to ensure palatability at the bedside.

Very little short-order cooking is performed in the hospital food service department. Such cooking is often called progressive cooking, which is an approach to food service that prepares smaller batches of food at regular intervals during the serving period. Although the main benefit of progressive cooking is improved freshness and palatability, many institutions have found the approach difficult to manage.

Cost savings have also been realized through changes in food technology that enable managers to schedule staff to work at times not specifically related to the next meal. For example, relatively new processes of food preparation include methods for packaging and freezing meal portions that may be heated in a microwave oven (in the department or on the nursing unit) just before being delivered. Another method called cook–chill allows the hospital to prepare foods overnight, either for the next day or to replenish inventory. This method is computer controlled, can save labor expense, and can maximize the return on capital investment when volumes are large.

Gourmet meals, where offered, must be carefully controlled to be sure that the department's normal routine is not interrupted and that costs are at least fully recovered. Gourmet meals can run the gamut from surf and turf to pizza from a local parlor.

Pressures to reduce hospital lengths of stay have resulted in new food service programs. Some hospitals have started preparing send-home meals for newly released patients. Recovering patients can then more easily handle meal preparation in their homes during the first few days after discharge.

Food Service and Delivery

According to the orders received, a meal tray is assembled for each patient. The vast majority of dietary departments use a centralized approach to tray assembly. Assembly-line procedures, often involving moving tray lines, are used. Quality control (food appearance, tray layout, and conformance with the menu) is routinely conducted by supervisory staff at the end of the line, just before trays are loaded onto their method of conveyance.

Care should be taken to ensure line balancing within the constraints of reasonable serving time periods. Line balancing may require the alteration of the number of workers, the number of stations, and/or the speed of the assembly line, depending on the menu. As a guideline, the number of trays that can be assembled per minute is 10 to 15.

Passing of trays is the term commonly used for delivering the trays to the patients. The serving times of the individual nursing units should be strictly adhered to because any deviation can disrupt the schedules not only of the nursing unit, but also of ancillary departments. Once the patient has finished the meal, the pickup of trays completes the delivery cycle. The duties included in the passing of trays may vary, and the responsibility may belong to either the food service or the nursing staff. Especially in hospitals where dietary employees pass out and/or pick up trays, the staff's personal appearance and grooming is very important.

Depending on the facility's size and physical constraints, a variety of delivery trays and equipment can be used, including dumbwaiters, tray trucks (or utility carts), insulated trays, pellet trays, and airline trucks (which have separate heated and refrigerated sections for hot and cold foods and bulk thermal containers for liquids). Also used, but only rarely, are hot bulk carts and portable kitchens. Hot bulk carts are heated carts that contain hot foods in bulk that are dished onto patient trays in the floor kitchen or in the patient floor corridor. Portable kitchens are carts containing open, heated, and refrigerated sections carrying the tray service items, portioned cold foods, and hot foods in bulk, permitting complete tray setting and food assembly in the corridor of the patient floor.

A typical one-way trip from the food service department to a nursing unit requires 7 minutes. The act of simply passing out and picking up the tray involves about 3 minutes per patient day. Preparing the patient and arranging the room before the meal and monitoring the meal require more time.

Cleaning and Sanitation

Dishwashing is typically the main part of the cleaning function. Most hospitals use a central dish line for all dishes, silverware, trays, and so forth. The cleaning function includes clearing trays, loading and unloading machines, and storing clean dishes. Some hospitals have dish lines that require cafeteria patrons to dispose of refuse and load dish racks. Pot washing is usually done by hand. Some hospitals have automated pot washers, but generally, they are not cost-effective.

Food service personnel also perform housekeeping and sanitizing functions that are not performed by the environmental services department. This may include the cleaning of exhaust hoods, stoves, ovens, dish racks, shelves, counters, refrigerators, and other equipment. Often, a split responsibility for cleaning exists. Environmental services may maintain the cafeteria dining area, but food service is responsible for cleaning the kitchen, storage, and serving areas.

Disposable food service supplies are sometimes used more widely than only for coffee breaks, precaution patients, and take-out services. The use of disposable dishware and utensils can have a significant impact on the cleaning function as well as other functions of the food service department. Relative cleanliness is seldom the deciding issue. With disposables, pilferage, loss, and breakage concerns are eliminated. Capital expenditure for equipment and space can be avoided. However, savings in dishwashing (labor, detergent, water, energy, and maintenance) are offset by increased storage, rubbish, handling, and disposal requirements. Major changes in the cost of cleaning and sanitation may be seen in the future due to the rising cost of water in some areas and the reformulation of disposables to eliminate harmful materials.

The hospital food service department is subject to local, state, federal, and JCAHO (Joint Commission on Accreditation of Healthcare Organizations) standards and inspections.

Situations and Problems

Patient admissions, discharges, and transfers can cause last-minute adjustments to meal preparation and delivery schedules, sometimes resulting in wasted food. Such last-minute changes may cause conflict among the food service, nursing, and admitting staffs. Anticipating the needs of other hospital departments and maintaining an effective communications system is the key to reducing such conflicts. In an institution with a well-run food service department, inpatient tray wastage should be virtually nonexistent. Bulk wastage can be reduced by offering unadvertised specials in the cafeteria or by incorporating leftovers into other menu items.

Conflict may also occur over whether nursing or food service staff should pass out and pick up patients' trays. Another potential problem may arise over the cafeteria prices for employee meals. In the past, employee meals have been priced below cost, and most hospitals continue this tradition. However, a change in policy to reduce hospital expenses may cause some resentment among employees. Different methods have been used to provide food services for employees on evening and night shifts.

It is difficult to provide a menu that pleases everyone, especially when costs must be contained. Restaurant menus, menu selection cards, and assistance from dietary supervisors can be effective in handling complaints and improving satisfaction. Some hospitals maintain a file on patient preferences.

Departmental Analysis

The application of management engineering techniques in analyzing the food service department is straightforward. Typical topics for departmental analysis include staffing, staff scheduling, meal delivery and tray pickup, evaluation of new equipment purchases, evaluation of alternative methods of food preparation and dishwashing, design of a communication system, evaluation of the purchasing system, and storeroom organization. The hospital coffee shop, employee cafeteria, or vending machine area might also be reviewed. Problems in other areas (for example, lengthy stays in the emergency department and requests for special trays) affect the department's work load. Recent MONITREND indicators for the dietary services functional reporting center are provided in table 9.

Table 9. HAS/MONITREND Data for Dietary Services: Six-Month Medians for Period Ending December 1988

Indicator	National Bed Size Groups							
	Under 50	50–74	75–99	100–149	150–199	200–299	300–399	400 and Over
Total meals per patient day[a]	6.71	6.72	6.88	6.81	6.46	6.38	6.40	6.12
Patient meals per patient day[b]	2.96	2.84	2.83	2.82	2.82	2.80	2.79	2.81
Paid hours per adjusted patient day[c]	2.01	1.72	1.65	1.49	1.40	1.37	1.38	1.31
Paid hours per 100 meals[d]	45.43	37.99	34.03	30.81	30.39	28.90	27.14	27.13

[a]Total meals per patient day = (dietary meals + other meals)/total patient days.

[b]Patient meals per patient day = (dietary patient meals/total patient days).

[c]Paid hours per adjusted patient day = dietary paid hours/(total patient days/overall RCC). The overall RCC (ratio of charges to charges) is an adjustment factor that is computed as follows: Overall RCC = gross inpatient revenue/gross operating revenue.

[d]Paid hours per 100 meals = dietary paid hours/([dietary patient meals]/100).

Source: HAS/MONITREND, 1988. Please refer to page x for more information about the data presented in this table.

Human Resources/ Personnel Department

Overview

The human resources/personnel department is responsible for the recruitment, selection, orientation, retention, and compensation (including worker's compensation and unemployment compensation) of all hospital employees. The department is also responsible for providing management and consultative services in employee and labor relations and in compliance activity regarding the laws and regulations that affect the employer–employee relationship. In addition, the department supervises the provision of employee health services and may supervise the provision of management engineering services, hospitalwide education and training, and volunteer services. Managers in the human resources/personnel department ensure that employee policies are developed and periodically reviewed, and they provide services to line managers in the areas of management development and conflict prevention or resolution, including but not limited to management education, employee and labor relations, and employee performance and productivity improvement systems. As hospitals become involved with mergers, acquisitions, and divestitures, the department may also be called on to undertake strategic manpower planning.

The activities of the human resources/personnel department are conducted in compliance with guidelines set forth by laws governing civil rights, wages and hours, labor relations, and employee health and safety. Department employees interact with all levels of hospital personnel, including the staff and governing board, as well as representatives from legal counsel, representatives of regulatory agencies responsible for compliance of organizations, advertising agencies, insurance companies, and the general public.

Employment

The human resources/personnel department recruits hospital staff using a variety of methods, including newspaper advertising, job fairs, college and school recruitment visits, employee referrals, open houses, and contacts with professional placement firms. Potential candidates are screened, interviewed, tested (if necessary), and referred to the hiring supervisor, in compliance with equal employment opportunity and affirmative action guidelines. Department personnel set up an employment physical and conduct reference checks for those applicants being considered for employment. New employees receive an orientation to the hospital (which may include an employee handbook) and are asked to complete all appropriate tax and benefit forms. For employees leaving the hospital, the department coordinates termination interviews and reviews the results of the interviews to assess recruitment and retention problems.

Compensation and Benefits Administration

The human resources/personnel department is responsible for establishing and maintaining an equitable and competitive compensation program that will be useful in attracting and retaining competent employees. Part of that compensation is a comprehensive package of relevant benefits such as a pension plan, health insurance, life insurance, dental insurance, and long-term disability insurance.

Benefits have become a major cost for hospitals. This is primarily because of increasing Social Security payments, government-mandated changes in pension plans, and rising employee health insurance costs.

Laws such as the Employee Retirement Income Security Act (ERISA) have added to administrative costs because they require extensive reporting to government agencies and to employees participating in the benefit plans. In addition, recent federal laws and regulations deal with the equitable nature of fringe benefits applying equally to highly paid health care executives as well as to support personnel. [See section 89 of the Internal Revenue Code (nondiscrimination testing for health and welfare plans).] As a result, the human resources/personnel department is continually reviewing benefit plans in terms of their cost and relevance as well as different methods of financing to ensure their competitiveness and to adapt to changing employee demographics and budgetary considerations.

Labor Relations

In 1974, hospital employees became a covered class under the federal Labor Management Relations Act (also known as the Taft–Hartley Act), which is the body of laws governing collective bargaining between unions and management in the private sector. Prior to 1974, many states had laws allowing hospital employees to bargain collectively; however, the number of hospitals experiencing organizing activities accelerated with the enactment of the Taft–Hartley Act. Today, many hospitals have one or more bargaining units, while others have their entire work force organized with the exception of a few management and administrative personnel.

The human resources/personnel department is responsible for handling the day-to-day interpretation and application of the provisions of the labor contract negotiated between the hospital and the union. Problems that arise with the contract or with employees covered by the contract are addressed by following an established grievance procedure. This procedure, which usually has several steps, is clearly explained in the contract.

In most cases, the director of human resources is designated as management's representative at some stage of the procedure. In some hospitals, the director of human resources is the hospital's chief negotiator with the union. In others, human resources staff may assist a professional outside negotiator (usually a labor attorney) with the preparation of necessary material and information to be used during negotiations.

The department plays a direct role in helping the hospital to avoid union organization. It works with top-level management, department heads, and supervisors to communicate the hospital's position during an organizing campaign.

Organization

The organizational structure of the human resources/personnel department varies with the size of the hospital. In small institutions, the director of human resources works with only one or two clerical assistants and, in addition to being responsible for employee matters, may have other responsibilities such as handling public relations. To look at all the different facets of human resources management, it is necessary to look at its function in a large hospital.

Generally, the director of human resources (or vice-president of human resources) reports directly to the hospital's chief executive officer or chief operating officer (or executive vice-president). The director usually has an assistant director or manager of human resources who oversees the department's day-to-day operations and assumes some of the director's responsibilities during his or her absence. The department's staff also includes such positions as wage and salary administrator, employment supervisor, benefits administrator, training director, manager of labor relations, and director of employee health services (usually a part-time physician). These positions in turn have employees who report directly to them, including job analysts, interviewers, benefits analysts, instructors, and employee health nurses. Each of these persons in turn works with human resource assistants, secretaries, receptionists, and employee records clerks.

Models and Systems

The functions performed by the department revolve around finding and retaining competent employees to staff the various areas of the hospital. However, in some hospitals, managers in nursing services are responsible for recruiting their own staff.

Recruitment and Hiring

A request for employment is generated by the department seeking the employee. The human resources/personnel department reviews the request, checking for proper title and pay grade and confirming that the position is budgeted and has the necessary approvals. Oftentimes, the hospital has a policy of promoting from within, and the position is posted to give current employees the chance to apply. When the position is not filled from within, the human resources staff conducts external recruitment procedures, which might include newspaper advertising, college and school recruitment, and contacting professional placement firms.

Job applicants are screened to ensure that they have the skills required to perform the job, and then they are referred to the hiring supervisor for an interview. Preemployment testing may include screening for substance abuse. The human resources/personnel staff checks references and previous work histories on candidates the supervisor is interested in hiring. The successful candidate is contacted by the human resources/personnel department and offered the position. Final hiring is contingent on the candidate's supplying proof of his or her U.S. citizenship or approved immigration status. The responsibility for ensuring compliance is the employer's.

A new employee's starting salary is based on established salary ranges and is usually determined by the hiring supervisor after a discussion with the human resources/personnel department. The department also conducts an orientation session for new employees that usually consists of a general overview of the hospital's operations, an explanation of policies and procedures, information on benefit plans, and completion of tax forms and appropriate personnel forms.

Compensation and Performance Evaluation

The hospital's compensation program is administered by the human resources/personnel department. Typically, the program consists of the development of individual job descriptions that explain the primary functions of each position. Positions are evaluated to determine their relative worth in comparison to all other positions in the hospital.

Although there are a great many evaluation systems, hospitals usually employ the point-factor system. Under this type of system, each position is evaluated according to an established group of factors, such as the amount of education required, the amount of experience needed, the number of people supervised, and so forth. Individual factors are segmented into levels and assigned a point value. For example, the education factor might be valued at 10 points if the position required two years of education beyond high school or 40 points if a master's degree were required. Once the position has been evaluated under each factor, the total number of points is added, and depending on the total, the position is assigned a particular grade. The human resources/personnel department conducts compensation surveys of other hospitals and nonhospital employers to determine comparable positions. On the basis of the data received, a pay range is established for each position. Each range has a minimum, or entry-level, rate and a maximum rate (the highest amount paid to a person in that range).

Once an employee is hired, a personnel record is set up and maintained throughout his or her tenure. A human resources information system keeps track of the dates employees are due for performance evaluations and, as appropriate, salary increases. The human resources/personnel department issues evaluation forms to supervisory personnel, who complete the forms and return them with recommendations for pay increases. The human resources staff reviews the forms and proposed salary increases to ensure their accuracy and to ensure that the salary adjustment falls within the limits established by the compensation program and budget restrictions. When all is in order, the appropriate paperwork is forwarded to the hospital's payroll department for processing.

Grievance Procedures

The human resources/personnel department develops and recommends policies for the mediation and documentation of grievances, disciplinary actions, and termination problems. Employees' problems are usually addressed through a grievance procedure. In a nonunionized hospital, the procedure typically begins with the employee bringing a complaint or problem to his or her immediate supervisor. When the problem cannot be resolved by the supervisor and employee, the issue is brought to the department head and then, if necessary, to the assistant director or vice-president of the division.

When it reaches this level, an unresolved problem is brought to the director of human resources; however, the director may have been consulted and may have provided advice during any of the preceding steps. The final step in the procedure involves the hospital's chief executive officer, whose decision is final.

The grievance procedure in a unionized hospital follows similar steps, and the union business agent or assistant business agent participates in the final steps. When the matter cannot be settled at the chief executive level, it is submitted to arbitration, where a final decision is made.

Education and Training

In most hospitals, nursing services and human resources share the responsibility for in-house training. Nursing's in-service education program, on the one hand, is designed to provide continuing education in patient care. The educational aim of human resources, on the other hand, is to provide training in administrative subjects, such as performance evaluation. In addition, the hospital's tuition assistance program for employees enrolled in educational programs outside the hospital is administered by the human resources/personnel department.

Productivity Management

Traditionally, the human resources/personnel department has been responsible for the management of the hospital's position control program. Recently, the department has also become more active in coordinating productivity studies by internal and external consultants and in producing reports from the productivity-monitoring system.

Today, the department is very active as a partner in attempts to maximize productivity and quality within the institution. This includes the implementation of programs to minimize employee turnover, the development of incentive programs, and the management of cost-containment programs.

Other Responsibilities

The department is often responsible for the employees activities committee. The committee's function is coordinating, sponsoring, and conducting a wide variety of morale-building and employee recognition programs. These extracurricular activities might include bowling or softball leagues, trips to sporting events, discounts at area shops and restaurants, and so on. Many of those activities are financially underwritten at least in part by the employer.

A developing trend in hospitals is to have the human resources/personnel department coordinate voluntary legislative and political activity among employees. An example would be encouraging employees and their friends and relatives to write Congress to support the American Hospital Association's "Elect to Protect Medicare" campaign.

Situations and Problems

Employees' attitudes about the hospital, their individual departments, and their own particular jobs are constantly changing. The human resources/personnel department must maintain a current awareness of their changing attitudes and recommend the steps administration should take to correct any potential or developing problems.

The increasing complexity of hospital services, brought on in part by rapid technological changes, can result in communication problems between employees and the administration. Usually, these problems occur in communication channels flowing from employees up to top-level management. When employees believe they are being ignored, they may seek a labor union to represent them.

In most hospitals, employees meet with a representative of human resources to discuss work-related problems, personal problems that affect work performance, discrimination issues, questions about their employment, and countless other issues that arise in a work environment. Many hospitals have employee assistance programs that offer employees confidential assistance with personal or family problems.

The human resources/personnel department acts as an employee advocate, sometimes at the request of employees, but also in matters that may involve an employee being discussed without the employee being aware of it. An example of this behind-the-scenes advocacy role might be when a position opens up in a department and the supervisor requests assistance from human resources in deciding whom to promote. The human resources/personnel department might discuss factors such as seniority, results of previous performance reviews, and other information that would help ensure that all employees are being considered fairly.

The responsibility for ensuring the fair treatment of employees, compliance with state and federal laws prohibiting discrimination, and promotion of equal employment opportunities for women and minorities rests with the human resources/personnel department. Every hospital should have an affirmative action plan (a plan to improve the representation of women and minorities in the hospital's work force), and the human resources/personnel department is generally responsible for the plan's development and implementation. Compliance with other laws involving the employer–employee relationship is also the department's responsibility.

Departmental Analysis

The effectiveness of the human resources function can be analyzed in a variety of ways; however, conducting a survey of employees' attitudes is probably the most effective. When it is properly designed and administered, an attitude survey can identify employee opinions, both favorable and unfavorable, on a variety of subjects including compensation, benefits, management, working conditions, morale, intradepartmental relations, and so forth.

Once the survey is completed, it is essential that management communicate the results to employees, including what actions management plans to take to rectify problems that were identified or an explanation of why no action is to be taken.

Computerization has led to the consolidation of a variety of employee-related information maintained by human resources. Data on employees—such as age, sex, earnings, skills, educational level, and address—can be extracted and analyzed to determine such things as the best geographic areas from which to recruit new employees, the relevancy of benefits provided versus the needs of the employees, and the identification of individuals already employed who may have the education and work experience to handle higher positions within the organization.

Information Systems Department

Overview

The information systems department — also called data processing (DP), management information systems (MIS), information systems (IS), and other similar titles — is one of the newest and most dynamic departments in the hospital. The principal objective of information systems is to improve the speed, scope, and quality of information capture and dissemination throughout the hospital. The central focus of this area has become the use of computer-based technologies to aid in this capture and dissemination role.

The information systems department was originally created to automate the financial accounting areas, but as the cost of computer technology has decreased, usage has spread from the financial areas to virtually all departments. The operating demands of the hospital for more accurate and timely information have also been a strong motivating force in expanding the presence of information services outside the traditional fiscal role. This revolution in use has even expanded to the point of care (the patient's bedside). The integration of special purpose or dedicated computer information systems into comprehensive information systems has also become very common. Many hospitals are also linking their systems to physicians' offices and other geographically separate operating entities. The variations in use of information systems in hospitals today do not generally fall into rigid models but rather follow general concepts of operation and functionality according to the individual needs and priorities of the hospital.

Organization

The six basic groups of personnel found in the information systems department are:

- Administrative personnel
- Systems analysts and/or computer programmers
- User coordinators
- Operators
- Data-entry staff
- Rounds technicians

Figure 7 depicts the organization of a typical information systems department.

Administrative personnel are responsible for the daily operation of the department, for long-range planning, and for the interface with administrative personnel from other departments. They are also involved in the make-or-buy decisions associated with software development.

Figure 7. Organization of a Typical Information Systems Department

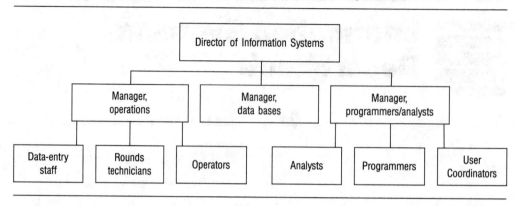

The head of the department is often called the director of information systems. Managers within the department supervise the operations and programming staffs and maintain the integrity of the various hospital data bases.

Systems analysts design the systems the hospital needs for processing its data. They interact with hospital personnel to find out how a need can best be met or a problem solved and then draw up a set of specifications that identify which data need to be processed and what type of processing should take place.

Computer programmers use these specifications as the basis for designing, writing, testing, and implementing new or replacement programs that direct the computer processing. The background and number needed of these technical staff members are determined by the degree to which the hospital uses turnkey or ready-to-use software and the degree to which this software is customized to the unique needs of the hospital. The larger the in-house systems development program is, the larger and more highly trained the programming and systems analyst staff needs to be.

User coordinators are responsible for training hospital personnel to use the information systems. These coordinators also act as liaisons between user departments and the technical staff of the information systems department. Coordinators may be trained in computer science, or they may be hospital professionals who have technical skills in information systems.

Operators are responsible for operating and maintaining the equipment. In most hospitals, shifts of operators keep the system in operation 24 hours per day, 7 days per week. The operators are also responsible for backing up files to guard against information loss and for maintaining equipment and doing preventive maintenance.

The *data-entry staff* usually includes keypunch operators who are responsible for entering information from other departments that do not have direct access to the information systems. The size of the data-entry staff is largely dependent on the number of on-line terminals available in other departments.

Rounds technicians replace faulty equipment throughout the hospital and carry out an ongoing preventive maintenance program.

The reporting relationship of the information systems department depends on the scope of services provided. In most hospitals, the head of the information systems department reports to the chief financial officer. With the expansion of the information systems department to include applications in areas outside finance, however, the trend has been for the department to report to an administrator other than the chief financial officer.

A recent development in medium-size and large-size hospitals is the creation of the position of chief information officer (CIO). The CIO generally oversees the work of the information systems, telecommunications, and management engineering staffs. At present, CIOs may be known by a number of titles, for example, vice-president for information systems.

Scope of Department

The information systems department is a service department. In addition to the financial applications that most hospitals run, the information systems department may be responsible for other applications, such as departmental systems and office automation. Because of the increasing complexity of systems and the need for communication among systems, it is preferable that the information systems department be actively involved in planning for all systems applications. Figure 8 shows the most common systems applications.

Some applications, such as results-reporting or order-entry systems, are called hospitalwide applications. (They may also be called hospital information systems or medical information systems.) Their purpose is to automate the flow of information among requesting departments (such as nursing units) and ancillary departments (such as the laboratory and radiology). In addition, hospitalwide systems applications enable the capture of charge information as a by-product of the order-entry process. These systems can be expanded to maintain additional medical information so that they act as clinical tools. One of the more common systems applications is the automation of the nursing service's medication profile for each patient.

Laboratory and pharmacy systems are the two most common departmental systems. A sophisticated laboratory system automates the capture of information from the clinical instruments once the information is entered. Other departments in which automation is becoming more prevalent include radiology, materials management, medical records, food service, and the surgical suite.

Departmental systems may be operated in a variety of ways. The most common method is for large departments, such as the laboratory, to install a separate computer. In technically advanced hospitals, such systems are interfaced with the financial and hospitalwide systems so that manual intervention is not required. In small hospitals, departmental applications may be run on the same computer that maintains the financial system. They may be kept separate from the financial and hospitalwide applications, or they may be integrated with them.

The use of office automation, including word processing, is common in many departments throughout the hospital, especially the medical records, radiology, and administrative areas. It is sometimes found in home health care and other remote departments. When properly implemented, office automation can significantly improve the productivity of hospital personnel. However, the hospital must carefully evaluate those functions for which office automation is used and examine the requirements for interfacing with any existing computer systems.

Figure 8. Common Information Systems Applications in Hospitals

Hospitalwide	Departmental	Financial
Admissions	Anatomical pathology	Accounts payable
Order entry	Food service	Accounts receivable
Results Reporting	Laboratory	Budgeting
	Medical records	Case mix
	Nursing service	Collections
	Emergency service	Cost accounting
	Surgical suite	Diagnosis-related groups
	Pharmacy	Financial modeling
	Quality assurance	Fixed assets
	Radiology	General ledger
	Tumor registry	Inventory
	Utilization management	Materials management
		Patient billing
		Payroll
		Preventive maintenance
		Time and attendance

Recently, many systems have been developed for hospitals with 200 or fewer beds. The availability of these systems has led to an increase in the use of in-house computers for small hospitals. There has also been a proliferation in the use of personal computers (PCs). Many of the departmental systems currently offered run on PCs. They are also used extensively in the financial areas and for office automation.

The evolution of automation in the hospital is reaching the point of care through the marketing of bedside computer terminal systems. These systems range in functionality and cost, but the more comprehensive systems can automate such functions as patient care order entry, medication charting, capture of patient charges, and reporting of test results directly from the laboratory or other ancillary services. Systems may also help the nursing service with staffing and care planning.

Three primary vendors have emerged with bedside systems, although many of the major hospital information systems vendors have developed or joint-ventured products with terminals at the bedside. A subset of the point-of-care systems are the intensive care unit bedside systems, which can transmit clinical data (such as a patient's vital signs) directly from the patient to the computer.

Models and Systems

As previously mentioned, most hospitals operate a 24-hour-per-day, 7-day-per-week information system. Throughout the day, the system is used by the various hospital departments, usually through access to on-line terminals. Data from nonautomated areas are collected on charge tickets or other source documents and sent to the data-entry staff. At a predetermined time each day, the day-end processing is performed (usually by the operations group), which consists of processing charges and backing up the daily files.

Another major activity of the information systems department is month-end processing, which usually involves backing up all files for off-site storage and preparing patient bills and third-party claims. Month-end processing also usually involves regenerating and updating the data base. In addition, tapes or disks can be created from departmental systems that do not interface with the billing system. Depending on the volume, charges from departmental systems may be processed on a daily basis.

Because of the rapidly changing nature of computer technology, hospitals meet their information systems needs through a variety of approaches. These approaches can be grouped into four basic types: shared services, turnkey systems, in-house development, and facilities management. The staffing and organization of the information systems department depend on which approach is used by the hospital. Because there are advantages and disadvantages to each approach, hospitals must evaluate their individual situations to determine the approach that best satisfies their needs.

Shared Services

The shared services approach is one in which the hospital utilizes computer support that is not uniquely dedicated to the single hospital. This may be in the form of a shared arrangement with another hospital or a group of hospitals. Another common shared services approach is the use of an outside commercial computer service that provides services to several hospitals out of common sites. This may be arranged by a for-profit service bureau or by nonprofit associations.

In different parts of the country, hospitals have joined together to take advantage of limited resources. Originally, this was a prevalent approach, but as the economics have changed, there has been a trend away from this type of service. The first major change affecting the use of shared services was the advent of improved computer hardware and lower costs that allowed individual hospitals to maintain dedicated computer equipment on a cost-effective basis. The second major change was the spread of automated information services activities into areas outside finance, especially within the clinical services of hospitals. The increased emphasis on clinically related systems places a heavy burden on remote systems to operate on a timely basis. Furthermore, increasingly specialized clinical information requirements have also resulted in a more widespread demand for unique information systems.

Shared services rely on a high degree of similarity among their users to maintain systems in a cost-effective manner. The general concept of shared services also imposes some operating limitations on new clients because of the need to maintain the level of standardization dictated by economic forces. This sometimes results in increased levels of user dissatisfaction with the artificial limits imposed and in an increased desire on the part of many hospitals to implement systems configured specifically for their individual needs.

Nevertheless, shared services tend to have a significantly lower risk factor associated with initial installations and tend to require shorter installation and operational training times. Depending on the size and complexity of the system, various levels of on-site support personnel may be required. Such on-site personnel may be employed by either the vendor or the hospital itself.

Turnkey Systems

Under a turnkey system, the hospital purchases a system that has been developed by an outside vendor. The vendor is responsible for installing the hardware and software but may or may not provide ongoing or maintenance support for the system. There is no generally accepted model involving the support of turnkey systems. Various levels of support may be provided depending on the hospital's resources and expertise in managing the system.

Some turnkey systems are purchased outright, and others may be implemented on the basis of a type of term lease. In most lease or operating license arrangements, the hospital does not acquire the outright ownership of the system (usually the software component) from the vendor. Rather, the hospital usually pays for some form of operating license that entitles the hospital to use the system for its own and directly associated use but that prohibits the hospital from using the system outside its own organization. Exceptions to this situation are sometimes found, but the general trend is toward some form of operating lease, license, or contractual support arrangement on software systems.

Lease or license arrangements are usually in force for a fixed period, with the hospital assuming some form of ownership of the hardware (outright ownership or a separate lease with another entity). This approach relies heavily on the vendor for ensuring that hospital personnel acquire the skills and expertise they need to operate the systems. Some technical (usually operations) personnel are required for various aspects of the computer system control and operations, but usually no in-house programming or systems analysis personnel are involved. Some vendors provide on-site personnel support, but this tends to be the exception rather than the rule.

In many settings, the difference between shared systems and turnkey systems is becoming less clear-cut. Although many vendors offer arrangements that have aspects of both approaches, the general differentiation between these two approaches tends to be whether the computer system is mostly on-site or off-site. Where it is off-site, the system is generally regarded to be a shared system; however, an on-site system under the control of the hospital is generally considered to be a turnkey system.

In-House Development

In-house development is the creation of new or replacement computer systems by analysts and/or programmers on staff at the institution. This approach to satisfying information systems needs tends to be used in large hospitals with extensive systems and a significant commitment to hardware and technical expertise. In some very small hospital settings, in-house development based on commercially available software may be attempted, but this is generally limited to circumstances in which information requirements and hardware (such as microcomputers) are on a small scale. Such small hospitals develop or purchase software packages and use their own technical staff to install and maintain them.

An advantage of in-house development is that analysts and programmers can customize the systems to meet the unique needs of the institution. The disadvantages include increased maintenance requirements and longer installation times.

Another major disadvantage of in-house development is that the hospital needs to make a large commitment of resources to keep the system current and to respond to changing internal and external information requirements. In the 1980s, this commitment caused many hospitals to move away from in-house development and toward other forms of information systems acquisition and operation. Today, large hospitals are generally the most likely locations of large-scale in-house systems. However, the external pressure to lower hospital costs has often resulted in the commitment of significantly smaller ongoing development resources to in-house information services.

Still another disadvantage of in-house development is that the hospital's internal expertise is much more susceptible to becoming obsolete than is the case with shared systems or turnkey systems. Every major advance in hardware capabilities results in the need to acquire new technical skills and experience from outside the hospital in order to make use of the new technologies. Therefore, in-house development carries the highest risk of any approach to information systems management.

Facilities Management

Under the facilities management approach, the hospital contracts with an outside service to provide on-site management and technical expertise for the department. This expertise may be supplied in the form of a manager or director, or it may be expanded to include the services of an entire staff. Therefore, in a properly managed contractual environment, the facilities management approach could conceivably be a highly cost-effective way of moving the hospital into a new level of information services without an ongoing commitment to recruiting and retaining scarce, technically qualified personnel. The level of services would determine the cost of the facilities management approach. However, this approach generally tends to be relatively costly and for that reason is not widely used.

Departmental Analysis

The topics for analysis in the information systems department range from planning to vendor evaluation and selection to benefits realization. Some typical areas of study are the following:

- *Long-range planning:* The typical long-range plan should cover a five-year time frame. A detailed plan is prepared for the first three years; years three to five are covered in more general terms. The plan should include such basic components as an evaluation of the current systems and a forecast of future needs for order-entry systems, financial systems, major departmental systems, personal computers, and office automation. Special attention should be paid to the present and future levels of expertise required of the information systems staff and to the need for, and sources of, external assistance.
- *Vendor evaluation and selection:* The basic vendor evaluation and selection process includes the identification of potential vendors and the selection of a vendor that satisfies identified needs. Vendors may need to be evaluated and selected for a hospital-wide system or for a specific departmental system. Hospitals should try to minimize the chance of selecting vendors that are likely to go out of business or alter or terminate a contractual relationship as a result of a merger or buyout.
- *Cost-benefit analysis:* Hospitals should analyze the benefits to be derived from purchasing automation systems. For example, the purchase of an order-entry system can

affect the work of every department in the hospital. A cost-benefit analysis enables the hospital to determine whether it should purchase the system and helps evaluate different vendors.

- *Benefits realization:* A program must be established for the hospital to realize fully the benefits associated with the system. In other words, once the system has been installed, manual support systems often must be redesigned in order for the hospital to use the information system properly.
- *Financial systems:* Hospitals could benefit from a work-flow analysis that would reveal ways for information systems to reduce the number of days of receivables outstanding. Other areas for improvement could include the identification of lost charges and the improvement of collections and third-party billing.
- *Response time analysis:* With the proliferation of on-line systems and the increasing use of existing computer capacity, increases in response time commonly occur just before lunchtime or at a shift change. In analyzing response time problems, both the size of the computer and the activities performed on it must be evaluated. Three ways to improve response time are upgrading computer capacity, restructuring the resource allocation or parameters of programs, and changing the operational procedures performed by user departments.
- *Physician's office linkage:* Hospitals are embracing the concept of clinical and demographic information flow between the hospital and physicians' offices. Many hospitals have recognized the marketing advantages of such linkages. The general rule is that if information on the patient exists in-house, it can be accessed at the physician's office. An analysis of the feasibility of such a linkage is one that should be conducted by the hospital information systems department.

As the information systems department increases its services and value to other departments in the hospital, its share of the hospital's operating budget is also likely to increase. In the past few years, budgets for information systems have continued to rise toward a level commensurate with expenditures in the general business community. This increase in expenditures also reflects a growing recognition that information systems can play an important role in ensuring a hospital's long-term viability.

Intensive Care Units

Overview

Intensive care units (ICUs) are specialty nursing units designed for treating patients facing life-threatening conditions. The size and type of ICU depends on the hospital's size. In a community hospital, an ICU may have 6 to 12 beds. Large community hospitals or teaching hospitals may have several ICUs with a total of more than 30 beds.

Brief descriptions of some types of ICUs are listed below:

- *Medical ICU (MICU):* Most large hospitals, whether community or teaching hospitals, have MICUs for treating patients with medical complications such as kidney, respiratory, or internal bleeding problems.
- *Surgical ICU (SICU):* Critically ill presurgical and postsurgical patients may be cared for in this type of unit.
- *Neuro ICU:* Patients with neurological or neurosurgical complications are cared for in a neuro ICU. Such specialty units usually do not exist in small health care facilities.
- *Pediatric ICU (PICU):* Pediatric ICUs specialize in the care of pediatric patients with medical, surgical, or other complications.
- *Neonatal ICU (NICU):* Neonatal ICUs are primarily responsible for caring for high-risk newborns, including premature babies.
- *Coronary care ICU (CCU):* This type of ICU treats patients with serious cardiac problems and is a common type of specialty ICU.
- *Respiratory ICU (RICU):* Some hospitals may provide respiratory ICUs for patients with respiratory complications. Such patients usually require ventilator support.

Other types of ICUs not commonly found in community hospitals include burn, trauma, transplant, and cardiothoracic ICUs. Such specialty ICUs are usually provided by teaching hospitals.

Some facilities have transitional units referred to as telemetry, intermediate care, step-down, or interim units. Patients are transferred to these units after their stay in the ICU and before going to a medical/surgical unit. Transitional units can also treat long-term critically ill patients.

Organization

Intensive care units are primarily staffed by registered nurses (RNs). Licensed practical nurses (LPNs), certified nurse's aides (CNAs), and/or other nonprofessional staff may or may not be used depending on the hospital's policy, the type of ICU, and the impact of the nursing shortage. Ward clerks or secretaries provide clerical and telecommunication support to the unit.

Intensive care unit staffing needs vary on the basis of census and patient acuity. A staffing ratio of one nurse to one patient is frequently necessary; however, the usual ratio is two patients to one nurse. In a step-down or intermediate care unit, a staffing range of one nurse to three or four patients is the target.

Intensive care units are administered by the nursing service, with nurse managers acting as department heads. Depending on the hospital's size and whether the management structure of the nursing service is centralized or decentralized, ICU nurse managers may or may not report directly to the director of nursing. In large hospitals and teaching hospitals with several ICUs, the nurse manager reports to an assistant director of nursing or a clinical director of critical care.

Depending on the size and complexity of the ICUs, nurse managers may or may not spend all their time on managerial duties. If they worked on the unit, they would perform the functions of the charge nurse—a registered nurse who usually has both clinical experience and staff seniority.

The charge nurse for each shift is responsible for the clinical coordination of the ICU for that shift. When there are problems or questions during the day, the charge nurse consults with the nurse manager. On off-shifts, the charge nurse consults or reports to the nursing supervisor on duty.

All ICUs have full-time or part-time medical directors. In a teaching hospital, a chief resident or a physician fulfilling a fellowship (that is, a physician completing specialty training in a specific area of practice) may also be assigned to a specific ICU. Generally, it is the responsibility of the medical director, chief resident, or fellow to monitor clinical practice and medical procedures. At teaching hospitals, numerous medical students, interns, and residents undergoing on-the-job training are accountable to the medical director.

Models and Systems

Clinical practice in the ICU is similar to that on other nursing units, but the severity of the patient's condition and ICU specialization require greater expertise of staff. Knowledge of special procedures and patient care expertise are very important. Frequently, a general flow sheet is used to combine all patient documentation for easy recording and reference.

Because the scope of practice in critical care is designed to provide highly specialized care, the orientation and education for newly employed RNs needs to be comprehensive. New employee training may include classroom study and clinical experience. It may be delivered in several modes, including preceptor orientation, unit-based training, hospital-based educational classes, consortium programs, buddy-assigned systems, or training with a clinical specialist. The ICU staff's continuing education requirements are similar to those of other RNs.

Capital expenditures for outfitting and maintaining a critical care area are higher than costs for other nursing units. Special monitoring systems (cardiac, respiratory, pulmonary artery, and intracranial) and support systems (IABP, CAVH, ventilators, and pacemakers) not only are expensive to purchase, but require continuous calibration, evaluation, and maintenance by the clinical engineering department. The nursing staff must be well versed in the operation of, and troubleshooting for, all equipment in these areas. New medical technology such as laser surgery, angioplasty, and drug therapy all have implications for special protocols and care delivery in ICUs, which may affect the resource allocation, staffing, and cost of the unit.

A variety of floor plans or layouts have been used for ICUs. The units are generally located close to the emergency department and surgical suite to provide faster access in crisis situations. Some of the popular floor plans may include U-shape or semicircular layouts that provide central work areas and monitoring observation areas for nursing personnel.

In newly designed ICUs, provision for overhead blood pressure equipment, patient-monitoring equipment, and oxygen gas lines for respiratory therapy greatly improves space utilization. Also, such arrangements facilitate access to patients. A special procedure room that can be shared by ICUs usually is equipped with fluoroscopy capabilities.

Situations and Problems

Because of the critical and unstable condition of patients and the urgency of care requirements, the ICU environment can be quite intense. Consequently, in view of the great demand for nurses' time, a management engineer may not command the staff's attention during departmental studies. Nevertheless, common problems can be predicted, such as the following:

- ICU RNs in general are highly motivated and particularly interested in their field. They are also likely to have strong relationships with physicians because of their close involvement with patient care. However, the fast pace and urgent nature of care may cause early burnout for some nurses and may result in high employee stress levels and turnover.
- ICU head nurses tend to have obtained their positions on the basis of their technical skill; as a result, they may lack administrative experience and managerial competence.
- In hospitals with old physical plants, lack of proper space in ICUs may result in inconvenience for patients, families, and staff and may adversely affect the staff's productivity.

An ethical problem with increasing financial ramifications is the maintenance of patients whose prognosis for recovery is poor. Although the staff must expend every effort to cure those patients who are curable, the question arises as to whether they should respect the wishes of those who do not wish heroic efforts to be made on their behalf. Because of such complex legal and moral issues, patients who are not being aggressively treated or who are not on life-support equipment usually are not treated in an ICU unit.

Departmental Analysis

When management engineering studies are performed in ICUs, the assignment of management engineering staff with clinical or ICU project experience can lend credibility to the process. Some examples of types of studies that could be conducted by management engineers follow:

- The development of patient classification systems could include traditional approaches; however, techniques for assessing the work load associated with special complex procedures and crisis situations must also be applied.
- Studies of workplace systems and procedures could often uncover areas where improved work methods, supply systems, or capital expenditures might improve efficiency.
- The evaluation of staffing needs must involve an analysis of the variability of demand for ICU services. Scheduling and staffing systems improvements designed to facilitate the flexibility of an ICU staff in responding to unpredictable work factors can result in better staffing coverage at reduced cost. Studies of staffing levels may benefit from reference to recent MONITREND data, such as those presented in table 10.
- An excellent opportunity to study means of gaining operational efficiencies is through staff involvement in the design or renovation of a unit.
- Information systems applications such as order entry and results reporting can have a significant impact on the efficiency of an ICU; monitoring systems can also show any significant variations in the amount of time required to maintain and observe this operation.

The ICU is a crucial part of the hospital's service capability. From the physician's point of view, good ICU capability can be a factor in deciding where to practice. The failure of the ICU service to contribute to the institution's image of providing good service and clinical competence can have major implications for the hospital's viability.

Table 10. HAS/MONITREND Data for the Medical and Surgical ICU: Six-Month Medians for Period Ending December 1988

Indicator	National Bed Size Groups							
	Under 50	50–74	75–99	100–149	150–199	200–299	300–399	400 and Over
Occupancy percent[a]	22.82	44.02	45.65	55.25	55.84	65.84	69.20	75.64
Average daily census[b]	0.91	2.25	2.74	4.60	6.06	10.46	13.99	26.48
Paid hours per patient day[c]	24.02	22.88	23.01	21.37	21.57	21.45	22.05	21.81

[a]Occupancy percent = (medical and surgical intensive care patient days/[medical and surgical intensive care beds × days in period]) × 100.

[b]Average daily census = medical and surgical intensive care patients days/days in period.

[c]Paid hours per patient day = medical and surgical intensive care paid hours/medical and surgical intensive care patient days.

Source: HAS/MONITREND, 1988. Please refer to page x for more information about the data presented in this table.

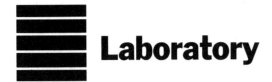

Laboratory

Overview

Recent advances in technology have brought medical care into what can be characterized as the era of laboratory medicine. Thirty years ago, laboratory determinations were done manually and centered on the basic diagnostic tests needed for patient assessment. Today, most laboratories are equipped with analytical equipment and information systems that greatly improve productivity and expand the scope of services. They are staffed with specialized personnel who provide laboratory services 24 hours a day. Studies conducted in major hospitals in the United States show that the number and variety of tests in most clinical laboratories are steadily increasing.

The laboratory is a major ancillary department of the hospital. It uses highly skilled personnel and can be a prime revenue-producing area. The primary function of the laboratory is to perform laboratory tests for all types of patients as ordered by physicians and as required by the hospital's patient population. In addition, the laboratory may also coordinate the purchase of tests from laboratories outside the hospital.

Organization

Typically, a pathologist, who is a medical doctor or osteopath, is responsible for the medical and technical aspects of testing within the laboratory. Large laboratories may employ assistant pathologists and laboratory scientists with doctoral degrees. The management structure also includes a chief medical technologist or laboratory manager who supervises technologists, technicians of various skill levels, and laboratory assistants. In many facilities, the laboratory manager also handles administrative and management matters. A medical technologist must have a bachelor of science degree and must meet the certification requirements of the American Society of Clinical Pathologists or a similar accrediting agency. The technicians may or may not have bachelor of science degrees.

The laboratory may be organized in subsections, each responsible for one or more of the following functions:

- *Anatomic pathology:* The primary function of this section is the processing of tissue removed during surgery or autopsy for both gross and microscopic examination. This is a labor-intensive operation. Equipment includes tissue processors, microtomes (used for cutting sections), cryostats (used to prepare frozen sections), and sometimes automated stainers.
- *Cytology:* This section processes various specimens (body fluids, smears, and so on) for microscopic examination to determine whether any abnormalities in cell structure

exist, such as malignant cells. The processes involve very little automation. Most laboratories use a cytospin or centrifuge to obtain a concentrate of cells from body fluid specimens. Cytology is not a major function of a typical laboratory, and specimens are often sent to another hospital for testing.

- *Chemistry:* This section of the laboratory analyzes serum and other body fluids for a variety of biochemical constituents such as electrolytes, glucose, protein, enzymes, hormones, and drug levels. Chemistry is a highly automated section that utilizes a wide variety of equipment. It is also one of the largest areas of the laboratory.

- *Serology/immunology:* This section tests various body fluids for detection of antigens or antibodies. Common tests look for signs of rubella and hepatitis infection. In community hospitals, this section is usually incorporated into other sections of the laboratory. A very limited amount of automation is available.

- *Hematology:* This section analyzes the cellular elements of blood such as the number, type, and morphology of red cells, white cells, and platelets. Tests usually include coagulation studies. The primary equipment includes a blood cell profiler and a coagulation analyzer. Hematology is one of the largest areas of the laboratory.

- *Blood bank:* The blood bank stores and distributes blood and blood components. This section contains very little automation. Activities include identification of blood type and Rh factor, cross-matching (compatibility testing), and related activities. Most blood banks possess a cell washer for preparing washed cells or deglyceralizing frozen blood. Responsibilities may also include donor recruitment and procurement of the actual blood supply. However, most institutions rely on regional blood centers for their blood supply.

- *Microbiology:* This section processes specimens for the isolation and identification of the microorganisms that cause infection (for example, bacteria, fungi, and parasites). Automation in microbiology is fairly recent. Blood cultures and isolates from routine specimens are now processed on automated equipment.

- *Microscopy:* This section analyzes body fluids, especially urine and to a lesser extent joint fluid, semen, and spinal fluid. Automation in this section is limited to the quantitative analysis of routine chemical constituents in urine.

- *Nuclear medicine:* In the laboratory, this section uses radioisotopes to test patient serum for various biochemical constituents. In most hospital laboratories, this section is part of the chemistry section. Equipment is limited to gamma counters, automatic samplers, pipettors, and dilutors.

The laboratory may also be responsible for general procurement and dispatch of specimens. In addition, a school of medical technology may be associated with the laboratory. Laboratory personnel may be cross-trained to perform a number of functions and so may work in several areas, especially in small hospitals. In large hospitals, each of these areas might constitute a small department that employs 10 to 30 people and provides around-the-clock coverage. In small laboratories, staff may be on call during less busy hours.

Models and Systems

The arrival of specific tests to be performed is almost random both in terms of time and in the distribution of work among types of tests. Because an order for multiple tests on a single patient may require activity at several workstations, the procedures for scheduling tests are similar to the procedures followed in a manufacturing organization that handles many small customer orders. These operational characteristics require the laboratory to be well organized to ensure efficiency and accuracy in two major areas: work flow and information flow. The laboratory also has one of the most formal statistical quality control systems used in the hospital.

Work Flow

The organization of work flow is determined by two basic functions. First, the procurement of the specimen and its delivery to the laboratory for analysis follow established procedures, which may or may not be the responsibility of the laboratory. Second, the laboratory tests are performed according to procedures established on the basis of the number and types of tests ordered, the time they are ordered and requested, and the availability of automated equipment. These factors determine the method by which the test is to be performed and how efficiently it can be done.

The major factor that determines work-load performance is the extent of automation in the production cycle. The type and sophistication of automated equipment in the laboratory varies from hospital to hospital. The most automated areas of testing are chemistry and hematology. At the very least, small hospitals have automated chemistry analyzers that fit on the bench top and handle high-volume procedures. Most laboratories have equipment that does low-cost profile testing, that is, it performs a preestablished set of a dozen or more tests from only one patient specimen. More sophisticated equipment can fill an entire room and do many tests in various combinations. The laboratory may have its own minicomputer that interfaces with the hospital's main computer for handling billing and demographic information and for reporting results.

Laboratory personnel generally favor as much automation as possible because it yields more accurate information than do manually performed tests, especially when laboratories are faced with rising work loads. A handful of manufacturers dominate the market, and the state of the art changes rapidly. Resources that provide detailed data on current equipment and technology include technical journals, professional societies, and vendors.

Information Flow

Information flow has two major phases. The first phase is a process whereby the test is ordered or requested. The order should indicate whether the result must be reported to the nursing station for inclusion on the patient's chart or to the requesting physician. The second phase of information flow is the logging in of the test and the actual reporting of the result.

The clinical laboratory processing system may be manual, partially computerized, or completely computerized. Whether manual or computerized, the statistical reporting procedure used by most laboratories to monitor work load and productivity is based on the College of American Pathologists' work-load recording manual.

When a *manual ordering system* is used, orders for procedures are received in writing or by telephone from nursing stations, physicians' offices, and the emergency department. Outpatients may also carry requests and specimens to the laboratory when instructed to do so by their physicians. The requests for tests are recorded in logs, and work requests are forwarded to the technologist. After the tests have been performed, the results are recorded on the report forms and transmitted to the physician or to the nursing station. The appropriate daily, weekly, and monthly statistical and management reports are also prepared manually from these logs and worksheets.

A *partially computerized system* using the hospitalwide computer system can greatly improve the efficiency of the laboratory's processing of information. The system generally uses minicomputers, with numerous data terminals located in the laboratory and throughout the hospital. The system is used for order entry and reporting and eliminates most paperwork. It also captures all charges at the moment an order is entered at the terminal, which helps to eliminate lost charges. The advantages to the laboratory of such a system are the following:

- Clerical time is saved.
- Response to emergency requests is faster.
- Order requisitions can be printed in the laboratory.

- Labels for specimen containers can be printed on the system, thereby improving identification of specimens.
- Daily statistical reports can be generated automatically.

A major shortcoming of such a partially computerized system is that although it can perform clerical tasks with efficiency, it cannot be used for work that is more specifically laboratory related, such as on-line capturing of results.

Fully computerized clinical laboratory processing systems are dedicated systems available as stand-alone minicomputers or as computer systems shared with other laboratories. The computer performs most of the clerical work that would otherwise be performed by the technical and support staff. The system organizes the laboratory's work flow, provides work assignments, reports data, and allows immediate access to data. It offers the following benefits:

- Increased production at a lower unit cost (not including computer cost)
- Improved response time
- Availability of comprehensive data and reports
- Expanded quality control in the laboratory

Other benefits of the system include its ability to provide computer printouts in place of manually compiled logbooks, detailed billing data, on-line acquisition of data from automated production equipment, and label printing. In addition, the system's ability to use customized software is a major advantage. The major disadvantage is that the cost of the comprehensive system may far exceed its benefits. This is one factor that encourages hospitals to develop shared laboratory services.

Shared Laboratory Services

A shared laboratory service is a clinical laboratory function that is common to two or more organizations and is used jointly by them in some way for the purposes of improving service, containing costs, and achieving economies of scale. Given appropriate facilities and personnel, a laboratory can perform work not only for inpatients, outpatients, and emergency patients, but also for local physicians and other hospitals. In general, all participating parties are held at risk.

Regardless of the organizational form, a comprehensive, shared laboratory program requires certain components:

- A group of pathologists providing clinical and anatomical services
- A group of supporting specialists performing a wide range of laboratory tests
- Adequate space and instrumentation to perform the procedures
- Modern methods of communication
- A reliable transportation system
- An effective management system that includes accounting, billing, and information processing
- The ability to process high-priority tests quickly

Sharing laboratory services is becoming increasingly common. The availability of automated equipment capable of processing a high volume of laboratory tests at a low unit cost has stimulated interest in expanding the laboratory's service beyond the hospital to take advantage of economies of scale. In addition, the use of computer systems for the storage and analysis of laboratory data and for the communication of clinical and management information has made sharing more feasible.

By participating in group practices, pathologists can serve several health care institutions in one area. This system also has facilitated the movement toward sharing services and consolidating laboratories.

Situations and Problems

When pathologists are in group practice and have a contract with a hospital, they may be paid a set fee for services, a percentage of the laboratory's revenue, or a combination of both. When pathologists are employed directly by the hospital, they may be paid a straight salary or a percentage of departmental revenue. Thus, pathologists may find that their compensation depends on the fluctuating quantity of laboratory work over which they have no control.

Because of hospital overhead, the need to provide 24-hour coverage, and the urgent care requirements of very ill patients, performing a laboratory procedure usually costs more in a hospital than in a commercial laboratory. Some hospitals try to be competitive by setting up a cost center that will function as a commercial laboratory or by setting up a separate corporation to provide laboratory services. However, when community physicians who have used the hospital laboratory refer outpatient tests to commercial laboratories outside the hospital, the pathologist and hospital may find their laboratory work load decreasing.

Appropriate test utilization continues to be a problem. Batteries of tests may be economical but are not always popular with physicians. Some physicians feel that test batteries may result in unnecessary testing, and others feel that they infringe on the physicians' medical judgment in deciding which tests are appropriate for their patients. Misuse of the laboratory's resources may occur when physicians order tests as stat requests when there is no true emergency.

Departmental Analysis

Among the many topics that could be studied in analyzing the operations of the laboratory, the major ones include staffing, feasibility evaluations of equipment and information systems, and cost finding. Cost finding refers to identifying the basic cost elements (labor, supplies, and equipment) associated with testing. The purposes of such analyses are to determine when the majority of costs are increasing and to develop strategies to control costs, such as purchasing tests from other laboratories.

Staffing and Scheduling Evaluations

In order to measure how effectively staff members are being used, the number of worked hours required must be calculated on the basis of predetermined standards and compared to the actual number of hours worked during the same time period. This comparison is usually expressed as a ratio or as a variance and is called the staff/labor utilization variance.

In determinations of the number of worked hours required to handle laboratory work loads, all tests and procedures performed should be identified, and the number of tests performed in specific time frames should be tabulated and extended by the appropriate time standards. These standards are readily available from the College of American Pathologists, or they can be determined in-house by conducting various time and motion studies.

Standard times should include all the operations necessary to set up or prepare for a procedure, to perform the procedure, to shut down the equipment, and to clean and put away the apparatus used in the procedure. As stated earlier, standards are applied to the appropriate volume statistics, and required variable hours are accumulated. It should be noted, however, that variable hours are work load dependent; that is, when no tests are performed, no variable hours are recorded.

All hospital laboratories conduct routine quality control tests during the determination of various procedures. Quality control samples may be commercially prepared solutions with a predetermined answer or a pooled serum sample that has been analyzed previously. The solutions are generally placed with a batch of unknown or patient samples and analyzed in the same way and at the same time.

Many of the procedures in the chemistry area, as well as some in other areas of the laboratory, involve the use of standard samples, a different type of quality control sample used to check and recalibrate an instrument. As a result, the laboratory standard time is adjusted to include the time necessary to obtain, prepare, and run the standard samples.

In addition to the variable worked hours component, the constant work load (also called nontechnical time) is measured to include all functions that are not directly related to the processing of laboratory tests, including activities such as equipment maintenance and calibration, clerical work, payroll processing, meetings and seminars, and other nontechnical or administrative activities.

A third component to be measured is the hours required for specimen collection for each laboratory section. This measurement, combined with the required variable hours and the constant hours, indicates the total number of hours required for the operation of each laboratory section during a specified time period.

Nothing seems so simple at the outset and yet can become so confusing as the proper scheduling of hospital personnel. Labor laws, fringe benefits, hospital policies (or their absence), and personnel limitations must be considered. However, in order to provide optimal coverage with the proper mix of required skills, scheduling must be done carefully. Effective scheduling is key to ensuring good patient care and simultaneous cost-effectiveness. It requires advance planning and knowledge of personnel requirements, an awareness of all constraints (for example, weekend coverage policies and skill requirements), and a determination of the proper balance of full-time and part-time positions. Evaluation of staffing and scheduling may be aided by reference to the recent MONITREND data in table 11.

Equipment Feasibility Studies

Determining the feasibility of adding computer systems applications and other automated laboratory equipment requires close study. Although automation does not ensure complete reliability, it is necessary for a modern, competitive clinical laboratory. It affords the well-trained technologist more time to devote to the development of new methodologies and techniques, and it requires less time for repetitive, routine testing.

The basic objectives of a feasibility study are the following:

- To evaluate the state of the art in such automated equipment as clinical chemistry analyzers

Table 11. HAS/MONITREND Data for the Laboratory and Blood Bank: Six-Month Medians for Period Ending December 1988

Indicator	National Bed Size Groups							
	Under 50	50–74	75–99	100–149	150–199	200–299	300–399	400 and Over
Work-load units per adjusted patient days[a]	53.10	50.04	40.67	48.05	43.65	44.39	46.16	50.98
Paid hours per adjusted patient day[b]	1.30	1.25	1.17	1.27	1.22	1.15	1.31	1.48
Percent charged work-load units of total work-load units[c]	69.84	77.40	79.51	77.64	84.00	84.14	84.74	82.55
Paid hours per 100 work-load units[d]	2.52	2.62	2.74	2.58	2.88	2.70	2.84	2.71

[a]Work-load units per adjusted patient day = (laboratory charged + other work-load units).

[b]Paid hours per adjusted patient day = laboratory paid hours/(total patient days/laboratory RCC). The laboratory RCC (ratio of charges to charges) is an adjustment factor that is computed as follows: Laboratory RCC = laboratory inpatient revenue/(laboratory inpatient revenue + laboratory outpatient revenue).

[c]Percent charged work-load units of total work-load units = (laboratory charged work-load units/[laboratory charged + other work-load units]) × 100.

[d]Paid hours per 100 work-load units = laboratory paid hours/(laboratory total work-load units/100).

Source: HAS/MONITREND, 1988. Please refer to page x for more information about the data presented in this table.

- To determine the financial feasibility of conversion to automated equipment (renting, leasing, buying, reimbursement, cost finding, and so on)
- To evaluate the economic impact of the various types of equipment available in terms of total life-cycle costs, projected revenues, capital expenditures, leasing charges, labor costs, maintenance costs, supply costs, and so on

Determining feasibility usually includes journal research, visits to hospitals, discussions with vendors and trade associations, reviews of sales literature, analyses of the current and projected work load, and preparation of cost analyses for the various alternatives.

Cost Finding

The laboratory is usually a revenue-generating department for the hospital. The prices of various tests reflect direct costs as well as indirect expenses, which include services provided by other hospital departments. The cost of performing high-volume tests is often used as a benchmark in pricing. The procedure for cost finding has two major components: analysis of the cost of high-volume procedures and examination of the impact of pricing on current hospital revenues.

The procedure for analyzing the cost of high-volume tests includes the following steps:

- Select the highest-volume procedures from all laboratory sections.
- Develop a standard cost analysis format that includes the costs of direct labor, materials, equipment, and indirect labor.
- Determine the various costs for each procedure and the average cost per procedure.
- Evaluate the cost impact of processing stat tests requested on all shifts and determine the feasibility of imposing a charge for stat tests.

The effect of pricing on current revenues can be examined by determining what financial impact, if any, could be expected if current charges for the tests analyzed were adjusted to reflect the actual cost of the procedures or if certain tests were offered in combination with automated equipment profiles at a reduced charge.

In analyzing any facet of the laboratory's operations, the following general standards of the College of American Pathologists and the Joint Commission on Accreditation of Healthcare Organizations should be kept in mind:

- The pathology and clinical laboratories should have sufficient space, equipment, and facilities to be able to perform the required volume of work with optimum accuracy, precision, efficiency, and safety.
- There should be sufficient, conveniently located bench space for the efficient handling of specimens and housing of equipment and reagents.
- Work areas should be arranged to minimize problems in transportation and communication and should be lighted to facilitate accuracy and precision.

Professional Organizations

Laboratory personnel may be members of a professional organization. The American Society of Clinical Pathologists is a professional society for pathologists, laboratory technologists, technicians, and personnel in related fields. The society conducts various certification programs. The College of American Pathologists (CAP) is open for membership only to board-certified pathologists. It was created over 30 years ago by the American Society of Clinical Pathologists. The two organizations meet twice a year.

In addition to publishing professional journals, the College of American Pathologists offers the following services. The Product Evaluation Committee certifies that equipment performs according to the manufacturer's specifications; however, the committee does not recommend laboratory equipment. The Workload Recording Committee has developed a workload recording and reporting system that assigns unit values to various laboratory procedures. Each unit value is equal to one minute of technical, clerical, and aide time required to accomplish one laboratory procedure. In most cases, these values are based on detailed time studies. The College of American Pathologists work-load recording manual is updated annually.

The Hospital Administrative Services of the American Hospital Association and many state regulatory agencies now require that statistics be reported using work-load recording units. The college offers an optional computerized work-load recording system that reports detailed productivity data for the hospital laboratory.

The Clinical Laboratory Management Association provides resources for the strategic development and business management of laboratories. The association holds educational programs, teleconferences, and an annual meeting; it also publishes a journal.

Laundry Department

Overview

Simply stated, the hospital laundry department is responsible for the processing, distribution, and storage of washable linen, garments, and other such items. These activities are similar to those in the laundries of hotels, dormitories, and other institutions; however, the hospital laundry handles specialty items and tasks not needed in other settings.

The basic laundry tasks include washing, ironing, pressing, folding, and mending. Most hospital laundries are also responsible for pickup, delivery, and storage of the linen. The laundry may be responsible for the inspection, mending, and fabrication of specialty items that require special handling because they must be sterilized and kept sterile before they are used.

The standard measure of performance for laundries is the weight of the materials processed, usually expressed in pounds per month or pounds per patient day. For example, a 200- to 250-bed hospital may process 100,000 pounds of laundry per month. Costs per pound vary according to the acuity of patients, the level of automation, the amount of specialty processing required, and whether an in-house or commercial laundry is used. It is important to define the unit of measure carefully (the pounds may be wet or dry, clean or soiled, and so on); it is also important to monitor the volume against a relevant statistic (number of patient days or surgical cases).

Organization

The laundry operation is usually managed by a laundry manager or supervisor, who may report to the hospital's assistant administrator or associate administrator, to the materials manager, or to the executive housekeeper. It is becoming more common for the laundry manager to report to the materials manager or the administrator for support services. Although training programs exist for laundry managers, many managers have come up through the ranks.

Laundry personnel may be assigned to teams that perform the various functions. There may be section supervisors. No formal training is required for laundry personnel, and most learn their responsibilities on the job. In general, these unskilled positions are low on the wage scale.

Many hospitals operate laundries for their own facility, but many others use a commercial laundry or a shared service plan. The most commonly used alternative to operating a laundry in the hospital is securing laundry services through a contract with a commercial company. In general, a commercial laundry picks up and delivers the laundry at the hospital's loading dock. Hospital personnel then organize the linen for use in the hospital and distribute it. Special tasks, such as the inspection of surgical and sterile linen goods, are usually performed at the hospital. The fee for commercial laundry services is usually based on pounds of laundry processed. Shared facilities and joint ventures are also alternatives to a hospital-operated laundry. Laundry facilities may be located at one of the hospitals in the joint venture or at a separate site. In many respects, the shared laundry service is similar to a commercial service. For example, the laundry must be transported to an off-site location. Unlike a commercial service, a shared service can provide consolidated storage, inspection, and mending of linen. Standardization of linen among the various users can yield cost savings.

Models and Systems

The laundry operation can be divided into the following three categories of materials management functions:

- *Processing:* Presorting and postsorting, washing, ironing, pressing, folding, inspection, and mending
- *Distribution:* Collection of soiled laundry from points throughout the hospital; delivery of clean linen to the point of use; pickup and delivery of laundry at a central point for off-site processing
- *Storage:* Maintenance and control of both active and backup inventories

Processing

Processing is the primary function performed by the laundry, and it generally includes sorting, washing, drying, ironing, pressing, folding, inspection, and mending. The actual methods and the sequence of steps used in a particular laundry are determined largely by the type of equipment available. A description of laundry activities follows:

- *Presorting:* Removing the soiled linen from laundry bags, sorting it, and placing each bundle in a conveyance for transportation to the washing area
- *Washing:* Weighing and recording the weight of the soiled linen; loading, operating, and unloading the washing machines; checking loads for quality of washing and pH levels
- *Extracting:* Removing excess water from washed linen by using an extractor or a combination washer/extractor
- *Conditioning:* Placing linen in a machine that separates tangled linen by agitation and that may remove moisture
- *Shaking out and postsorting:* Separating damp linen into categories according to the drying, ironing, pressing, and inspection processes it will receive
- *Tumbling:* Placing extracted linen in a machine that completely dries it by exposure to heated air
- *Laying up flatwork:* Smoothing and arranging the linen for loading into the flatwork ironing machine or onto an automatic spreader, which feeds the flatwork iron
- *Flatwork ironing:* Using automated or semiautomated flatwork ironing machines, manually loaded and unloaded, for sheets, pillowcases, blankets, gowns, aprons, and surgical linen in order to dry, press, and in some cases automatically fold flatwork linen (these machines pass the items between dry, heated metal rollers)
- *Pressing:* Placing items on and operating a press machine and placing finished items on hangers or folding them (commonly used for uniforms, presses are used on one item at a time and employ steam and pressure to finish the item)
- *Tumble-dry folding:* Folding items that are not flatworked or pressed, sorting, and stacking them in categories or using a twofold drying/folding operation by tumble-drying and running the items through a flatwork ironing machine
- *Inspecting:* Passing sterile gowns, sheets, drapes, and so on over a light table so that flaws can be spotted

- *Mending:* Repairing damaged linen with stitching or patches; making specialty pieces (such as surgical drapes) and labels (hospital name and department)

The control of expenses for laundry supplies and processing involves two areas: the linen/laundry itself and the materials needed to clean it. For each area, once purchase decisions are made, vendor relationships tend to remain constant.

Ideally, the procurement of the individual linen/laundry items is coordinated by an efficient purchasing department. All concerned departments should be involved in the process because the ramifications of purchasing decisions can be greater than anticipated. For example, plastic-coated vinyl tablecloths might seem like highly desirable items from the food service department's point of view, but they may not be easy for the laundry to process unless they are handled in special batches, which increases laundry costs. In another example, the purchase of surgical drapes and wrappers should probably involve the medical staff, surgical suite staff, infection control staff, central supply staff, quality assurance staff, and housekeeping staff as well as the laundry department and its inspection and mending staff.

The nature of backup or safety stocks is not consistently defined. Variously, such stocks can represent enough materials to get through the weekend because no processing is done Saturday and Sunday, stock on hand for periodic replenishment of the system, enough stock to cover the hospital's needs in the event of an equipment breakdown (whether in-house or at a contract service's facility), or disaster supplies. The hospital's definition of backup or safety stock determines where it is stored and who controls it.

In terms of controlling the expense of cleaning materials, the most significant operating cost that is usually under the control of the laundry manager is the cost of detergents, softeners, conditioners, and other chemicals used in the department. Utility unit costs cannot be controlled, but utility usage itself can be reduced most significantly at the time of equipment replacement. The current trend is to install equipment that automatically dispenses the correct amount of detergent into the system at the proper time. Vendors of equipment and detergent are usually eager to offer an analysis of these systems. Generally, their claim is to reduce costs not only by eliminating the judgmental factor associated with manual dispensing, but also by reducing pilferage of cleaning supplies. These systems also reduce employees' exposure to caustic chemicals through inhalation.

Distribution

The distribution of clean linen throughout the hospital may be performed by laundry personnel or through consolidated materials management distribution methods. Both systems use requisitions, par-level maintenance (in which shelves are refilled to a predetermined level based on historical usage rates), and/or exchange carts. Systems for the collection of soiled linen vary. Many hospitals use laundry chutes. Bags of soiled laundry are placed in the chute, and the laundry distribution personnel unload the chute from the bottom. One potential problem with this method is that it is difficult to identify specialty linen. For instance, if a bag of surgical linen were halfway up the chute and were needed for washing and immediate use, half the chute would have to be emptied to retrieve the bag. Many hospitals have mixed systems of chutes and hampers. Direct pickup of hampers allows for immediate processing of more urgently needed linen.

The current trend in linen distribution is to process laundry on a daily basis. However, a five-day week plus a half-day on Saturday may still be scheduled in some hospitals. This practice is based on the assumption that reduced patient census and curtailed services (surgery, radiology, and so on) on weekends allow for reduced weekend laundry coverage. Such a schedule requires nurses to make do through Sunday and change linen only when absolutely necessary. In reality, the hoarding of linen in anticipation of weekend shortages can result from this schedule. In addition, the laundry experiences heavy work loads on Monday and possibly Tuesday. Higher inventory levels and storage space are also required.

Storage

The storage function includes the maintenance of adequate stock at the points of use. In addition, storage includes the planning and control of both the active and backup inventories.

A stratified inventory system is often used to plan and maintain the inventory. Such a system assumes that for every piece of linen in use, four others are being processed. Therefore, the active inventory should consist of the number of items used daily multiplied by five. For example, for each hospital bed in use, one pillowcase or patient robe is located at any given time in each of the following places:

- In use on the bed or worn by the patient (soiled)
- In a linen closet or on an exchange cart (clean)
- In a laundry chute or hamper (soiled)
- In the laundry process
- In storage as backup for emergencies and replacing active linen (clean)

An important factor to consider in planning the inventory is the loss of inventory items, which is inevitable in a laundry system. Losses can result from wear and tear, pilferage, and transfers of patients to other facilities. When the active inventory becomes depleted to the point at which daily operations become difficult, the inventory must be replaced. A method that smooths this transition is to calculate a loss factor and replenish the active inventory on a regular basis, that is, weekly or monthly. An additional advantage to such an approach is the need for a smaller backup inventory. When reliable usage rates are known, cost-saving purchasing arrangements, such as drop shipments or standing orders, can be made. The result can be a minimum amount of money committed to the inactive or backup inventory.

Another factor to consider when planning inventory is the schedule for changing linen. Many hospitals change all bed linen every day for every patient. With all but incontinent patients, the traditional procedure is to strip the bed, use the used top sheet as the new bottom sheet, and remake the bed. This procedure should be kept in mind in determining correct linen supplies. Problems in maintaining adequate inventory may occur when this procedure is not followed or when the demand for fresh linen increases during summer months.

The mending operation is important not only because it can reduce the cost of replacement items, but also because it can eliminate the unnecessary reprocessing of clean items such as gowns without a tie string(s), which may be immediately placed in a soiled laundry bag by nursing staff after they are drawn from the supply shelf.

Situations and Problems

In general, the two groups most involved in laundry operations are the laundry, which is the provider, and the nursing units, which are the primary users. Cooperation and understanding between these groups is important. The nursing units need to be assured of having adequate stock, whereas the laundry needs to maintain strong inventory control to keep processing costs low and to prevent the loss of linen. Consequently, a problem may arise when the laundry thinks that the nursing units use too much linen or when the nursing units think that they do not receive enough linen. The result may be that the laundry cuts back on the amount of linen it delivers or that the nursing units hoard linen supplies. With such lack of control, some nursing units may have an overabundance of linen while others do not have enough. In addition, such hoarding reduces the usable active inventory. Accurate information regarding linen usage should be provided to the nurse managers. These data should be tied to volume data to generate a pounds per surgical case or pounds per patient day trend.

The use of disposable linen may also be a controversial topic. Some disposables commonly used are facecloths, patient gowns, and surgical gowns, drapes, and sheets. Problems may arise when physicians and surgeons disagree with the use of disposables. Patients may also have complaints. The cost of disposables is also a factor in determining whether they should be used.

In the near future, the implementation of universal precautions will have a direct impact on laundry operations and costs. Treating all items as potentially contaminated increases the need for gloves, gowns, and eyewear. Segregation practices and their associated costs will also change.

Future increases in the cost of water, sewer service, electricity, and other utilities will have a significant impact on the costs of laundry operations. Vendors are beginning to respond to these situations, and more hospitals are considering early replacement of equipment, the digging of new wells, the reuse of water, and the installation of thermal oil and heat-recovery systems.

Departmental Analysis

An analysis of the operation of the laundry might include the following topics:

- *Department staffing:* Determination of the appropriate staffing level by skill, position, and shift
- *Department utilization:* Evaluation of current use of the department and determination of its capacity
- *Distribution:* Design and implementation of appropriate distribution systems and quotas, possibly in conjunction with the analysis of a total materials management distribution system
- *Storage of inventory:* Determination of an inventory control plan and of appropriate levels of inventory
- *Equipment:* Cost analysis for potential new equipment purchases
- *Alternative laundry services:* Cost analysis of other laundry services, such as a shared service or a commercial service
- *Reporting:* Review of statistical reporting systems and development of a usable management reporting and monitoring system
- *Layout:* Review of layout, especially when revising distribution areas

Recent MONITREND data for the laundry and linen functional reporting center are provided in table 12. The staffing needs of the laundry depend on the systems, volume, equipment, and services provided. High productivity (95 to 100 percent) is to be expected from the laundry as a production department. Therefore, several hospitals have instituted productivity bonuses or incentives in this area.

Table 12. HAS/MONITREND Data for Laundry and Linen: Six-Month Medians for Period Ending December 1988

Indicator	National Bed Size Groups							
	Under 50	50–74	75–99	100–149	150–199	200–299	300–399	400 and Over
Total pounds processed per patient day[a]	20.81	20.59	20.07	19.08	19.54	19.48	19.43	20.84
Contract pounds processed per patient day[b]	17.88	19.08	17.16	17.13	16.68	16.18	15.17	17.33
In-house laundry paid hours per 100 pounds[c]	3.84	3.39	3.04	2.81	2.57	2.27	2.31	1.86

[a]Total pounds processed per patient day = (laundry in-house + contract pounds processed)/total patient days.

[b]Contract pounds processed per patient day = laundry contract pounds processed/total patient days.

[c]In-house laundry paid hours per 100 pounds = laundry in-house paid hours/(laundry in-house pounds processed/100).

Source: HAS/MONITREND, 1988. Please refer to page x for more information about the data presented in this table.

Maintenance Department

Overview

The maintenance department (also commonly called plant services, plant operations, or plant engineering) is responsible for the performance and coordination of facility operations, plant and equipment maintenance, and related services. The department is taking on an increasingly important role in the successful operation of hospitals because of the introduction of new technology and the increase of costs related to plant, equipment, and utilities.

The performance of the department is reflected in the physical condition of the facility, which is a factor in shaping the attitudes of visitors, staff, and patients toward the hospital. The department also plays a key role in the hospital's interaction with external organizations, including fire marshals, building inspectors, insurance underwriters, and regulatory agencies such as the Joint Commission on Accreditation of Healthcare Organizations (JCAHO).

Organization

The organization of the maintenance department varies according to the size of the hospital and the scope of services for which the department is responsible. In most hospitals, the maintenance department reports to an administrator, assistant administrator, or vice-president. In a small- to medium-size community hospital, the department generally includes the following personnel:

- *Department manager or chief engineer:* Usually a skilled craftsman who may have been promoted from within the department; may be a working supervisor
- *Maintenance supervisor or assistant chief engineer:* A working supervisor who is responsible to the chief engineer and assists in planning and directing the department (the position may not be necessary in a small hospital)
- *Skilled craftsman:* Usually a craftsman proficient in one or more trades or skills (and usually licensed by the state in his or her trade) who performs duties in some or all of the following areas:
  - Heating, ventilating, and air-conditioning (HVAC)
  - Plumbing
  - Carpentry
  - Boiler operation
  - Electricity
  - Biomedical electronics

- *Helper (an entry-level position):* An unskilled or semiskilled person who assists the skilled craftsman and performs some tasks independently (for example, changing light bulbs or air filters); may operate an incinerator
- *Painter:* A semiskilled person who works under close supervision and is usually given little or no authority in determining what to paint or which type or color of paint to use

The maintenance department of a medium- or large-size hospital might include some or all of the following personnel:

- *Department director or manager:* Person primarily responsible for the planning and development of physical facilities; advises on structural additions or modifications to the hospital; coordinates energy programs; acts as a staff adviser to the administration; and may also be responsible for laundry, housekeeping, safety, and security; may be a professional engineer with a degree in mechanical, electrical, or civil engineering
- *Engineering supervisor:* Usually a nondegreed skilled craftsman who has been promoted from within the department; is responsible to the director for equipment and craftsmen assigned to various specialty areas; assigns, reviews, and inspects work; ensures that work orders are carried out promptly; is sometimes a working supervisor; and may be one of several engineering supervisors
- *Skilled craftsman:* A mechanic or skilled artisan who is responsible to an engineering supervisor for performing assigned work in specific specialty areas; assists in another trade or craft as required; and has skill in one or more of the following areas:
  - Heating, ventilating, and air-conditioning (HVAC)
  - Plumbing
  - Carpentry
  - Boiler operation
  - Electricity
  - Painting
  - Biomedical electronics
  - Groundskeeping
  - Preventive (or scheduled) maintenance engineering
  - Locksmithing
- *Assistant mechanic (helper):* A person who assists the skilled workers as assigned by the engineering supervisor
- *Utility worker:* An entry-level person who may operate the incinerator and who runs errands
- *Secretary:* A clerical worker who performs secretarial functions, assists in the operation of the work-order system, and assists in the maintenance of required documentation
- *Stockroom clerk:* A clerical worker (usually employed in large hospitals) who maintains the inventory of spare parts, special tools, and manuals; assists in maintaining accurate departmental records; and may be responsible for administering the hospital's preventive maintenance program (these tasks are often assumed by the lead workers, secretaries, or craft supervisors in smaller hospitals)

Depending on the hospital's organization, the maintenance department may be responsible for performing or coordinating the following activities:

- Routine maintenance of plant and equipment
- Preventive maintenance of plant and equipment
- Equipment installation
- Plant energy systems (heating, ventilation, air-conditioning)
- Equipment selection and acquisition
- Maintenance of interior appearance (painting, replacement of wall coverings and flooring, and other activities not including housekeeping)

- Maintenance of hospital grounds
- Plant, technology, and safety management (compliance with JCAHO requirements and other regulations)
- Monitoring of maintenance contracts with outside firms
- Energy conservation systems and energy management
- Computerized building automation systems
- Biomedical engineering
- Resale of maintenance services (revenue generation through provision of services for a fee to external organizations such as private physicians or clinics)
- Waste management
- Renovation and new construction
- Snow removal
- Parking
- Security
- Telecommunications
- Maintenance of hospital blueprints
- Medical gases
- Fire protection systems
- Disaster control and planning
- Utility usage
- Emergency power
- Nursing unit computerized monitoring systems
- Nursing call systems
- Pneumatic tube systems

Maintenance personnel generally do not have direct contact with patients, but they must deal extensively with the employees of all departments in the hospital and must exercise tact in doing so. Conflicts may easily arise between the maintenance department and other departments regarding the urgency of the situation and the timeliness or quality of the work performed. The maintenance department works especially closely with the housekeeping, laundry, food service, and nursing departments. In some hospitals, housekeeping personnel act as the eyes of the maintenance department. While performing their routine duties, housekeeps watch constantly for conditions that require the attention of the maintenance department (for example, burned-out light bulbs, broken windows, and faulty switches). Food service, laundry, and clinical areas rely on the maintenance department for prompt inspection and repair of essential equipment. Typically, the maintenance department is staffed 24 hours a day. Backup support is usually provided by on-call staff.

Operating Systems

The maintenance department receives requests for work to be done from a variety of sources. Generally, standard requests are submitted on a work-order request slip and are mailed to the department through the interoffice mail. In addition, the department usually accepts requests made by telephone.

In many hospitals, a maintenance department staff member is assigned to conduct inspection rounds each day. He or she goes to each department (especially the nursing units) and reviews a communications book that lists things that need to be fixed.

The department manager or a supervisor may also go on monthly safety and repair inspection rounds to identify what needs to be fixed and to identify safety problems. These inspections are sometimes held with individual department managers present. This allows for good communication and creates a service orientation image for the maintenance department.

Emergency maintenance requests are usually communicated by telephone and demand immediate attention. After the crisis has subsided, however, a written work order should be prepared to document the work performed. All essential personnel should be accessible by radio dispatch or beeper.

The department uses a variety of scheduling and category systems to monitor and control all the work requests. Work requests are categorized to facilitate prioritizing the work. Typically, work orders are classified as belonging to one of the following types:

- *Preventive maintenance:* Labor and materials are used to inspect, adjust, calibrate, clean, and repair a piece of equipment on a planned schedule to prevent breakdowns. The department should keep a detailed historical data base on maintenance costs to determine when equipment should be replaced.
- *Emergency maintenance:* Labor and materials are used to make immediate repairs on a vital piece of equipment that has unexpectedly broken down. Fires and floods are considered emergency maintenance situations.
- *Routine maintenance:* Labor and materials are used to make nonurgent repairs on a routine basis. Usually, such repairs include painting walls, replacing tiles, maintaining beds and equipment, and fixing stuck doors. These activities can be deferred until scheduling is possible.
- *Project work:* Labor and materials are used for completion of a one-time-only project or for the installation of a piece of equipment or renovation to an existing room area.
- *Contract maintenance:* Contracted labor and materials from an outside source are used to make equipment repairs.

All types of work except emergency maintenance are usually scheduled. A typical work-scheduling system might operate in the following way. *Preventive maintenance* is usually initiated by a card from the preventive maintenance card file. The card is given to the appropriate craftsman, and the work is performed. The craftsman initials and dates the card, and after all appropriate documentation has been made the card is filed. The supervisor should receive a report of outstanding preventive maintenance jobs and of maintenance scheduled but not completed. Computerized systems are available that generate work orders and assist in determining staffing requirements automatically. Preventive maintenance reports may also note excessive wear, which should trigger more extensive repair before an emergency develops.

Routine maintenance can be initiated through a work-order system. The work order is initiated when a problem is noted on a nursing unit or in another area of the hospital. Requests are submitted to the maintenance department on a work-order form, which includes the following information: the location of the problem, the equipment identification number (if applicable), a description of the problems observed or the work needed, the person requesting maintenance, the date, and the time. The maintenance department records the request in a work-order and project log and classifies it according to its priority level (see table 13). The work order then is forwarded to the appropriate person for action. Upon completion of the task, a description of the work performed and the parts and labor used is transcribed to an equipment history record (if the repair was to a piece of equipment). The work is indicated on the work-order and project log as having been completed. The work order and the equipment history record are then filed appropriately in a preventive maintenance historical file.

Table 13. Priorities for Classifying Maintenance Requests

Priority	Criteria
Emergency repair	Life is endangered. Hospital services would have to be curtailed if work were not performed.
Urgent repair	Emergency situation would probably develop if problem were not addressed.
Normal repair to patient area	Repairs should be completed within 8 working hours.
Normal repair to support area	Repairs should be completed within 2 working days.
Routine repair	Minor tasks should be completed within 7 working days.
Long-term maintenance	Maintenance is requested but not yet scheduled.

Project work includes such tasks as cabinet building, room renovation, carpet installation, and wall covering installation. A well-organized maintenance department asks that requests for such projects be submitted prior to the budget year so that consideration can be given to financial and labor allocations. The maintenance department helps those requesting work to estimate time and material costs and then forwards the request to the administration. At the beginning of the budget year, a project priority list should be established by the maintenance department and the administration. Projects can then be scheduled according to their priority.

Contract maintenance is performed by outside contractors either on a routine basis by a service contract or on an occasional basis. Contract maintenance is routinely used by many hospitals to perform maintenance or repairs outside the usual scope of the maintenance department's activities. Contract maintenance is also commonly used in areas that require special training, certification, or experience (or that require special repair equipment) that is not feasible for the hospital to provide. Some situations require outside contract maintenance because of insurance or governmental regulations or requirements. Examples of areas commonly handled under outside contracts include elevators, fire suppression equipment, telephone systems, emergency power generators, asbestos removal, boiler maintenance, and high-pressure steam systems.

The maintenance department often manages other departments' outside maintenance contracts as well as its own. Many contracts allow for a discount (up to 10 percent) to be applied when the maintenance department routinely reviews the problem before calling in the outside organization. This can prevent outside services from being brought in for small problems such as blown fuses.

Although the maintenance department is not thought of as a revenue-producing department, the resale of services to other hospitals, clinics, and physicians' offices has a relatively long history. In some areas, this practice has been expanded to schools, libraries, and other institutions. Such practices may not only generate revenue from underutilized resources, but they may allow hospitals with an expanded number of specially trained staff to respond better in cases of emergencies, staff turnover, and absences. Not-for-profit institutions, however, should consult legal counsel before offering services to other institutions because revenue from such services is likely to be declared unrelated business income by the Internal Revenue Service.

Maintenance expenses for the hospital are usually allocated into the revenue-producing departments. Various regulatory agencies specify methods of allocation such as costed work orders or square feet. However, internal cost allocation methods that may be used for diagnosis-related group cost analysis may require alternative allocation methods to truly identify these costs. The maintenance department should be held responsible for monitoring all maintenance expenses in the hospital. This will generate a consolidated review of maintenance expenses and help in identifying when equipment should be replaced.

Staffing and Productivity

The work-load requirements of the maintenance department relate to both the amount of fixed activity (boiler tending, preventive maintenance, painting, and so on) and the number of work orders received and filled. However, many hospitals do not maintain a work-order system with enough detail to determine relative work-load requirements. Therefore, departmental standards may be expressed in relation to patient days, calendar days, the square footage of the plant, and the number of beds.

The size of the maintenance department staff depends on many factors, including the following:

- Amount and sophistication of equipment (for example, pneumatic tube system, centralized vacuum system, automatic cart system, and so on)

- Total square footage of the plant to be maintained
- Age of the facility
- Layout of the facility (centralized or decentralized)
- Whether a major construction or renovation project is in progress
- Number of service contracts
- Extent to which outside contractors are used for renovation, construction, or other work
- Number of patient days of care (that is, the utilization rate of the facility)
- Specific areas of responsibility assigned to the department
- Efficiency of the work-scheduling system
- Effectiveness of supervision
- Whether it is a teaching or nonteaching hospital

In maintenance, the variety of equipment used in the hospital and the hospital's physical layout are extremely important factors in staff productivity. Delays and increased utility costs may be caused by the following situations if not anticipated and dealt with effectively:

- Waiting for tools and/or elevators
- Waiting for other tasks to be completed
- Waiting for help and/or instructions
- Following union work rules
- Traveling to get tools, parts, and/or instructions

In each of these situations, a decentralized facility would have a higher delay factor associated with it than would a centralized facility.

There is wide variation in the staff size of various maintenance departments. Generally, there is about one maintenance person (full-time equivalent) for every 12 to 22 beds. Another comparison is 11 to 16 paid hours per 1,000 net square feet. Each institution needs to be reviewed in terms of the services that are provided and the satisfaction of administration and department managers.

Situations and Problems

The maintenance department plays an important role in the hospital by providing services to virtually all departments. This role also places the department in a difficult situation that is not always easy to manage. The following are potential problem areas that a hospital may encounter:

- The maintenance department's primary responsibility is in maintaining the current facility at optimal operational performance. As a result, the preventive maintenance program at the hospital is critical to the long-term goals of the department. A well-run preventive maintenance program should reduce the wear and tear on equipment through periodic maintenance as well as identifying when equipment should be replaced. Many maintenance departments are heavily involved with construction projects. This can be a problem because construction projects tend to be very labor intensive, and preventive maintenance projects are not always followed up on.
- Many institutions have a high staff turnover rate. In addition, it is often difficult to attract qualified skilled craftsmen. This is due primarily to the fact that hospitals usually have a lower pay scale than other employers.
- Often, it is difficult to find a qualified director to manage the department. This is particularly true for small institutions. A contract management firm may be retained to manage the maintenance function.
- The relationship that the maintenance department has with other departments is key to the success of the department. As mentioned earlier, the department must deal

extensively with personnel in other departments. Conflicts may easily arise over the urgency of a problem and the timeliness or quality of the work performed. Because housekeeping personnel can act as the eyes of the maintenance department, it is especially important that the maintenance department have a strong working relationship with the housekeeping department.

- The main concern that user departments usually have concerning the maintenance department is the turnaround time of requests. This time needs to be monitored by the department, and goals should be established that are understood by the departments and the maintenance staff.
- The satisfaction of user department managers is critical to the success of the department. All department managers need to understand what is reasonable to expect from the maintenance department as well as what they need to do to request work.
- Many departments do not have a detailed work-order control system. The work order is the main documentation that the department needs to maintain to evaluate the quantity of work performed by the department. Many good control systems are available and can be implemented either manually or through a computerized system.
- The department needs to keep detailed records on costs of repairs that are performed in the institution. All maintenance work on equipment should be filed in a master preventive maintenance historical file that helps identify when it is justifiable to replace equipment. In addition, detailed records are required to determine the costs associated with construction projects and repairs.
- The maintenance department needs to have management reporting that will communicate to the administration on the following items: volume of work requests by area and type; number of open and completed requests; list of pending major projects.

Departmental Analysis

The maintenance department is taking on an increasingly important role in hospitals because of its ability to affect the productivity of other departments. Through the introduction of new technologies and increases in costs related to plant, equipment, and utilities, it is important that this department run effectively.

As mentioned earlier, the department's performance can be evaluated on the basis of the physical condition of the facility. This is important because the facility's condition is a factor in shaping visitors' and patients' attitudes toward the hospital.

Some major topics of traditional systems analysis for the maintenance department include the following:

- Staffing determination by skill and shift (this study may be aided by reference to recent MONITREND data, such as those provided in table 14)
- Establishment or review of a preventive maintenance program

Table 14. HAS/MONITREND Data for Plant Operations and Maintenance: Six-Month Medians for Period Ending December 1988

Indicator	National Bed Size Groups							
	Under 50	50–74	75–99	100–149	150–199	200–299	300–399	400 and Over
Square feet per bed[a]	1138.15	1205.22	1202.03	1183.75	1311.66	1263.30	1354.01	1269.06
Paid hours per 1,000 square feet[b]	12.61	11.77	13.03	12.94	12.60	13.19	13.15	13.35

[a]Square feet per bed = building gross square feet/total beds.

[b]Paid hours per 1,000 square feet = plant operation paid hours/(building gross square feet/1,000).

Source: HAS/MONITREND, 1988. Please refer to page x for more information about the data presented in this table.

- Establishment or refinement of the work-order and documentation systems
- Establishment of a quality assurance program
- Review of service contracts
- Cost analysis of equipment and facilities
- Review of layout changes and remodeling of hospital areas
- Energy audit

■ Marketing

Overview

The approaches hospitals take to the functions of marketing vary widely depending on how management defines and values the functions and the extent to which funds are available. According to Kotler and Clarke (p. 5), a marketer would define marketing in the following way:

> Marketing is the analysis, planning, implementation, and control of carefully formulated programs designed to bring about voluntary exchanges of values with target markets for the purpose of achieving organizational objectives. It relies heavily on designing the organization's offering in terms of the target markets' needs and desires, and on using effective pricing, communication, and distribution to inform, motivate, and service the markets.

The performance of marketing functions within a hospital, however, does not necessarily indicate that the hospital has adopted a marketing orientation. Kotler and Clarke (pp. 28–32) contrast the marketing orientation against three other orientations that an organization might have (though noting that no hard-and-fast lines among these orientations exist and that the hospital as a whole may be made up of different departments, each with a different orientation):

- *Production orientation:* Holds that the major task of an organization is to pursue efficiency in production and distribution
- *Product orientation:* Holds that the major task of an organization is to deliver products it thinks would be good for the market
- *Sales orientation:* Holds that the main task of the organization is to stimulate the interest of potential consumers in the organization's existing products and services
- *Marketing orientation:* Holds that the main task of the organization is to determine the needs and wants of target markets and to satisfy them through the design, communication, pricing, and delivery of appropriate and competitively viable products and services

Depending on the extent of a hospital's philosophical and financial commitment to a marketing orientation, those responsible for marketing may perform a wide range of functions, including:

NOTE: The author of this profile acknowledges a debt for significant portions of the chapter's substance to *Marketing for Health Care Organizations* by Philip Kotler and Roberta N. Clarke (Englewood Cliffs, NJ: Prentice-Hall, 1987). Page references are provided wherever specific material is quoted, but readers in need of more in-depth information are urged to consult the full original text.

119

- Evaluation of the hospital's existing situation with forecasts for the future as a basis for planning
  - Analysis of past patient data, including range of services with utilization data and classification by payer
  - Analysis of competition, including other area hospitals as well as alternative delivery sites such as physician-owned surgicenters, and estimation of market share
  - Identification of key variables affecting patient volume and consumer choice of provider
  - Analysis of the hospital's strengths, weaknesses, opportunities, and threats (known as a SWOT analysis) (an analysis of internal capabilities and past performance will reveal the hospital's strengths and weaknesses, and an analysis of the external environment will reveal opportunities for new products/services or new markets for existing products/services as well as threats or barriers to success)
- Assessment of marketing opportunities
  - Analysis of percentage of the total population that forms the potential market for a given product/service
  - Segmentation of markets to define those targets of marketing efforts most likely to meet the hospital's objectives
  - Forecasts of potential current and future demand for new products/services
  - Analysis of medical staff composition and existing technology and participation in efforts to acquire needed clinical expertise or requisite technology, including physician recruitment activities
  - Analysis of consumer and payer behavior and preferences with a view to adapting products/services
- Development, implementation, and evaluation of the marketing plan
  - Development of products/programs (may focus on a new product or some reformulation of an existing product)
  - Structuring of distribution/referral system, including evaluation of sponsorship of, or participation in, managed care plans (health maintenance organizations, preferred provider organizations, and their hybrids) or joint ventures (may also involve corporate restructuring)
  - Formulation of pricing strategies
  - Creation of promotional strategies
- Marketing communications
  - Image management
  - News media relations
  - Payer relations
  - Community relations
  - Advertising
- Internal marketing
  - Patient relations (patient representative programs, patient education and health promotion, and service orientation programs for employees) and customer satisfaction research
  - Medical staff relations (forging alliances for the mutual benefit of the hospital and its physicians through consistent communication and through a variety of physician practice enhancement activities)
  - Employee relations
- Product line management and territory management
- Sales and sales management
- Fund-raising (may be the primary function of a development office with participation from marketing as well as public relations)

Kotler and Clarke (p. 28) suggest that hospital marketing could bring a revolution in hospital management over the next 10 years:

1. Hospitals will be much more sensitive and knowledgeable about community health needs.
2. Hospitals will abandon the attempt to be all things to all people and will seek differentiated niches in the market. Each hospital serving a community will focus on providing those services that are most needed and/or that are competitively viable.
3. Hospitals will be quicker to drop services and programs in which they have no competitive advantage or distinctiveness.
4. Hospitals will be more capable of developing and launching successful new services.
5. Hospitals will create more effective systems of distributing and delivering their services.
6. Hospitals will develop more creative pricing approaches.
7. Hospitals will create more patient, doctor, nurse, and employee satisfaction.

As suggested in the situations and problems section of this profile, this view of the promise of marketing is counterbalanced against some opposition to the application of consumer product industry principles to the health care delivery system.

Organization

As indicated in the overview, the placement of marketing within the hospital varies from hospital to hospital. Unpublished studies conducted by SRI Gallup Hospital Market Research for the Society for Healthcare Planning and Marketing (SHPM) of the American Hospital Association in 1985 and 1987 (and reported in an unpublished paper entitled "State of the Art of Marketing: Lessons from a National Survey" by Roberta Clarke and Judy Neiman, presented at the 1988 American Hospital Association Convention) indicate the following structures, ranked in order of prevalence:

1. Marketing, public relations, and planning in a single department
2. Marketing and public relations in a single department; planning in a separate department
3. Marketing and planning in a single department; public relations in a separate department
4. Marketing, public relations, and planning in three separate departments

The 1987 study found that the last option has decreased in popularity since the 1985 study and attributes the phenomenon to the fact that this option requires the greatest commitment in human and financial resources. Especially in small hospitals, the chief executive officer frequently assumes management of all three functions. The SHPM studies indicate that the responsibility for marketing may also lie with an assistant or associate administrator, the chief financial officer or vice-president of finance, the vice-president or director of nursing, the chief operating officer, or the chief of the medical staff. The 1987 study also found that the budget for marketing is higher when combined with planning than it is when combined with public relations and that the combination with planning tended to place marketing at a vice-presidential level whereas the combination with public relations more often placed marketing at a director's level or lower.

In many organizations, budgetary constraints as well as resistance to the creation of a new senior-level position lead some hospitals to place marketing with an existing function. Hospitals that emphasize the communications and promotional aspects of marketing may be led to place the function with public relations. Hospitals that emphasize the analytical and strategy development aspects of marketing may be led to place the function with planning. The choice of placement may have distinct implications for the effectiveness and efficiency of the marketing effort. The background of personnel and the mission of the existing department may skew the marketing effort toward certain aspects of marketing. For example, a public relations practitioner could overweight promotional aspects, and a hospital planner could overweight analytical aspects with inadequate support for promoting and selling the products that emerge from analysis. To offset possible problems, the objectives management sets for marketing must be clearly communicated, and the person charged with management responsibility must be given the training, support, and authority to fulfill those objectives.

The creation of a separate marketing department directed by a qualified hospital marketer is complicated by the relative newness of the subspecialty of hospital marketing. In recruiting for marketing positions, the hospital frequently chooses one of the following options: (1) to promote or retitle someone already in the organization, (2) to hire a marketing professional from another industry, or (3) to hire a marketing professional from another health care organization. With respect to the first of these options, the SHPM study found that 39 percent of the marketing executives surveyed had been promoted from within the hospital, chiefly from public relations or planning positions. When the hospital chooses the second option, recruiting a marketer from another industry, training and adjustment to the characteristics of the health care environment are needed. The hospital also needs to be aware of certain risks. For example, marketers from other industries may quickly become disillusioned with the often lengthy approval process that involves the medical staff and the governing board, and they may find the compensation offered in health care less desirable than that offered elsewhere. The final option, recruiting a marketer away from another health care institution, offers limited possibilities, given the number of such professionals who may be available, but it does offer the advantage of securing a person who has both marketing and health care experience.

Beyond the decision about where to place marketing are decisions about staffing. Kotler and Clarke (pp. 151–52) present a generic chart of a marketing organization and generic marketing position descriptions, reproduced here as figures 9 and 10. However, as indicated in table 15, the commitment in human resources to the marketing, public relations, and planning functions in hospitals does not begin to approach the vision suggested by Kotler and Clarke.

The organizational structure and staffing of the marketing function also depends on available budget. The SHPM studies found that, unlike consumer product industries that may spend from 10 to 25 percent of the budget on marketing, hospitals are spending well under 5 percent, with most spending less than 2 percent.

Staffing constraints may be greatest with respect to market research. Depending on the internal capabilities of hospital staff, the objectives and complexity of the research effort,

Figure 9. Generic Marketing Organization

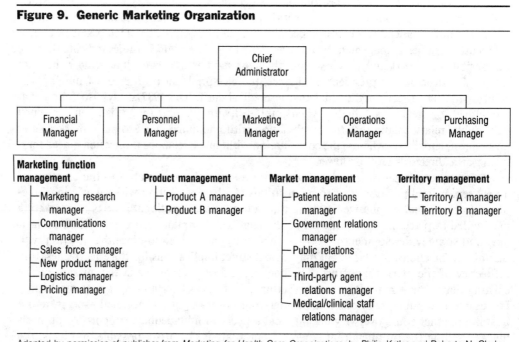

Adapted by permission of publisher from *Marketing for Health Care Organizations,* by Philip Kotler and Roberta N. Clarke, figure 5-3, p. 151 (Englewood Cliffs, NJ: Prentice-Hall, © 1987).

Figure 10. Generic Marketing Positions

Marketing manager

The marketing manager heads the health care organization's marketing activities. Tasks include providing a marketing point of view to the top administration; helping to formulate marketing plans for the organization; staffing, directing, and coordinating marketing activities; and proposing new products and services to meet emerging market needs.

Product manager

A product service manager is responsible for managing a particular product, service, or program of the health care organization. Tasks include proposing product objectives and goals, creating product strategies and plans, seeing that they are implemented, monitoring the results, and taking corrective action.

Marketing research manager

The marketing research manager has responsibility for developing and supervising research on the organization's markets and publics, and on the effectiveness of various marketing tools.

Communications manager

The communications manager provides expertise in the area of mass and selective communication and promotion. This person is knowledgeable about the design of commercial messages, media, and publicity.

Sales force manager

The sales force manager has responsibility for recruiting, training, assigning, directing, motivating, compensating, and evaluating salespeople, representatives and agents of the organization, and coordinating the work of the salespeople with the other marketing functions.

New product manager

The new product manager has responsibility for conceiving new products and services; screening and evaluating new product ideas; developing prototypes and testing them; and advising and helping to carry out introduction in the marketplace.

Logistics manager

The logistics manager has responsibility for planning and managing the distribution systems that make the organization's product and services available and accessible to potential users.

Pricing manager

The pricing manager is responsible for advising and/or setting prices for those services and programs for which the health care organization controls the price.

Patient relations manager

The patient relations manager has responsibility for managing patient services and handling patient complaints.

Government relations manager

The government relations manager provides the organization with intelligence on relevant developments in government and manages the organization's program of representation and presentation to government and regulatory organizations.

Public relations manager

The public relations manager has responsibility for communicating and dealing with various publics in matters involving the organization's image and activities.

Third-party agent relations manager

The third-party agent relations manager provides the organization with information on trends and new policies of third-party agents and manages the organization's program of representation and presentation to third parties.

Medical/clinical staff relations manager

The medical/clinical staff relations manager is responsible for managing medical/clinical staff services and handling medical/clinical staff complaints.

Territory manager

The territory manager has responsibility for managing the organization's products, services, and programs in a specific territory or service area.

Reprinted by permission of the publisher from *Marketing for Health Care Organizations*, by Philip Kotler and Roberta N. Clarke, table 5-1, p. 152 (Englewood Cliffs, NJ: Prentice-Hall, ©1987).

Table 15. Mean Full-Time Equivalents for Marketing, Planning, and Public Relations by Hospital Bed Size and Ownership

Bed Size/Ownership	Marketing	Planning	Public Relations
Total (mean)	1.67	1.50	1.90
Bed Size			
Under 150	0.93	0.97	0.94
150–249	1.74	1.47	1.88
250–349	1.58	1.69	2.11
350–449	3.16	1.45	3.21
450+	2.97	2.83	3.61
Ownership			
Investor owned	1.16	0.94	1.18
Nongovernment, not-for-profit	1.90	1.62	2.11
Government, nonfederal	0.94	1.29	1.23

Source: Society for Healthcare Planning and Marketing of the American Hospital Association, July 1985. Unpublished study conducted by SRI Gallup Hospital Market Research, Lincoln, Nebraska.

and the availability of staff time and budget, market research might be undertaken by a qualified external consultant under the direction and supervision of the person responsible for marketing functions.

Models and Systems

The processes by which marketing functions are carried out flow from the definition of the hospital's mission and goals, which in turn is translated into definitions of specific strategies. When the hospital's mission statement clearly defines the purpose of the organization, the scope of its activities, and its future direction, marketing planning and marketing communications can be structured to support these definitions, as well as to *refine* them in light of market research findings of customer and stakeholder needs and expectations. Hospital goal statements articulated as specific, measurable action statements also provide the necessary superstructure for setting the goals and objectives of marketing activities.

The development of a marketing plan may begin with the statements of a hospital's goals. Market research and an assessment of both the hospital's internal capabilities and the external environment are used to determine where the hospital currently stands and what directions it might take. Out of this stage the marketer seeks to define achievable objectives that address the hospital's larger goals and the strategies that can be used to achieve those objectives. The strategies will also be tested to ensure that the cost of implementation and follow-up are in acceptable proportion to the benefit to be derived.

The marketing plan focuses on what are known as the four *P*s of the marketing mix:

- *Product:* Decisions about the service offerings of the hospital based on its mission and the genuine needs of the markets it currently serves or could potentially serve. Some hospitals have instituted the concept of product line management, clustering clinical services (such as the range of diagnostic, clinical, and therapeutic services for cancer care) under a person responsible for planning; service, program, and/or product development; and marketing of the clustered services.
- *Price:* Decisions about rates for services growing out of an examination of such factors as the hospital's costs, payer mix, and revenue/patient margin objectives. Decisions may be influenced by the need to increase utilization, to provide disincentives to channel patients away from certain options and toward others, and to address competitive position issues. Strategic pricing decisions might be decentralized for some areas of the hospital, but especially with the need to negotiate discount schedules for managed care plans (health maintenance organizations, preferred provider organiza-

tions, and direct contracts with major employers) and the need to balance the hospital's overall performance, there is a need for centralization and a cooperative relationship between the marketing and the financial management functions.

- *Place:* Decisions that affect consumer access to the hospital's services. Questions about access include how patients enter the system (referral processes) and where they go for services (the main hospital, satellite centers, and so on). Access may also involve decisions about a range of convenience factors such as when patients want services (hours of operation, average waiting time) and the atmosphere in which they would prefer services (facility design, accessibility to parking, accommodations for the handicapped). Access questions and the marketing strategies that address them dictate the involvement of all affected departments in the decision-making process. In some areas, questions of access may lead to a need for collaborative planning efforts with other health care institutions in the service area and the formation of some form of shared service arrangement or referral network.
- *Promotion:* Decisions about the nature of public and community relations, advertising, telemarketing, sales strategies, and patient education that will bring providers and consumers together.

In structuring the marketing plan, those responsible for marketing must safeguard themselves against an organization that expects marketing to stimulate demand for existing products/services without first having ascertained that demand exists and that goals of increased utilization are attainable. As the marketing plan is developed, appropriate consensus-building activities also become important to the success of the ultimate plan.

Situations and Problems

Marketing is a relatively new phenomenon in health care, having been introduced in the late 1970s, and it has been the object of considerable criticism. Any management engineering study of operational effectiveness and efficiency must therefore include an assessment of the extent to which barriers or management, medical staff, or public resistance exist.

In *Marketing in Small and Rural Hospitals* (Chicago: American Hospital Publishing, 1989), Carolyn C. Roberts and Eugene C. Beck quote an article by W. J. Winston (Why do the majority of marketing programs in hospitals fail? *Health Marketing Quarterly* 2(1):xvii–xxi, Fall 1984) that suggests six major factors that contribute to failures of marketing programs:

1. Most marketing programs are not based on a formal marketing plan.
2. Most marketing programs do not target their efforts to specific audiences but instead use a shotgun approach.
3. Marketing programs often do not have the support of the hospital's board, administration, and medical staff.
4. The majority of marketing programs are directed by people who lack broad marketing knowledge and experience related to the marketing of hospital services.
5. Administrators have unrealistic expectations of what marketing can do for their hospitals. Marketing should be a part of a long-term strategy, not a short-term solution to operational problems.
6. Internal marketing is often overlooked. Internal marketing means the development of an organizational marketing philosophy and staff support for marketing. According to Winston, "Employees must understand that the patient is a client where an exchange is occurring and the client cannot be taken for granted."

An unpublished paper by Roberta Clarke and Judy Neiman entitled "State of the Art of Marketing: Lessons from a National Survey," referred to earlier, suggested that the problems hospitals may have in setting expectations for marketing and marketers may come up in any combination of the following:

1. The marketer is hired to "market the hospital," although what that term entails is never specified. Objectives are not spelled out. It is therefore difficult to judge the marketer's performance because there are no objective benchmarks against which to judge performance.

2. Objectives are set, but they are totally unreasonable. For example, one hospital, operating at a 50 percent census in maternity, gave its new marketer two years to bring the maternity census up to 90 percent. However, the marketer was given no significant resources and no authority to change the outdated physical facility, nursing staff, or practice of the obstetricians. Another hospital's marketer was told he was expected to increase the whole hospital's census 15 percent within one year.

3. Objectives are set on too many fronts: improve the image of the cardiology service, attract a better financial mix of patients to the emergency services, increase the number of babies born at the hospital, increase the number of businesses using the hospital's employee assistance program, keep enough beds filled in pediatrics so that the hospital can justify keeping a pediatric service open, develop a package of services to attract the elderly, and so on. And all of these objectives are set within one to two years. This is not a matter of unreasonable objectives as much as it is an unreasonable number of objectives. It is irrational to expect all or most of the hospital's problems and opportunities to be addressed effectively within a short time period.

4. The objectives are reasonable, but the marketing efforts are underfunded or under-supported. No matter how small the objective, some resources will be necessary to achieve it. In addition, some change in the practice of hospital personnel or physicians may be required, as might facility, structure, or system changes. The marketing plan for each objective should spell out what funds, resources, and support are needed to achieve each objective. If these cannot be provided, the objective should be dropped until they can be provided.

5. A small number of reasonable objectives are set and are well budgeted and supported, but no one measured the effort before and after the implementation to determine its effectiveness. The measurement and evaluation of marketing effectiveness are not without cost, and yet almost nothing in the SHPM data suggested that hospitals were budgeting for the cost of evaluating marketing efforts. How then are hospitals to know whether their marketing efforts are working?

Kotler and Clarke (pp. 21–27) describe six major criticisms leveled against marketing. Such criticism may exist within the hospital or its medical staff as well as in the external environment, and such criticism limits both the effectiveness of the marketing function and the breadth and nature of the activities subsumed under marketing. The criticisms also inject a note of caution to hospitals as they seek to find applications of marketing in the unique environment of health care delivery. For example:

- Marketing wastes money.
- Marketing is intrusive.
- Marketing is manipulative.
- Marketing lowers the quality of health care.
- Marketing causes health care institutions to compete.
- Marketing creates unnecessary demand for health care.

Additional criticism of, or resistance to, a hospital's marketing strategies can come from the medical staff. Inasmuch as the medical staff has its own management structure, conflict can be avoided only when the hospital-based marketing department routinely invites medical staff participation, especially in new product development decisions. With the growth of hospital outpatient services, marketing plans can be viewed as hospital competition for services offered within the physicians' private practices. Some hospitals have sought to avoid such conflicts by hiring marketing managers who have a clinical background and who will therefore meet with easier medical staff acceptance or by placing the marketing function within the medical staff management structure.

Beyond not getting clear communication of realistic objectives, marketers may meet with less than success when they are not working with an adequate budget and an adequate information system. As indicated earlier, budget allocations may be extraordinarily modest and yet may be paired with extraordinarily high expectations for results. The hospital information system, too, may not be sophisticated enough to trap the necessary data and perform the analysis of the factors that underlie marketing research.

Departmental Analysis

Management engineering studies of marketing are seldom undertaken. Because of the administrative nature of marketing, no nationally recognized productivity standards or measures have been developed or accepted. The size and personnel composition of the function is a largely discretionary issue from institution to institution. The scope of activities and responsibilities also varies significantly among facilities, which also effectively prevents the development of a standard activity profile on which productivity measurement can be based.

In some cases, clerical or administrative work load may be measured to determine the utilization of clerical time. Such studies might be performed by audit (yielding generalizations) or by work sampling (yielding more exact data). However, the management of the qualitative aspects of marketing is difficult to quantify and is generally dealt with by a subjective evaluation of performance and staffing needs.

In the absence of any nationally recognized standards or any consistency in the organizational structure and range of activities, one is left with performing an audit against self-determined and institution-specific objectives. The marketing audit may seek to ascertain whether, how, and by whom information is gathered and decisions are made about competitive position, product/service mix, pricing, distribution, and other aspects of marketing detailed in this profile.

Materials Management Department

Overview

In the contemporary sense, materials management encompasses the movement of all goods, supplies, equipment, and people for an organization. The function may be called materials handling, purchasing, or support services. The scope of materials management can be wide and can be defined in many ways. A model that organizes materials management activities can be described according to the following types of activities:

- *Acquisition:* Purchasing, vendor negotiation, lease and rental arrangements, shipping and receiving, and equipment acquisition; materials evaluation
- *Warehousing:* Storage of goods, supplies, and equipment; inventory control
- *Distribution and transportation:* Materials handling, delivery and pickup of goods and supplies, equipment waste management, messenger and mail service, and patient escort and transportation system
- *Processing:* Activities that directly relate to support services for patient care units, such as sterilization, sorting and wrapping of instruments, laundry, and housekeeping

Traditionally, such areas as the laboratory and the nursing units performed their own materials management because of the uniqueness of their needs. For example, the radiology department might transport its patients to and from the nursing units, as well as negotiate the price of film with a vendor. However, as the need for, and the complexity of, supply systems and hospital systems have grown, special departments have evolved. For instance, a purchasing department may be created, the central service department may perform sterilization for surgery and for the radiology and emergency departments, and general storerooms may hold commonly used supplies.

With the development of materials management as a recognized concept, the problems that many hospitals experienced with excessive decentralization in materials-related activities have begun to be addressed. These problems include duplicated inventories, lack of standardization among areas, undue vendor influence, and loss of quantity or contract purchasing power. With increased computerized automation to assist the materials manager in meeting the hospital's materials needs, the acceptance of materials management as a necessary capability has drastically increased.

Organization

Materials management may follow any of several organizational models. Whether or not there is actually a materials management department, there are generally both formal and informal links among many departments. Together, these links make up the materials management function. The departments typically involved are purchasing, general storage, shipping and receiving, central service, delivery and transport, laundry, housekeeping, mail and messenger service, and patient escort. The maintenance and food service departments may also be involved. In some organizational structures, all of these departments may be coordinated by one manager or administrator. In other organizational structures, the departments may report to different managers. The significant advantage of the combined approach is that one manager can coordinate or consolidate programs and resources, thereby preventing costly duplication of efforts. For instance, central service personnel may report to a nursing manager, but the storeroom may be the responsibility of another manager. Yet, both typically perform similar supply and delivery functions; therefore, the consolidation of functions could produce savings. The duplication of many activities under a decentralized system also reduces the effective coordination of similar activities throughout the hospital. Reduced coordination generally results in high inventory levels and a noticeable lack of standardization in items commonly used in more than one department.

The personnel involved in materials management have various degrees of education and training and various credentials and certifications. Frequently, the staff members have acquired their skills by beginning at the entry level in the department and advancing as they gained experience. Although materials management is gaining acceptance through the efforts of professional societies, it has not reached the level of common certification or professional standards development on a broad basis.

Typical positions within a materials management department are as follows:

- *Receiver:* Reviews the paperwork for an order, verifies that the items received match the order (quantity, items, and so on), and checks that there is no damage to the order
- *Storeroom clerk:* Issues storeroom items and completes the appropriate paperwork to track issues; may deliver stock to a specific department
- *Purchasing agent/buyer:* Coordinates with hospital staff the specifics of the items needed (that is, quantity, type, size, model, delivery date, and so on) and negotiates with vendors for hospital purchases
- *Central service technician:* Cleans and sterilizes equipment and supplies used in the hospital
- *Transporter:* Transports equipment, patients, and supplies to appropriate locations
- *Supervisor/manager:* Directs and coordinates specific functions within the materials management department (supervisory positions are typically found in such areas as central service, storeroom, transport, and purchasing)
- *Director:* Coordinates the overall activities of the department; may function as the line manager of a subarea

Figure 11 illustrates an organizational chart for the materials management department.

The department's hours of operation depend on the size of the facility, the organization and physical layout of the department, the services provided, and the work loads of other departments. Typical operational hours are:

- Storeroom: 8:00 a.m. to 4:30 p.m., Monday through Friday
- Central service: 8:00 a.m. to 4:30 p.m., Monday through Friday
- Purchasing: 8:00 a.m. to 4:30 p.m., Monday through Friday
- Transport: 7:00 a.m. to 7:00 p.m., seven days a week

Many hospitals manage materials programs on an in-house basis, using hospital-employed managers or administrators. Others use contract management programs. There is no generally accepted approach that would meet the needs of all hospitals. The most common factor is the overall administration concept used, as well as the availability and accessibility of trained and experienced personnel in the various materials functions.

Figure 11. Organization of a Materials Management Department

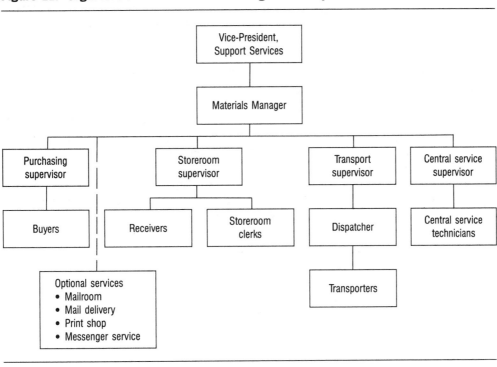

Models and Systems

The following conceptual models are typically employed when studying materials management systems:

- *Centralized:* A centralized materials management network focuses on each activity, assigning a department or team to provide a specific function for the entire hospital. For example, the admitting department or the nursing service may be able to request service from a centralized patient escort and transportation pool instead of sending their own staff to escort patients.
- *Decentralized:* A decentralized materials management model is one in which each area or department performs the various materials management functions itself. Decentralization is generally found in areas where common activities or unity of action with other departments is not common. In other cases, the tasks or actions involved would not be frequently performed, thus making the task of cross-utilizing personnel among departments difficult. When the facility covers a large area, movement among departments for common activities may reduce the efficiency of centralization to such an extent that the decentralized approach is more cost-effective.

Materials management systems rarely follow a purely centralized or decentralized model. Rather, using a combination of both systems is common because the materials management function needs to change and evolve in response to the physical layout and facilities of the hospital, the organization of the staff, and the needs of the hospital.

The general trend in recent years in hospitals has been toward centralization of the materials management function. One reason for this movement has been the effect of increased materials-related expenditures on the total hospital budget. The cost of many kinds of supplies and materials radically increased, and with the increased technology available within medicine, many new medical supplies and products are now available. In general terms, hospitals are spending proportionally more on materials and supplies than they did in earlier decades. The potential for better utilization of resources has supported the acceptance of this concept in many hospitals.

The centralization of the entire materials management program can yield cost savings as well as facilitating more efficient and effective service provision. Centralization can enable hospitals to consolidate and control services as follows:

- *Purchasing:* Centralized purchasing can eliminate uncontrolled purchases from such areas as the laboratory, respiratory therapy, nursing units, and the food service department. A reduction in prices can be realized through improved purchase analysis and group hospital arrangements.
- *Distribution (including supplies distribution, messenger services, and escort services):* Deliveries and other trips can be combined to reduce duplication of effort and save staff time. Distribution systems can be streamlined.
- *Warehousing:* Centralized warehousing can result in reduced inventory costs, more organized purchasing, and improved allocation of space.
- *Processing:* Possible improvements in processing include better use of staff, increased control over such things as sterilization and batch numbering and enhanced quality control.
- *Charging:* A charge system analysis for supplies might show that the cost to process chargeable items may be more than the revenue gained. Quantitative profiles and cost analyses can be used to develop break-even points for determining what is a chargeable supply and how much the charge should be.
- *Cost accounting:* As hospitals monitor the expenditure of resources used for patient care, the impact of materials and supplies becomes a major focus. Under many reimbursement models, the amount the hospital receives for the care it delivers is controlled, and the hospital must concentrate on the monitoring of resources committed to the care process. Automation within many hospital materials management systems and patient accounting systems is enabling hospitals to identify the consumption of supply resources on a patient-by-patient basis. This trend has developed apart from the need to capture charges for supplies. It is a related issue, but cost accounting and management of care have become common themes in many hospitals. Through that effort, the most effective resource usage is achieved for all patients.

The physical facility affects the materials system to be used. Older hospitals without suitable storage space are particularly limited in their ability to adopt centralized materials management systems. Many mechanical features within hospitals such as corridor widths, elevator access, patient transport routes, and other systems (for example, pneumatic tube systems), all have an impact on the options the hospital has open to it. The most common problems are lack of suitable space for location of sufficient inventories or exchange carts near centralized use areas (for example, patient care units, emergency rooms, convenient care centers, and surgical suites). In many cases, cabinets, closets, or small storage spaces are used because of the lack of suitable sites. This can result in problems with supplies being scattered throughout a large area, as well as the duplication of supplies at multiple locations throughout one department.

Of equal concern is the common problem of lack of central space for management of a materials program. When space in the central warehouse is limited, supplies are often distributed immediately to the ordering department once they are received from suppliers. This fosters a feeling of independence and places the burden of inventory-level monitoring on the individual departments. Once the individual departments become the custodians of their own supplies, the hospital loses many of the benefits of quantity purchasing, group contracts, product standardization, and other related systems.

Situations and Problems

For some time, the materials management functions in many hospitals have been delegated to individual departments. Therefore, efforts to change over to a centralized organization of services may be met with resistance. Unless the hospital is willing to effectively address the major issues and components associated with conversions to a centralized concept, the departments may not cooperate and may even begin to hoard supplies.

The most common challenge in implementing the centralization process is getting individual departments to believe that their needs will be met in a timely manner through a centralized system. Because so many departments have controlled the entire supply process for a long period of time, they each feel that they have developed considerable expertise in dealing with ordering and inventory balancing. Such expertise is an asset that the hospital should safeguard as much as possible. To do so, the technical knowledge and experience involving the specific needs of each department should be transferred to the materials management department over a reasonable period of time. This will ensure that cooperation is developed on the basis of successful performance and trust rather than on an arbitrary schedule of forced transition.

The centralization of many common supplies may uncover information revealing supply misuse or pilferage. A typical pilferage pattern found in the supply system is the autumn back-to-school run on office supplies. Efforts to control office supplies (such as requiring the return of an empty pen in order to get a refill) may cause resentment among employees. Under all circumstances, the level of control and accountability must be consistent with the cost of that control as well as the benefits to be gained. In many hospitals, the majority of effort is expended on controlling items of low cost (for example, paper and pencils), while at the same time no control or accountability exists on the use of items costing many hundreds of dollars (for example, procedure trays). For materials management to be an effective operating concept, materials managers must be sensitive to such issues as well as to the human relations issues involved with increased supply control. Incentives for reducing the cost of materials and supplies may be developed through cost-containment plans and suggestion boxes.

Departmental Analysis

The scope of analysis projects that can be conducted in materials management is wide, from a general overview to a detailed analysis of a specific materials management area (such as purchasing).

An analysis begins with an overview and evaluation of all materials management functions throughout the hospital. Existing systems, their overall effectiveness, the relationship among departments regarding materials functions, and the adequacy of the facilities should be evaluated. The results of an overview of the existing system may be the identification of the strengths and weaknesses of the system, the development of alternatives for organizing and improving the materials management function, and suggestions for further studies.

Specific studies are detailed analyses of the performance, statistics, staffing, systems, and facilities of a particular area. Some examples of detailed analysis techniques include profiling the waiting and service time of the messenger and escort services and conducting a cost analysis of the stock control system to make such decisions as whether to make or buy sterile solutions. Such specific studies of various departments or functions can be an integral part of a materials management program. Typical topics of study are purchasing, patient escort and transportation systems, messenger service, and central service. For a hospital initiating a materials management program, specific studies can be beneficial in improving specific functions, as well as in gaining insight into the entire network. Specific studies can also be part of an overall plan through the evolution of a total materials management program. Areas of specific study include:

- *A-B-C analysis of inventory:* Identifying and managing aggressively the high-cost, high-usage items (*A* items are high-dollar, high-usage items; *B* items are moderate-dollar, moderate-usage items; *C* items are low-dollar, low-usage items)
- *Analysis of inventory versus special order practices:* Identifying the appropriateness of adding items to the inventory (or deleting items from the inventory)
- *Time-of-day service analyses:* Identifying the hourly service demands on the department
- *Individual supply item redundancy:* Identifying similar or duplicate items maintained in the inventory
- *Economic order quantities (EOQ) computation:* Determining whether it is more economical to order items as needed rather than carrying them in the inventory
- *Vendor price analysis of common or interchangeable items:* Comparing prices on the same item from different vendors, similar items from the same or different vendors, and/or different brands
- *Staff productivity and utilization:* Analyzing productivity and scheduling by activity within the department
- *Customer satisfaction/responsiveness surveys for services provided:* Conducting surveys of the materials management department's customers and the individual departments to assess their perceptions of the quality of supply services

Medical Record Department

Overview

The medical record department, sometimes called the health information department, maintains records and documents related to patient care. In addition to filing, indexing, and retrieving records (described later in this section), the department performs, coordinates, or assists with the following tasks:

- *Record processing:* Record processing includes the following activities:
  - *Admission:* Upon admission, the medical records of previously admitted patients are retrieved, or a medical record number is assigned as the first step in establishing a record for each new patient. A log or out guide is used to document the location of the record (usually the name of patient care unit) when it is removed from the department.
  - *Discharge:* The completeness of the record is checked, the record is routed to holding areas for dictation or physicians' signatures, and so on. The existence of a record for every patient on the discharge list is confirmed.
  - *Transcription:* Reports dictated by physicians—such as discharge summaries, histories, physical findings, operative reports, and so on—are typed and physicians' signatures are obtained.
  - *Coding:* All diagnoses and operations are coded according to *ICD-9-CM (International Classification of Diseases, Ninth Revision, Clinical Modification)* coding principles for statistical purposes.
  - *Abstracting:* For statistical purposes, an abstract form is completed from data available in the record. The statistics are used for profiling hospital utilization and may be compiled by using manual or computerized in-house systems. Statistical services that provide computerized data reduction and information reporting systems may also be used.
  - *Correspondence:* Copies of some or all of a medical record may be made available as documentation for birth certificates, court cases, insurance claims, personal requests, patient transfers to other health care facilities, and physician review.
  - *Record storage:* State regulations vary regarding the minimum length of time medical records must be maintained. For example, Massachusetts state regulations mandate a 30-year retention period for medical records, but Vermont requires only 10 years.
- *Reimbursement:* The effect of diagnosis-related groups (DRGs) and the prospective payment system (PPS) on medical record functions has been significant. Most reimbursement systems, whether based on DRGs or not, require coded information from

the medical record department on diagnosis, surgical procedures, length of stay, and other factors as a basis for calculating payment. This has led to an increasing demand for coders, especially those with some background in medical procedures. It also places greater emphasis on coding and reinforces the need for timely completion of records. Some activities required by the new reimbursement policies are the following:

— Instituting accurate and consistent coding policies, procedures, and practices
— Monitoring and following up on problem DRGs (cases that are hard to group or whose diagnoses do not match the surgical procedure, and so forth)
— Monitoring length of stay (LOS) and outliers (cases in which the LOS is outside the normal range for that DRG)
— Analyzing patterns for physicians and services by DRG
— Serving as a member of a DRG committee
— Educating physicians regarding DRGs and reimbursement, coding, and the effect of their timely (or otherwise) completion of medical record documentation
— Coding of ambulatory care visits for reimbursement (under some systems, coding may be done by the medical record department)

• *Quality assurance:* The department provides the data or medical records needed for a quality review of the care delivered. Sometimes quality assurance and medical records personnel report to the same manager.

• *Utilization management:* In order to control health care costs, utilization management (UM) ensures that the appropriateness of all admissions is reviewed as well as the appropriateness of the length of stay, discharge planning practices, and tests and procedures ordered for the patient. Review activities take place before admission (prospective review), at the point of admission and during the course of the hospital stay (concurrent review), and after discharge (retrospective review). Among the objectives of these activities are these:

— To identify areas in which hospital resources are being underutilized, overutilized, or perhaps utilized inefficiently
— To help providers identify and eliminate services that are medically unnecessary
— To improve the relationship between the hospital and third-party payers by reducing the amount of billed services
— To ensure that appropriate data are available for responding to questions from clients, regulators, and others
— To improve the hospital's ability to compete in the marketplace

Medical records personnel may coordinate fact gathering and data management for these review activities. Often, quality assurance and utilization management are under one manager. Either or both functions may report to the director of medical records.

• *Tumor registry:* Some hospital medical record departments maintain tumor registries, either manually or on computers. In some hospitals, this function may be a separate department, or it may report to oncology.

Figure 12 is a flowchart showing the record-processing and reimbursement tasks performed by the medical record department in a typical medium-size hospital. This basic archival function is performed for inpatients, outpatients, and emergency patients. Traditionally, the three types of patient records have been handled separately; however, the merging of all of a patient's records into one unit record is recommended. It should be noted that outpatient records are generally maintained only for outpatient clinic or ambulatory care patients and are not kept for private referral patient services, for example, outpatient radiology or laboratory services.

The medical record department's typical hours of operation are from 7 a.m. to 10 p.m., seven days per week. The department generally has procedures for access to records between 10 p.m. and 7 a.m.

Figure 12. Flowchart of Work Performed by the Medical Record Department in a Medium-Size Hospital

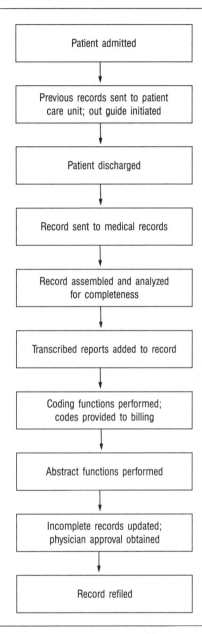

Organization

The department generally consists of a medical record administrator or manager and supervisors (depending on the size of the department) for the major functional areas of transcription, coding and abstracting, filing and indexing, discharge analysis, medical audit, and utilization review.

Two credentials are recognized in medical records. An accredited record technician (ART) has completed either a two-year college program or a comparable independent study course. Accredited record technician training programs emphasize technical training for medical records functions, with limited emphasis on management skills, although a qualified ART could move into management or supervision. A registered record administrator (RRA) has completed a four-year baccalaureate program that puts less emphasis on technical training and more emphasis on management.

Both credentials require medical record experience and an examination administered by the American Medical Record Association (AMRA), which serves as a strong national professional organization for ARTs and RRAs. The association is also responsible for setting standards for and approving ART and RRA programs, as well as credentialing. Both ARTs and RRAs must meet continuing education requirements every two years in order to keep their credentials.

According to the Joint Commission on Accreditation of Healthcare Organizations (JCAHO) standards for hospital accreditation, the manager responsible for medical record administration is required to hold at least an ART credential. Certain small hospitals may forgo this requirement if they employ an ART or RRA consultant to supervise the department. Large hospitals should have RRA managers. Medical record personnel other than managers do not necessarily need to be either an RRA or an ART. Rural areas may face a shortage of RRAs.

The majority of personnel employed by the department are clerical staff trained on the job. The clerical staff may perform the retrieval, filing, assembly and analysis, and correspondence functions.

The medical record department is responsible to the hospital's administration. The medical staff must also have a medical record committee, which provides a forum for professional input from physicians, and the medical staff is responsible for reviewing the records of peers and ensuring that the hospital's medical records meet JCAHO and other professional standards. The department often is responsible for the medical library, which is maintained primarily for physicians. This is especially true in small hospitals.

The department, usually represented by the director, must deal extensively with the medical staff regarding such problems as tardy record keeping. Because the department provides medical record information for parties engaged in liability cases, good communication is necessary among the director, the physicians, and their lawyers.

Models and Systems

Various models and systems can be used for the following functions: assembling, numbering, filing, indexing, and dictating and transcribing.

Assembling Systems

The medical record department may use a unit record model or a traditional record model, although most departments are converting to unit records on the basis of the JCAHO's recommendation. The unit record model consolidates and retains a patient's record for all services in a single unit. Thus, emergency department, inpatient, and outpatient records make up the patient's unit record. Generally, unit records are indexed according to a numbering system, with a permanent number assigned to each unit record. With a traditional record model, each record of a patient visit is independent. The primary advantage of the unit record is that it consolidates all the patient's records so that the patient's complete history can be quickly and easily reviewed.

The two most common methods of assembling the medical record are to assemble it chronologically by source of information or section (physician's notes, nurse's notes, laboratory record) and to assemble it chronologically without regard to source. A third method of organizing the medical record, which is relatively new and not widely used, is to assemble it chronologically by topic or problem. Each problem section includes records from all sources (physicians, nurses, and others). The preparation of problem-oriented records is currently being taught in medical schools and may become more common in the future.

Numbering Systems

Various systems for numbering medical records are used, including unit and serial numbering, depending on the needs of the hospital and the location of the admissions/registration, medical record, and outpatient departments.

The unit numbering system is generally recommended and is usually used in conjunction with the unit record system, in which one medical record is maintained for each patient. Assigning a single, permanent number for each patient helps to ensure accurate identification. The permanent number can also be used to identify X-ray films, accounting records, and other materials that are not part of the medical record. The system is especially good for hospitals in communities with a stable population because patients are likely to return to the hospital for ongoing medical care.

When serial numbering is used, a new number is assigned each time a patient is admitted. The previous record should be retrieved and merged with the new record under the new number. An empty folder, or dummy, replaces the old record file and includes a reference to the new number. Alternatively, the old record may be left in its original file location, but this system is not recommended. Under this system, the old and new files must be cross-referenced so that the complete history of the patient can be traced. The serial numbering system allows a number to be assigned immediately without reference to the index.

Filing Systems

The type of filing system to be used could be chosen without considering which numbering system is in use, but each works better with a suitable numbering system. Under the terminal digit filing system, sequential numbers are filed within categories ending with the same digit or digits. For example, all numbers ending in 9 or 29 are placed in one section. The system can be coupled with a color-coded label so that misfiled records can be easily spotted. This system works well with the unit numbering system, equalizes the amount of space required for subdivisions, and allows for uniform expansion of the files. When serial numbering is used, straight numerical filing may be the most workable, although there may be problems when the file becomes very large.

The advantages and disadvantages of a unit record system coupled with a unit numbering system are as follows:

- Advantages
  - All data are combined in one record.
  - The record usually has a permanent number for indexing.
  - The fewest possible file folders are used.
- Disadvantages
  - Records must be merged.
  - Additional record retrieval is required.
  - Round-the-clock staffing is needed to assign numbers.
  - Control and security problems may occur.

The advantages and disadvantages of a traditional record system coupled with a serial numbering system are as follows:

- Advantages
  - Inactive records are continually purged.
  - There is less retrieval of old records.
  - The medical record number usually corresponds to the business office's file number.
- Disadvantages
  - Additional retrieval for complete patient records may be required.
  - Empty file folders are left in the file.
  - Dummy folders require time to fill out.

Indexing Systems

The medical record department maintains a master patient index. For each retained record, an index card lists the dates of admission and the file numbers. Two indexing systems are used: alphabetic, which files by the last name, first name, and middle initial; and phonetic, which files by phonetics and is generally useful for ethnic names that sound alike but may be spelled differently. Alphabetic indexing is more common. Automation for indexing is available.

The types of technology used for indexing are as follows:

- *Manual:* File drawers hold 3-by-5-inch cards. This type of system is very time-consuming to maintain.
- *Motorized:* Power-assisted file cabinets save space and are commonly used.
- *Batch computer output:* Alphabetic index listings on computer printouts or computer output microform save space, but they are somewhat costly. This system requires regular updating, and new data must be kept on a manual system until the data are batch processed. The service is offered as part of some shared service financial computer systems.
- *On-line computer indexing:* Computer files with on-line entry, retrieval, and locator (sign-out) capability are expensive, but they require the least number of staff to maintain and allow such remote areas as emergency or admitting to search and retrieve medical record numbers. They also allow universal numbering for both medical records and radiology.

Dictating and Transcribing Systems

Various types of dictating and transcribing systems are available. Equipment should be selected carefully to accommodate the specific needs of the hospital, and it should facilitate dictation in locations distant from the medical record department. Transcription can then be performed in a central location. The department may provide transcription services for all physicians and support staff who make entries in the medical record. Some hospitals have a charge-back system whereby a specific department, such as pathology or radiology, is charged for these services.

Departmental Analysis

An analysis of the department can serve to identify problem areas and to develop solutions to those problems. Topics that may require study include the following:

- *Staffing:* Analyze all positions, functions, task assignments, and work-load balance; use established time standards; determine task frequency and real time; determine project staffing requirements for new programs or system changes. (See table 16 for recent MONITREND data for the medical records functional reporting center.) The impact of DRGs and other recent reimbursement systems based on coding has increased the need for staffing analyses in many institutions.
- *Record-processing systems:* Make a flowchart of basic procedures, determine bottlenecks, and review detailed procedures for highly repetitive tasks such as indexing and logging. Analyzing flows and delays has become increasingly important because of the significance of accurate and timely coding to reimbursement.
- *Timeliness of record processing:* Sample the flow of records through the system, and determine its timeliness and responsiveness in meeting requirements (for example, determine how discharge diagnoses are communicated to accounting for billing purposes).
- *Filing space:* Measure the available filing space, determine the requirements for future growth, plan for possible change in the system, and conduct a cost analysis.

Table 16. HAS/MONITREND Data for Medical Records: Six-Month Medians for Period Ending December 1988

Indicator	National Bed Size Groups							
	Under 50	50–74	75–99	100–149	150–199	200–299	300–399	400 and Over
Discharge units per calendar day[a]	7.41	13.92	18.13	28.20	38.06	54.16	70.05	106.33
Charts per calendar day[b]	16.82	35.70	41.25	66.09	90.32	122.89	149.27	207.53
Discharges per medical records FTE[c]	22.22	26.00	26.74	28.26	30.10	31.10	31.31	33.86
Paid hours per 100 charts[d]	104.55	103.78	104.39	110.69	113.10	99.56	126.09	110.59
Paid hours per discharge unit[e]	2.77	2.47	2.50	2.53	2.38	2.38	2.51	2.50

[a]Discharge units per calendar day = discharge units/days in period.

[b]Charts per calendar day = medical records charts/days in period.

[c]Discharges per medical records FTE = discharges/medical records FTEs.

[d]Paid hours per 100 charts = medical records paid hours/(medical records charts/100).

[e]Paid hours per discharge unit = medical records paid hours/discharge units.

Source: HAS/MONITREND, 1988. Please refer to page x for more information about the data presented in this table.

Additional areas of study include the following activities:

- Plan the implementation of new systems (unit record, index systems, department move, microfilm) when necessary.
- Evaluate and recommend software and hardware for DRG grouping and analysis.
- Analyze costs and benefits of services or equipment, such as microfilm, dictation equipment, filing, and shelves.
- Analyze whether the layout of the department accommodates work-flow requirements and minimizes travel time.
- Analyze utilization review procedures.
- Analyze the feasibility of in-house transcription.

Typical results of departmental analyses include the following:

- The record-processing system is improved to minimize delay time in processing. Improvements may include the performance of completeness reviews before the patient is discharged.
- Staff assignments are designed to reduce delays or bottlenecks.
- Record purge and retrieval policies are implemented to reduce work load. (For example, only the most recent record may be retrieved for admitted patients.)
- Space allocated for record filing is sufficient enough to store four to five years worth of records. This system minimizes the relocation of files because of a shortage of storage space.
- A cost-effective microfilm filing plan is determined.
- Redundant indexing and filing systems (for example, as in the admissions/registration department) are eliminated.
- Record processing is reduced by matching the medical record file format with the floor-chart format when possible.

A medical record department that produces high-quality discharge data in a timely fashion benefits the financial status of the institution by reducing accounts receivables.

Medical Staff Office

Overview

The medical staff office is involved in liaison and support activities between the hospital and its medical staff. A small department reporting directly to the hospital's administration, the medical staff office is an important link between the hospital's administration and its physicians. There is typically a direct day-to-day relationship between the director or chief of the medical staff and the medical staff office. The personnel in this office must possess a high level of maturity and credibility if a positive link between administration and the medical staff is to be maintained.

The responsibilities of the medical staff office include the following:

- Physician credentialing, which includes verifying specialty certification and coordinating each physician's appointment to the medical staff
- Coordinating physicians' reappointments to the medical staff (usually every two years)
- Coordinating medical staff committees and medical staff meetings
- Maintaining updated medical staff rosters
- Maintaining hard-copy files for each physician
- Assuring compliance with Joint Commission on Accreditation of Healthcare Organizations standards that apply to the medical staff
- Maintaining, reviewing, and revising medical staff bylaws

The medical staff office is also responsible for managing and maintaining a central data file or data base for all hospital physicians. This data base is usually maintained on a microcomputer and must be updated continually.

Some medical staff offices must also maintain files and certifications for the hospital's allied health professionals, which include physician's assistants, certified registered nurse anesthetists, and others.

Organization

The medical staff office is usually organized as a one- or two-person department that reports directly to the hospital administrator or chief operating officer. In some hospitals, this function also reports directly to the chief of the medical staff. The medical staff office is usually managed by a medical staff coordinator. This position has evolved tremendously in recent years, and many coordinators hold a national certification in this field (certified medical staff coordinator).

Models and Systems

Medical staff meetings are coordinated and attended by medical staff office personnel. The office's responsibilities include scheduling, notifying participants, attending, and preparing minutes for all medical staff meetings and committees. Other activities related to meetings include maintaining membership rosters, tracking individual attendance, and following up on committee actions.

Appointments to the medical staff are also handled by the medical staff office. After a physician has completed the application for appointment, the medical staff office assembles information on references, malpractice insurance coverage, and verification of credentials and puts together a package for committee review. The results of the review are reported to the applicant, and a file is initiated.

Most hospitals reappoint medical staff members every other year. Reappointment involves evaluations of continuing education, medical records, incident reports, dues, meeting attendance, and delineation of privileges.

Physician reappointment is a cumbersome process that requires a great deal of information to be submitted and verified for each physician. Many hospitals have 200 to 500 physicians who must be reappointed to the medical staff every two years. All information for each physician must be completed and updated before reappointment can be finalized. The medical staff coordinator must initiate all forms and correspondence for this process and must effectively manage and coordinate the completion of each physician's reappointment.

Disciplinary actions are also handled through the medical staff office. Some state boards require the medical staff office to report annually on medical staff credentialing and disciplinary issues.

The medical staff office must also maintain an accurate and up-to-date listing of each physician's delineation of privileges. The delineation of privileges identifies the specific services and procedures that each physician is authorized to perform at the hospital.

Many medical staff offices use personal computers or some other form of automation to maintain an automated data base for all hospital physicians. Commercial software packages are available that are custom-tailored for medical staff office operations. The information maintained on these systems usually includes the following:

- Physician's name, address, and office address
- Medical service/specialty
- Medical staff status (active, courtesy, emeritus, and so on)
- State medical license number(s)
- Drug Enforcement Administration (DEA) certification number
- Dates of appointment and reappointment
- Committee memberships and attendance
- Continuing medical education (CME) credits
- Hospital utilization statistics (admissions, procedures, and so on)
- Disciplinary actions and information
- Delineation of hospital privileges
- Board certification(s)
- Medical malpractice information

Such automated systems allow for the efficient management of vital information and also provide for easier generation of reports, listings, and mailing labels. The use of word-processing systems has also enabled the office to function more efficiently, allowing it to generate personalized form letters to the medical staff and to update and change the medical staff bylaws.

Often, departmental linkages exist between the medical staff office and utilization review or quality assurance. Many software products used for utilization review and quality assurance also have medical staff components. However, these products commonly address only a portion of the medical staff office's information needs.

Departmental Analysis

The analysis of medical staff office operations focuses on improvements in methods and application of office automation. Information flow, forms development, data security, information storage, and information retrieval are the systems that typically require review. The implementation of basic time management principles often improves the functioning of this department.

Nursing Service

Overview

The nursing service (also called the department of nursing) is directly responsible for the continuing care of the hospital's patients. Nursing is usually the largest single department in the hospital, often constituting approximately half the hospital's employees. The salaries and wages account for 25 to 30 percent of the institution's total costs. The department is headed by a director of nursing, or vice-president of nursing (patient care) services, who usually reports directly to the hospital's chief executive officer.

The purpose of the nursing service is to provide a broad spectrum of direct and indirect patient care activities, including management of nursing (patient care) units for routine and special services for both inpatients and outpatients. Nurses assess, plan, implement, and evaluate patient care as well as help to educate patients and recommend policies and procedures. The success of the nursing service is measured in the patient outcomes resulting from patient care services and treatments during a hospital visit.

Organization

The role and responsibilities of a nurse are defined according to the type of position on the hospital staff. Although the positions vary somewhat from one institution to another, the usual hospital nursing positions, in ascending order of responsibility, are staff nurse, charge nurse, head nurse/nurse manager, shift supervisor/nursing supervisor, assistant/associate director of nursing, director of nursing, and vice-president of nursing services. A short description of the duties of each is as follows:

- *Staff nurse:* A staff nurse provides nursing care for patients on his or her assigned unit according to established standards and practices.
- *Charge nurse:* A charge nurse is a registered nurse (RN) who manages all nursing activities of a nursing unit for one shift. He or she reports to the head nurse or shift supervisor, depending on the organizational structure of the nursing service in the hospital.
- *Head nurse/nurse manager:* A head nurse or nurse manager is a first-line manager who is responsible on a 24-hour basis for patient care, operations management, and staff development for one or more nursing units.
- *Shift supervisor/nursing supervisor:* A shift supervisor or nursing supervisor directs and supervises nursing service functions and activities during the day, evening, night, or weekend shifts. This supervisor keeps the director of nursing fully informed of department activities during those shifts.

- *Assistant/associate director of nursing:* The assistant or associate director of nursing is responsible for managing several units and may serve as the evening, night, or weekend supervisor of several units for as many as eight shifts.
- *Director of nursing:* The director of nursing manages several units or an entire department or service.
- *Vice-president of nursing:* The vice-president of nursing reports to the chief executive officer of the hospital and administers all nursing activities in the hospital.

The nursing service may also administer the nursing care provided in the emergency department, the surgical suite, ambulatory care, rehabilitation, central service, home care, and long-term care.

The nursing staff is usually organized according to one of two basic structures: centralized and decentralized (illustrated in figures 13 and 14). A centralized structure focuses management responsibility and decision making on the shift supervisor and director of nursing. This tends to divide the functional organization by shift. A decentralized structure places management responsibility at the nursing unit level, with the head nurse assuming 24-hour responsibility for the unit. This structure tends to divide the functional organization by nursing unit.

In either structure, it is essential to have well-developed communication patterns between the head nurse and the shift supervisor. Currently, the trend in nursing departments is toward decentralization, where head nurses at the unit level define policy and procedure through

Figure 13. Centralized Nursing Service Structure

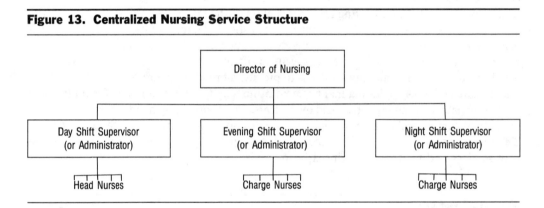

Figure 14. Decentralized Nursing Service Structure

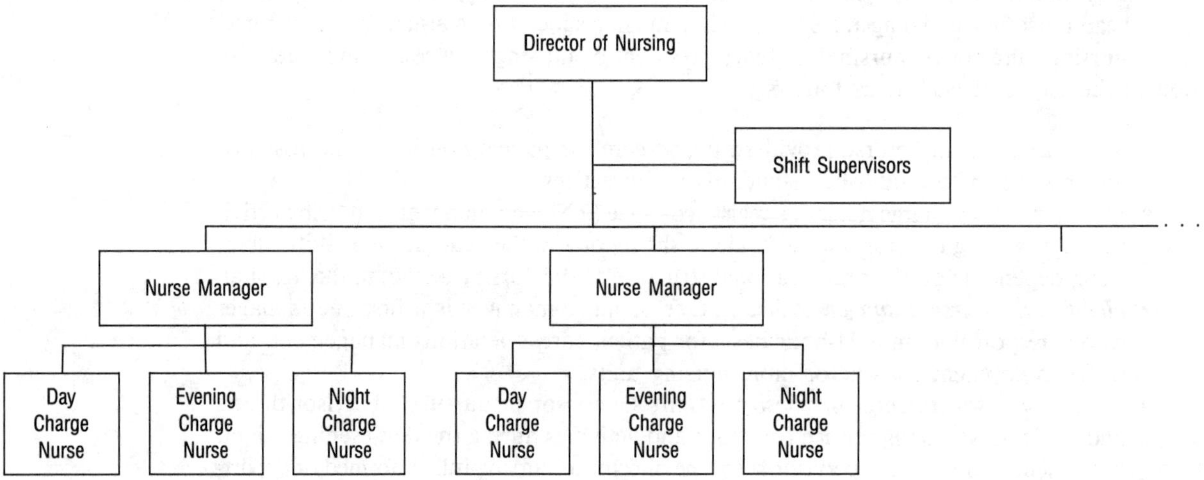

line relationships with nursing directors. The role of the shift supervisor in a decentralized organization is to carry out these policies during off-shifts and report problems or variances to the head nurse. The day shift supervisor is usually eliminated in a decentralized structure.

Within the nursing organization, staff members assume clinical, managerial, or educational roles. Some nursing departments have developed criteria for each of these roles through their employee evaluation system or, more formally, through a career ladder program. Such criteria require that nurses take advantage of management training courses, seminars, and in-service training to maintain and improve their skills.

A variety of staff roles and credentials exist in nursing:

- *Nurse practitioner:* A nurse who provides advanced nursing care and performs some functions historically performed by physicians. A nurse practitioner has completed a certification program and may hold a master's degree. This position is not commonly seen in a hospital.
- *Registered nurse (RN):* A nurse who has passed a state licensing examination and who holds a bachelor of science (four-year) degree from a college or university, a three-year diploma from a hospital-based school of nursing, or a two-year associate's degree from a community college. Although most nurses do not currently hold a bachelor's degree, the bachelor of science program is becoming more and more common. Many hospitals are closing their schools of nursing because of cost and staffing considerations, and increasing emphasis is being placed on more comprehensive education for nurses. Registered nurse administration titles could include vice-president of nursing services, director of nursing, assistant director of nursing, clinical director, supervisor, head nurse, nurse manager, charge nurse, in-service educator, and quality assurance coordinator, with many institutions using the same title for vastly different roles.
- *Licensed practical nurse (LPN):* A nurse who has earned a diploma from a one-year program (usually hospital affiliated) and who is licensed by state examination. State licensure strictly controls what types of patient care activities may be performed by the LPNs.

Nonprofessional staff members who serve in the department include nurse's aides, orderlies, patient care technicians, ward secretaries, and unit managers:

- *Nurse's aides and orderlies:* Nurse's aides and orderlies are trained on the job to assist the nursing staff with various routine patient care activities.
- *Patient care technicians:* Patient care technicians are trained and credentialed by the nursing department to provide an expanded level of support compared to nurse's aides. The technician's functions are closely related to the unit specialty (orthopedics, cardiac, surgical, and so on) and include tasks such as performing phlebotomy and electrocardiography.
- *Ward secretaries:* Ward secretaries are allied health care employees who provide nurses with clerical, medical record, and information system support.
- *Unit managers:* On large units, several ward secretaries may report to a unit manager who is responsible for a broad range of administrative activities. The unit manager may be responsible for more than one unit.

Models and Systems

There are five major models of nursing care delivery that are currently used by most hospitals: functional, team, modular, primary, and total patient care. Functional and team nursing are delivery models that utilize paraprofessionals to deliver much of the nursing care, with a few registered nurses to supervise and evaluate the outcomes of care. Modular and primary nursing and total patient care utilize registered nurses more intensively in all aspects of clinical care, assisted by a few paraprofessionals and support staff. A sixth delivery model, case management, is also followed in some hospitals.

Functional Nursing

Functional nursing takes a task-oriented approach to patient care. Each staff member is assigned to do one or several specific tasks for all patients in an entire nursing unit rather than a variety of tasks for specific patients. Traditionally, the task assignments are determined by the head nurse, and each task is assigned to the staff member with the lowest skill level appropriate to the task. This model accomplishes the most work in the shortest amount of time.

Team Nursing

Team nursing was developed in the late 1940s as a means of individualizing patient care and personnel assignments. In traditional centralized organizations, a team is a group of licensed and nonprofessional staff headed by a professional nurse team leader who reports to the charge nurse. A written nursing care plan is developed as a means of managing and planning nursing care for a large number of patients because a team leader's contact with patients is usually limited and ancillary services staff (for example, respiratory care and physical therapy) and nonprofessional staff are providing many facets of care to the patient.

Modular Nursing

In modular nursing, each member of the team has a broader responsibility for the care of specific patients under the direction and coordination of a nurse (RN) leader. The LPNs and nurse's aides in a module deliver all patient care within the limitations of their roles, receiving clinical support from the module leader. This type of structure provides continuity of care at the individual patient level.

Primary Nursing

In primary nursing, an RN is responsible and accountable for specific patients during their entire stay in a particular nursing unit. The primary nurse is responsible for the assessment, planning, implementation, and evaluation of the patient's plan of care while on the assigned unit. Associate nurses carry out the plan of care when the primary nurse is not on duty. However, the primary nurse retains 24-hour responsibility for his or her patient and is expected to be available for consultation. Discharge planning—including patient education, family involvement, and appropriate referrals—is an integral part of primary nursing. Primary nursing usually has a higher registered nurse skill mix than other care models.

Total Patient Care

Total patient care is sometimes confused with primary nursing. In total patient care, an RN assumes total responsibility for only an eight-hour shift, receiving assistance from nonprofessional staff, centralized support, and ancillary functions. This RN usually cares for a group of four to six patients, depending on how acutely ill each patient is.

Case Management

Case management extends the patient-level responsibility defined in primary nursing to cover a patient's entire hospitalization. An RN case manager is responsible for planning and coordinating the care as a patient progresses from unit to unit, such as from intensive care through acute care and into rehabilitative services. Case management models usually include a collaborative practice forum among physicians, intensive care nurses, medical/surgical nurses, and rehabilitation nurses. Case management models are typically organized around clinical specialties or diagnosis-related groups (DRGs).

Design of the Nursing Unit

Many different floor plans or layouts of nursing units have been designed. One design objective is to minimize the distance between nurses' stations, supply areas, and patients' rooms. It has been estimated that travel time occupies about one-sixth of the nurses' time. The most commonly used layouts are the racetrack, the spoke design, the control center concept, and various hybrid systems.

The most common floor plan resembles a racetrack. The nurses' station, utility and supply rooms, and conference areas are centrally located. Usually, a single, long corridor with patient rooms on both sides extends in two directions from the nurses' station. Variations of the racetrack floor plan are the single-corridor, double-corridor, and T-shape configurations.

The spoke design resembles a wheel. The support service areas are located at the hub as a central core. Several corridors with patients' rooms on both sides extend from the nurses' station like spokes from a hub. Each corridor is shorter than the corridors in the racetrack design so that the distance between extreme points is minimized. The design provides flexibility in the use of beds, and divisions between units can be adjusted to the demand for accommodations of a certain type. Going from room to room on different spokes does present a problem, however.

The control center concept, also known as Friesen design, eliminates the necessity of having nurses' stations on each unit. Instead, units are served through an administrative control center staffed by an administrative aide. Patients' rooms are equipped with special facilities such as pneumatic tube stations, passthrough cabinets for linen supplies and medications, and a work-space alcove. In this system, nearly everything needed for the care of patients is prepared centrally and transported to rooms as automatically as possible, thereby freeing physicians and nurses from travel time and permitting more time for personalized patient care.

Information Flow

The nursing department must manage a tremendous amount of information. Some of the many reports involved are census reports, test requisitions, and requisitions and stock records for supplies, linens, and medications. In addition, the nursing unit must manage information related to patient transport, medical records posting reports, nursing notes, discharge planning, patient education, in-service training of personnel, and patient conferences.

The size of the nursing units and the complexity of the hospital determine the type of personnel needed to manage the flow of information. Large institutions usually have one ward secretary on each unit for each shift to perform routine clerical activities such as ordering tests, handling telephone inquiries, typing, and so on. As mentioned earlier, large units employ several ward secretaries who report to a unit manager.

A manual system of information requires the extensive use of multipart forms and telephones. Frequent trips away from the nursing unit to other service areas are required. In contrast, computerized systems eliminate much of the paperwork, cut down on trips away from the unit, and increase the timeliness, quality, and quantity of the data made available for patient care and management. This is especially true when the computer system includes terminals to be located at each nurses' station. Some sophisticated hospital information systems enable physicians to use the terminals. These systems save clerical time, decrease the use of forms, prevent lost charges, reduce the number of clerical errors, eliminate duplication of work with other hospital departments, and are perceived as beneficial by nurses and physicians.

Bedside terminal or point-of-care systems are receiving significant attention from software and hardware vendors. The next major step in the improvement of efficiency and the integration of information systems will come as a result of the implementation of point-of-care systems and the elimination of all manual clerical systems. It is still too early to assess completely the impact of these new systems; however, paperless systems are on the horizon.

Staffing and Productivity

Staffing and productivity issues are central to the effectiveness and efficiency of the nursing service.

Patient Care Requirements

The standard index for measuring the level of nurse staffing is the number of hours per patient day (HPPD). This measure is simply the number of hours of care provided in one 24-hour day for one patient. In evaluating HPPD levels within and among institutions, one must assess whether the nursing service is responsible for patient transportation, supply procurement, housekeeping duties, and so on because these nonprofessional duties affect comparative HPPD levels.

Budgeted and actual HPPDs express the amount of nursing care planned or delivered. Required hours per patient day are determined by a patient assessment or classification system. There are three primary types of classification systems used in the industry: subjective, acuity, and intensity. Each tool is used to identify the required HPPD for patients based on each nursing unit. Factors affecting the type of nursing care required are the patient's diagnoses and the acuity of the patient's condition; the age, sex, and emotional state of the patient; and the amount of family support available.

A subjective system of patient classification groups patients into categories utilizing broad descriptive statements of the patient's requirements or conditions. These systems are easy to set up but hard to control and difficult to audit.

An acuity system of patient classification identifies objective criteria that are associated with categories of care. The highest criterion selected during the assessment determines the appropriate category. This type of system is easier to control than a subjective system; however, sometimes a patient with a high acuity level will have lower actual care requirements and vice versa.

Intensity systems use objective criteria that are time-weighted indicators and cover all aspects of patient care requirements. A patient's assessment involves summing the weights of appropriate indicators. Intensity classification tools are more accurate at an individual patient level and have structured audit criteria, thus making them more popular under DRG-based prospective payment systems.

In all the patient classification systems, time is associated with the patient assessment. There are two methods of making this time conversion: the discrete conversion method and the continuous conversion method. The discrete conversion method places patients into categories and associates an HPPD standard with each category. In the continuous conversion method, mathematical formulas (that is, linear regression) are used, and patients are not grouped into category ranges. Each type of conversion is designed to add indirect care activities not specifically described by the assessment tool.

Validation of the time conversion is usually performed through data collection. The goal of data collection is to compare the required care predicted by the tool to the actual care delivered. Two techniques commonly used in this evaluation are activity sampling and frequency studies.

A patient assessment or classification system does not yield direct information on skill mix requirements. Skill mix requirements are affected by the model of care delivery, the design of the nursing unit, and the philosophy of the nursing service.

Nursing departments vary on the method of communicating the patient's plan of care. Intensity classification measures can be formulated to be consistent with these methods, which include nursing process and nursing diagnosis.

Nurse Scheduling

An overall analysis of the nurse scheduling function can be useful for improving the hospital's staffing effort, particularly in relation to staff assignment and utilization. To accomplish such an analysis, detailed evaluations of centralized and decentralized scheduling and of current scheduling policies and parameters should be undertaken. Factors that should be evaluated include policies regarding weekend duty, holidays, sick leave, vacation, time staff rotation, skill levels, shifts, and full-time and part-time schedules.

There is an increasing use of computers in the area of staff scheduling. Most of the computer applications have developed along similar lines. Scheduling applications are most often found for microcomputers or microcomputer networks. Shift staffing decision support systems exist in both microcomputer and order-entry environments; however, unit-level access to data is better when the staffing system is part of order entry.

Nursing managers decide on patient care assignments on the basis of the patient's requirements and the availability of staff. This decision process is complicated by changes in census, patient requirements, sick calls, and emergencies. Frequently, float pools, per diem staff, and flexitime are utilized to respond to these variables. Optimal utilization of the nursing staff is directly related to the management of these programs. A daily staffing system should provide input to a comprehensive nursing management data base. Typically, these daily staffing systems are manual; however, automation of daily staffing systems is becoming popular.

Currently, there is a nursing shortage in health care. The shortage is not just a matter of unfilled positions but often indicates a lack of qualified nurses to provide patient care on the days, times, and specialties that are required. Some institutions are closing beds and delaying elective surgeries to decrease the demand for nursing services.

The causes of the nursing shortage include expanded career opportunities for women, increased demand for nursing services, decreased college-age population, decreased interest in health care careers, and decreased funding for nursing education. Retention strategies include reviewing salary ranges, evaluating job design and work load, increasing the use of information and systems technology to support patient care, and implementing nurse recognition programs.

Management Reporting/Budgeting

Management reports and budgets are derived from the nursing management data base and from payroll systems data. Nursing management should have access to information pertaining to the following parameters: census, care hours per patient day, staffing levels, benefit time, and cost. Budgeting organizes the forecasts pertaining to these parameters. Patient classification data are also utilized by cost-accounting and case-mix-reporting systems to analyze costs by DRGs or product lines.

Quality Assurance

The Joint Commission on Accreditation of Healthcare Organizations (JCAHO) requires every hospital to establish a program of quality assurance designed to review, evaluate, and improve the delivery of patient care. Many nursing departments have a full-time position and a committee devoted to maintaining a quality assurance program.

A management engineering analysis of the nursing service should consider staffing levels, staff scheduling, organizational effectiveness, development and validation of patient classification systems, and budget development. Other related topics include management reporting, position control systems, and interaction with other departments.

Pharmacy

Overview

Hospital pharmacy departments provide services not only to patients, but also to physicians, nurses, and hospital administrators. These services focus on the purchase, distribution, and control of all pharmaceutical agents within the institution. For example, a hospital pharmacy performs a dispensing function by filling medication orders received from physicians. The pharmacy also maintains records of the dispensing of medications; maintains and controls the inventory of medications at all nursing units, including the emergency department; and provides intravenous solutions, with medications added (when prescribed), to the nursing units. The goals of the pharmacy may include improving the efficiency of drug distribution and increasing the effectiveness of the pharmacist's influence on drug therapy decision making.

Pharmacy purchasing and inventory control systems generally minimize drug acquisition and distribution costs and ensure that drugs are efficacious and of acceptable quality. Because many new drugs are formulated and marketed each year, physicians and pharmacists are continually assessing and purchasing many of these new drugs. Such ongoing product assessment, and the constant need for a large amount of drugs and supplies in the pharmacy, may necessitate that the pharmacy, and not the materials management department, handle the purchasing function.

Directors of pharmacies may participate in group purchasing arrangements to obtain volume discounts. Pharmacy directors may also establish prime vendor arrangements in which the hospital agrees to purchase the majority of its pharmaceutical products from a local wholesaler at a contract price obtained through competitive bidding.

Other functions of the pharmacy may include the following:

- Providing services for such special drug therapy programs as chemotherapy (oncology)
- Providing pharmacy services to satellite clinics that are physically remote from the hospital (for example, outpatient clinics, nursing homes, and regional offices connected with the hospital)
- Compiling, storing, retrieving, and disseminating drug information
- Educating and training the hospital staff in pharmaceutical matters
- Performing research and participating in the evaluation of investigational drugs
- Maintaining a teaching affiliation with pharmacology colleges for student work-study programs
- Providing pharmacy services, such as drug and health information, to the public as part of occupational health programs
- Providing services to ambulatory and home care programs

155

- Performing therapeutic equivalence assessments on drugs in order that equally effective but less expensive drugs may be put on the hospital formulary (a list of drugs approved by the medical staff for hospital use) and kept in inventory
- Performing drug utilization review

Pharmacy departments in large teaching hospitals may perform many or all of the listed functions, while departments in small hospitals may fulfill only a few of these functions.

Organization

The pharmacy is usually managed by a director or chief pharmacist. The director is responsible to the clinical administrator of the hospital and may also be responsible to a hospital pharmacy committee. The pharmacy committee may include members of the pharmacy, administration, and medical staff; it provides a mechanism for the review of drugs used in the hospital.

The pharmacy staff may include the following positions:

- *Pharmacist (including the director):* The minimum educational requirement for this position is a bachelor of science degree in pharmacology. Master's and doctorate degrees are also available. Professional registration as a pharmacist is usually required for the director and preferred for the staff.
- *Pharmacy technician:* A pharmacy technician may attend hospital-based and other types of training programs, although many are trained on the job. Certification is available. A technician performs tasks such as filling medication orders under the direction of the pharmacist.
- *Pharmacy aide:* A pharmacy aide may be trained to become a pharmacy technician, but no specific education or training is required. He or she performs unskilled tasks such as stocking intravenous solutions, taking inventory, and making deliveries.
- *Pharmacy clerk:* A clerk is not required to have specific training and usually does filing, record keeping, general clerical work, and charging.

The usual hours of operation for a hospital pharmacy are 7 a.m. to 11 p.m., seven days per week. Small hospitals may have more limited coverage, and large hospitals may have more extended coverage. After-hours coverage is usually staffed on an on-call basis. Because of the decreased activity on weekends, some hospitals reduce the hours of operation and staff coverage for the pharmacy on Saturdays and Sundays.

The cross-training of pharmacists in all functions of the department and the use of technicians to assist the pharmacists are important in ensuring proper coverage during regular business hours. Depending on the hours of operation, many pharmacies require the pharmacist staff to work 10- or 12-hour shifts. Many departments give nurse supervisors access to the pharmacy department after regular business hours. This decreases the need for on-call pharmacists to report to work to perform the dispensing function. The nurse supervisor obtains the needed medication and generally signs a log book noting the name of medication and the name of the patient.

Many hospitals are utilizing pharmacy technicians to perform functions historically performed by pharmacists. This allows more time for the pharmacist to provide clinical services to patients, physicians, and nurses. The ratio of pharmacists to technicians is generally one pharmacist to 0.8 technician.

The required staffing levels for the pharmacy vary by level of service provided. For example, functions such as intravenous additive programs, clinical services, and ambulatory services must be considered when evaluating staffing levels. Usually, staffing guidelines are based on the bed size of the institution. See table 17 for guidelines on staffing by skill level.

Table 17. Staffing Guidelines for the Hospital Pharmacy (Annual Paid Hours per Patient Day)

Skill Level	Bed Size of Institution					
	50–99	100–199	200–299	300–399	400–499	Over 499
Pharmacist	0.34	0.31	0.27	0.27	0.27	0.26
Technician	0.30	0.26	0.23	0.24	0.23	0.19
Support staff	NA	NA	0.07	0.07	0.07	0.06

Note: NA means not applicable.

Models and Systems

The role of the pharmacy differs among hospitals. Common models are the dispensing pharmacy, the clinical pharmacy, and more commonly, the dispensing–clinical pharmacy. The dispensing pharmacy is largely dedicated to dispensing prescriptions as ordered by physicians. With the exception of monitoring drug incompatibilities, the dispensing pharmacy takes no role in determining what to order; the physician alone decides. The clinical pharmacy, usually found in large hospitals and teaching hospitals, becomes involved in the determination of what to order. Thus, clinical pharmacists become part of a team effort to determine treatment.

In the dispensing–clinical pharmacy, the pharmacist may perform not only the dispensing function, but also clinical functions as well. The clinical functions could be limited to medication therapy review based on acceptable clinical standards established by the department. Consultations among pharmacists and physicians are also possible. It is a common belief among pharmacists that when the pharmacist actively participates on the pharmacy committee and has frequent interaction with physicians, he or she may have a significant effect on medication use in the hospital.

Medication-Dispensing Systems

Two medication-dispensing systems are prevalent: the traditional system and the unit dose system. The main difference between the two systems is the assignment, either to nursing or to pharmacy, of preparing the precise dose to be administered.

The traditional pharmacy system has the following characteristics:

- According to a physician's order, the pharmacy sends a supply of the medication (labeled for the patient) to the nursing unit. The supply usually is placed in a medicine cabinet.
- The supply may be enough for several days, depending on the packaging quantities and the expected usage.
- The nursing unit prepares the individual dose from the supply in the medicine cabinet.
- Any remaining medication is returned to the pharmacy.
- When the supply is depleted, the nursing unit requests a refill from the pharmacy.

The unit dose system has the following features:

- The system usually utilizes a cassette mechanism. A cassette is a small chest (located in each nursing unit) that stores medications in a number of drawers. One drawer is designated for each patient.
- Some unit dose systems use an exchange cart concept in which two cassettes are utilized. With this system, one cassette is located in the nursing unit and one is located in the pharmacy for replenishing medications. When the cassette drawers are replenished, the full cassette is sent to the nursing unit and exchanged for the empty cassette. This cycle is repeated each day.

- Cassette refills are scheduled, usually according to a 24-hour supply cycle.
- The doses supplied in drawers have already been measured or packaged by the pharmacy so that the nursing unit only administers the medication.
- Medications used as needed (PRN) by the patient are provided in sufficient quantities much as in a traditional pharmacy system.
- Floor stock items not dedicated to individual patients are usually maintained on cassette carts.

More than 90 percent of pharmacies utilize the unit dose distribution system.

The procedure for using unit dose cassettes follows a cycle. First, the physician order is removed from the chart located at the nursing station. Next, the medication card index record in the pharmacy is updated by the pharmacist from the physician's order. As scheduled, the cassette is exchanged by the technician and then refilled. A quality check is performed by the pharmacist. Finally, the cassette is ready for exchange the next day. Thus, each nursing station, pharmacist, and technician performs a specific function in the cycle.

Some factors to be considered include the following:

- The unit dose system is recommended by the JCAHO.
- The unit dose system reduces the amount of time required of nursing personnel and increases the time required of pharmacy staff.
- The unit dose system reduces medication errors.
- The unit dose system increases the control and recording of medications by the pharmacy.
- The unit dose system increases the predictability of the pharmacy's work load.
- The unit dose system increases communication between the pharmacy and the nursing units.
- The unit dose system requires more frequent delivery of carts.

However, the following factors should also be considered:

- The decreased involvement of the nursing staff may not result in direct measurable savings. Most comparative studies show that the unit dose system results in fewer errors but higher costs.
- A traditional pharmacy may be more realistic and practical on specialty units such as pediatrics, intensive care, and obstetrics.
- Already-packaged unit doses can reduce the amount of time for dispensing, pouring, and counting from bulk.
- The increased control and recording of medications by the pharmacy allows for easy reconciliation of the patient's administration record with the dispensing record or profile.
- The patient's dispensing record or profile may be used to capture patient charges (costs).

Both systems use administration records for keeping track of medication. However, the unit dose system requires a patient medication profile (maintained by pharmacy staff) that contains the patient's current medication orders.

The unit dose system is made more efficient through the use of computerization. Computerized patient profiles are provided in nearly 50 percent of all hospitals, and they are capable of providing computerized patient billing information. Also, many computerized systems are designed to generate a medication administration record, which can be used by the nursing staff to document the medications administered to the patient.

Intravenous Solutions Systems

Two systems are prevalent for intravenous (IV) solutions: the traditional and the IV additive. The systems are similar to the traditional and unit dose systems. The activity involved is the mixing of medications with IV solutions.

With the traditional system, IV solutions are stocked by the nursing unit. Medications are sent to the nursing unit, where the medication nurse mixes or adds medication to the solution. Partially filled solution bottles are often used.

With the IV additive system, medications and IV solutions are mixed in the pharmacy. The completely mixed bottle is sent to the nursing station. Some factors to be considered regarding this system are the following:

- It centralizes the process, thus increasing hospitalwide control.
- It increases the predictability and improves the scheduling of the pharmacy's work load.
- It reduces nursing time but increases pharmacy time.
- It may improve the mixing technique being used.

In addition, the following factors should be considered:

- Batch processing and refrigerated stock can reduce pharmacy time.
- Cost savings result from batch mixing of quantities so that lower priced bulk solutions can be purchased instead of more expensive partial fills.
- Direct labor savings in nursing time may not be measurable.
- Intravenous product standardization allows the use of commercially prepared products that may reduce waste, medication errors, and work load.

Regardless of whether the traditional or IV additive system is in use, the pharmacy rather than nursing unit usually performs hyperalimentation, which is the administration of nutrients to patients through intravenous feeding. Hyperalimentation is required only for a small number of patients.

Paperwork and Record Keeping

Numerous paperwork and record-keeping systems are employed during the pharmacy cycle, from ordering medication by a physician to documenting the administration of medication. Typical physician ordering systems use shingled carboned sheets, with copies being distributed to the appropriate departments (or a secretary transcribing the order onto charge tickets and records). Another system uses tear-away requisition forms, which are then transposed to a recording sheet and so do not require transcription by the secretary.

Medication administration records often use a card index format. The records involved are the nursing unit medication file, the pharmacy medication file (sometimes called the profile), and the medical chart. The nursing unit may place a copy in the patient's medical record or transcribe the card index information onto the patient's chart. This system results in a redundant record, it can be time-consuming, and it may lead to errors in transcription.

Computerized interdepartmental communication systems can improve the paperwork systems and record keeping of the pharmacy. Computerized systems eliminate the carbon paper syndrome through direct order entry and communications. Records are also kept as part of the order-entry system. Lost charges and transcription errors may also be reduced. Automatic pricing with such a computerized system requires extensive and detailed information for each drug stocked by the department. Inventory control systems may be a spin-off of order entry, and dispensing labels may also be printed on computer terminals. Less sophisticated paperwork improvements can be made by using automated label printers and magnetic card typewriters.

Departmental Analysis

The range of topics to be covered in analyzing the pharmacy includes specific analyses of such tasks as implementing the unit dose system, as well as full studies of clerical systems and batch processing. Other topics for analysis include the following:

- *Staffing:* Time studies of current and expected activities and work load, analyzed by skill and shift, are conducted. Staffing depends on the service level of the department and varies according to the volume of medications dispensed by the department. Recent MONITREND data for the pharmacy functional reporting center are provided in table 18.
- *Layout:* For unit dose of IV additives, a workstation analysis is valuable.
- *Purchasing and inventory analysis:* Stock levels and purchasing procedures are reviewed.
- *Charging:* Charging procedures and charge policy are reviewed and lost charges are analyzed.
- *Paperwork and record keeping:* Paperwork and record-keeping procedures and their effectiveness are analyzed, as is the design of appropriate systems.

Still other topics for consideration in a departmental analysis of the pharmacy include these:

- The latest JCAHO requirements
- The applicable state and local community legal requirements
- Decentralized (satellite) pharmacy concept, featuring minipharmacy and pharmacist on the nursing unit
- Mobile decentralized pharmacy concept, which consists of a medication cart that is transported to nursing units for dispensing of medications while on the nursing unit
- Pharmacy inventory and turnover (turnover is defined as yearly purchase dollars divided by average inventory dollars)
- Direct data phone-ordering systems with vendors
- Installing effective computer systems that may increase the efficiency and accuracy of the medication delivery system
- Evaluation of alternatives for drug procurement (that is, group purchasing and prime vendor arrangements)
- Development of a formulary to control the number of drugs in each therapeutic category

The costs associated with the purchase of drugs account for as much as 70 percent of total pharmacy expenses. Therefore, the greatest cost savings in a pharmacy can be realized by focusing on drug purchasing and inventory.

Table 18. HAS/MONITREND Data for Pharmacy: Six-Month Medians for Period Ending December 1988

Indicator	National Bed Size Groups							
	Under 50	50–74	75–99	100–149	150–199	200–299	300–399	400 and Over
Work-load units per adjusted patient day[a]	6.59	27.12	13.65	16.72	15.20	14.39	17.20	26.07
Paid hours per adjusted patient day[b]	0.59	0.60	0.61	0.61	0.59	0.58	0.59	0.69
Paid hours per 100 work-load units[c]	8.69	2.89	4.24	2.99	4.19	3.65	3.07	2.79

[a]Work-load units per adjusted patient day = pharmacy work-load units/(total patient days/pharmacy RCC). The pharmacy RCC (ratio of charges to charges) is an adjustment factor that is computed as follows: Pharmacy RCC = pharmacy inpatient revenue/(pharmacy inpatient revenue + pharmacy outpatient revenue).

[b]Paid hours per adjusted patient day = pharmacy paid hours/(total patient days/pharmacy RCC).

[c]Paid hours per 100 work-load units = pharmacy paid hours/(pharmacy work-load units/100).

Source: HAS/MONITREND, 1988. Please refer to page x for more information about the data presented in this table.

Physical Therapy Department

Overview

The physical therapy department provides a specialized rehabilitation function, which may be indicated as a result of surgery, trauma, stroke, or other functional impairment. Traditionally, this function was performed by nursing personnel; however, this specialty has evolved and has been separated from nursing primarily as a result of improving technology and the rising cost of equipment.

Physical therapy provides therapy services for inpatients, outpatients, and ambulatory and emergency patients. Most therapy sessions are scheduled. Therapy is conducted both in the department and in the patient's room. In addition, some physical therapy departments provide therapy through home care programs. A patient may receive one or more modalities, or methods, of treatment during a single physical therapy visit. Common examples of modalities include ambulation, whirlpool, wheelchair evaluation, and walker training.

The department is relatively small in most hospitals, although it tends to be larger in osteopathic hospitals. The size of the department is also related to the amount of orthopedic surgery and rehabilitation therapy practiced in the institution. Besides fulfilling their day-to-day duties, the physical therapy department's staff may participate on committees concerning continuing care, home care, behavior modification, and other matters.

Organization

The physical therapy department may be part of a rehabilitation service division including physical therapy, occupational therapy, speech and hearing therapy, recreational therapy, bracing, and prosthetics. Some hospitals have also included respiratory therapy under the rehabilitation services division. Physical therapy may also be part of a community health program, or it may be a freestanding department. Thus, the physical therapy department may be the responsibility of a director or vice-president of rehabilitation services who reports directly to the hospital's administration. Alternatively, it may be managed by an outside contract management firm.

The department is usually directed by a chief therapist or supervisor. The chief therapist may also be responsible for other therapy services such as occupational and recreational therapies. Medical direction is provided by a physiatrist or orthopedist.

In most cases, education and training for physical therapists consists of a four-year bachelor's degree program. Master's degree programs are also available. The widely accepted and generally required registration as a registered physical therapist (RPT) is usually obtained through an examination and work experience. Two-year programs and registration for physical therapy assistants also exist. Generally, the registered physical therapy assistant can perform most of the same functions as an RPT except patient evaluations.

The staff of the physical therapy department may include the following personnel, with specific credentials:

- The chief physical therapist is usually a registered physical therapist. He or she supervises staff, assigns and schedules staff, performs therapy, completes departmental administrative functions, and may participate on continuing care and rehabilitation committees.
- Staff physical therapists are usually RPTs who evaluate patients, provide treatment, maintain required records, and participate in in-service programs.
- Physical therapy assistants provide treatment, maintain records, and participate in in-service programs but do not provide patient evaluations.
- Physical therapy aides prepare equipment and facilities for treatment, assist physical therapists, and order supplies but are not required to have formal credentials.
- Secretaries perform standard clerical duties, may schedule patients, and may handle charging and billing procedures.
- Physical therapy students, used by many hospitals in educational programs, may perform aide functions.

Staffing guidelines by hospital bed size are difficult to predict because staffing requirements depend on several factors. These factors include the level of orthopedic services provided in the hospital, the availability of competing physical therapy services provided in the community, and the amount of confidence placed in the physical therapy by referring physicians.

The department's hours of operation generally correspond to regular office hours, five or six days per week. On-call coverage is not usually established for other times.

Models and Systems

The types of service generally provided by the physical therapy department are evaluation and therapy. Evaluation is the first step for most patients referred to the department by physicians. In some cases a specific treatment is designated by the physician. In others, evaluation is necessary before appropriate treatment is prescribed by the therapist. The findings of the evaluation and recommendations for treatment by the staff of the physical therapy department are documented in the patient's medical record.

The referring physician sometimes provides the patient with a specific set of exercises or treatments and sometimes describes the need to the therapist in general terms. In the latter case, the therapist evaluates the patient's needs and establishes a set of exercises and goals. The established set of exercises and goals is the therapy program. The therapy program specifies the frequency and the duration of a particular set of modalities and may state the patient's anticipated progress. Treatment and progress are documented in the medical record and on the physical therapy department's patient chart.

Specialty programs may also be available from the physical therapy department, including a cardiac program, chest therapy, and sports medicine. A cardiac program is a specially designed rehabilitation program for cardiac patients. Chest therapy is designed in close cooperation with respiratory therapy and deals with breathing and with drainage of fluid-filled lungs (this function may be the responsibility of physical therapy, respiratory therapy, or the nursing service). In some hospitals, chest therapy is provided by the physical therapy department on the day shift and by the respiratory therapy department on the evening shift. A sports medicine program includes rehabilitative therapy, including exercise equipment for patients recovering from sports injuries or orthopedic surgery.

Most hospital physical therapy charge systems are based on modalities. Printed tickets with assigned charge codes for specific modalities are commonly used. Alternatively, therapy may be charged on the basis of patient time units representing the duration of therapy (10-, 15-, and 20-minute units are common). This technique works well for hands-on therapies such as massage, exercise, and gait training. Some hospitals include an additional digit as a therapist code when submitting patient charges. This enables the physical therapy manager to identify the total work load processed by individual therapists at the end of any given period.

The scheduling of therapy sessions for patients may be done by either a secretary or a therapist. The time allocated per patient depends on the number of modalities per visit and their complexity. In addition, the number of patients that each therapist can handle concurrently may vary, depending on the type of therapy to be provided. When a set schedule is made for a patient throughout the course of treatment, this constraint may reduce the efficiency of a therapist's schedule. The availability of specialized equipment may also be a constraining factor for the schedule and the therapist's productivity.

In many departments, patients are assigned to specific staff therapists. In such cases, a staff therapist arranges, coordinates, and provides direct therapy for a patient, much as in the primary model for nursing care.

Situations and Problems

Most physical therapy patients, especially outpatients, receive treatment on a routine basis. For example, heat treatment may be scheduled once a week for three months. This repeating pattern may cause problems in the registration systems. To avoid such problems, some central registration systems for outpatients are designed so that patients register at a central desk each visit even though this step may be an inconvenience and perceived as a nuisance by routine patients. This repeating pattern also may cause problems in the billing systems. The hospital's financial billing cycles may occur every 30 days, requiring that partial bills be generated each month. In some hospitals, the physical therapy department maintains a running tally of charges and must maintain some form of tickler file so that bills can be generated.

Internal and operational problems of the physical therapy department may include a lack of coordination between the therapy schedule and an inpatient's schedule. For example, a therapist may arrive on a nursing unit to provide patient therapy at the bedside but find the patient is in radiology or is bathing and therefore unavailable for therapy. An effective escort service for inpatients can help ensure that schedules are met. Another possible problem may occur when a therapist needs a patient's medical chart while it is being used by physicians, nurses, or students.

The federal reimbursement system based on diagnosis-related groups has forced many hospitals to reconsider the rehabilitation process for some types of patients, such as patients with fractured hips and major joint replacements. The increased use of outside rehabilitation facilities for extended rehabilitation therapy has enabled many hospitals to ensure that the patients receive high-quality care at the same time that overall hospital costs are being reduced.

Recent regulations in the financial area have necessitated the use of statistical reporting systems that measure physical therapy department productivity. Relative value unit (RVU) and work-load unit (WLU) systems have been developed for such areas as physical therapy, radiology, respiratory therapy, and laboratory. In physical therapy, these RVUs and WLUs are essentially time standards based on predetermined indicators, with each modality assigned a predetermined value or time standard that reflects the amount of the therapist's time involved in a treatment. The time required for patient treatment may differ from the amount of the therapist's time because many modalities can be carried out by the patient without the constant involvement of the therapist. For example, massage therapy may require 15 minutes of both the patient's and the therapist's time; in contrast, a hot pack could require 30 minutes of the patient's time and yet only 15 minutes of the therapist's time inasmuch as continuous involvement is not required for a hot pack. The difference between the patient's time and the therapist's time can be confusing, and departments that bill on the basis of units of time must clearly delineate whether the time unit refers to the patient's or the therapist's time.

Departmental Analysis

Systems engineering projects generally focus on staffing requirements, patient scheduling, registration, charging, and layout. Other topics of study are the level of compliance with regulations for reporting productivity, the analysis of equipment to be purchased or leased, the feasibility of using shared or contracted physical therapy service programs, and the impact of competing private physical therapy providers on the hospital-based department. Samples of recent MONITREND data for the physical therapy functional reporting center are provided in table 19.

Table 19. HAS/MONITREND Data for Physical Therapy: Six-Month Medians for Period Ending December 1988

Indicator	National Bed Size Groups							
	Under 50	50–74	75–99	100–149	150–199	200–299	300–399	400 and Over
Patient time units per adjusted patient day[a]	0.44	0.35	0.35	0.29	0.35	0.40	0.50	0.46
Paid hours per adjusted patient day[b]	0.16	0.14	0.18	0.19	0.20	0.23	0.24	0.28
Treatments per adjusted patient day[c]	0.22	0.27	0.26	0.27	0.30	0.29	0.30	0.32
Paid hours per 100 patient time units[d]	39.30	52.60	43.30	63.87	55.34	59.76	61.21	72.26

[a]Patient time units per adjusted patient day = physical therapy patient time units/(total patient days/physical therapy RCC). The physical therapy RCC (ratio of charges to charges) is an adjustment factor that is computed as follows: Physical therapy RCC = physical therapy inpatient revenue/(physical therapy inpatient revenue + physical therapy outpatient revenue).

[b]Paid hours per adjusted patient day = physical therapy paid hours/total patient days/physical therapy RCC).

[c]Treatments per adjusted patient day = physical therapy treatments/(total patient days/physical therapy RCC).

[d]Paid hours per 100 patient time units = physical therapy paid hours/(total patient days/physical therapy RCC).

Source: HAS/MONITREND, 1988. Please refer to page x for more information about the data presented in this table.

▤ Planning Department

Overview

Strategic planning (referred to in a more global context as strategic management) has become an essential management tool for most large-size and medium-size businesses. Its importance as a tool has evolved in the past two decades as data have become more available and as analytical techniques have been refined. Strategic planning is one reflection of the information age that has contributed to dramatic changes in the U.S. economy.

The health care industry has been relatively slow to adopt strategic planning, but it has been involved in some sort of planning since at least the 1940s. In 1946, the so-called Hill–Burton legislation, which involved federal funding of new hospitals (primarily in rural areas), required the development of planning skills in the design and construction of hospitals, especially to determine the locations and sizes of the hospitals to be constructed. In the 1960s, with the passage of legislation for regional medical programs and comprehensive health planning, the focus shifted to program planning. This involved the design and development of clinical programs targeted toward certain services and diseases.

It was only in the 1980s that strategic planning came into the health care industry. The primary impetus for this change has been the shifts in federal policy that tend to emphasize competition among health care providers. The operative term in strategic planning is *strategic;* strategies apply only where competitors exist. Strategic planning does not displace the other forms of planning but rather provides a framework within which the other forms of planning occur. Thus, facility and program planning continue but take place within the strategic context.

As planning has evolved, so have the departments in which planning activities take place. Strategic planning, which usually has a 3- to 5-year time horizon, has recently given way to more operationally based planning with approximately a 12- to 18-month planning horizon. Planning specialists who have concentrated on strategy or the long-term realm have become more involved in implementation or the short-term realm. This phenomenon reflects the tightening financial situation for most hospitals and a recognition that, although planning may be sound, making plans a reality is a major challenge. As a result, in numerous settings, the orientation of planning departments has become focused more on line management and less on staff functions. The department responsible for planning has also often been expanded to include such disciplines as marketing, public relations, and communications, to name a few. It is also not uncommon to find the planning department actually providing new product development and product management for certain services during an "incubation" period.

One particularly important consideration in evaluating the planning department is that the discipline tends to cut across all levels of the organization. Strategic planning, for example, should involve input from board members and medical staff leaders in addition to management. The strategic planning process is primarily a top–down activity that must ultimately be translated into annual operating plans, that is, plans that according to John Abendshien translate "strategies into specific operational priorities, timetables, and responsibilities" (*A Guide to the Board's Role in Strategic Business Planning*, Chicago: American Hospital Publishing, 1988, p. 65). Annual operating plans, on the other hand, can often involve a bottom–up process starting with general guidelines consistent with the strategic plan.

Although planning departments in hospitals will likely continue to lag somewhat behind commercial industry, further change can be anticipated as the discipline evolves. Paralleling trends in business and industry, today's hospital has pared down its number of full-time planning staff, but if anything, it has heightened its expectations of the planning staff. The planning officer who originally guided the hospital through the maze of regulatory and legislative requirements of the 1970s may now be charged with contributing information on much broader and more fundamental concerns: What can the hospital do to compete and ensure its survival? What needs to be done to preserve a tax-exempt status? Should a merger, consolidation, or acquisition be considered? How can quality objectively be measured?

As the scope of health care planning has broadened, it has become increasingly important for effective planning officers to report directly to the hospital's chief executive officer, who functions as the organization's chief strategist. Although business unit managers often generate their own detailed plans for achieving short-term goals (often called business plans), the planning officer is still the manager of this type of planning process. In addition, it is still the planning officer, often with assistance from other internal staff and external consultants, who is responsible for writing a strategic plan that includes an overall assessment of the hospital's internal, external, and competitive environments. This strategic plan should clearly specify the organization's long-range goals and objectives and the actions necessary to achieve them.

How does the planning officer accomplish this? In *A Strategic Planning Process for Hospitals* (Chicago: American Hospital Publishing, 1985), Joseph P. Peters suggests that nine tasks constitute the strategic planning process:

1. Audit the current situation (the present mission and the long-term goals, strategies, and conditions that have obstructed the hospital's effectiveness in accomplishing its mission, goals, and past strategies).
2. Revise the hospital's mission, if necessary, to reflect the desired future situation or to provide a clearer sense of the institution's purpose.
3. Scrutinize the hospital and its environment to identify any outside forces that may affect the hospital, and assess its ability to manage these forces to its advantage.
4. Identify and evaluate the major issues, problems, opportunities, and threats that the hospital is or will be facing, and rank them in order of importance.
5. Choose appropriate goals and strategies, after reviewing various options, that balance the hospital's potential with the challenge of changing conditions. Take into consideration the hospital's mission, the values and desires of its board and management, its resource capabilities, and its social responsibilities.
6. Prepare a written plan to support and carry out the strategy.
7. Obtain approval(s) for the plan.
8. Carry out the plan.
9. Establish a procedure and a timetable to monitor the plan and to determine whether what is subsequently accomplished is what was actually intended. Revise strategies and plans if indicated.

Peters observes that it can take from 12 to 15 months to complete these tasks and that the plan is then revised as needed. He acknowledges that planning officers often receive many other assignments in addition to these.

What types of plans are produced during or through the planning process? In addition to the strategic plan, most organizations also prepare annual operating plans and budgets, as mentioned earlier. Other plans mentioned by Peters that may be part of an overall strategic planning process include the following:

- Capital expenditure plans
- Marketing plans
- Human resources plans
- Program and resource development plans
- Quality assurance plans
- Organization plans
- Physician recruitment plans
- Contingency plans

Usually, these individual plans are not included in the strategic plan, but rather flow from it. Even in an organization in which the chief executive officer (CEO) and/or planning officer tightly controls the writing of the strategic plan, the operational plan and other plans are more often than not written by the managers responsible for implementing them. In these cases, as a system of checks and balances, the CEO and planning officer still review and approve the plans. Figure 15 illustrates the steps taken during the strategic planning process.

Organization

The planning function has undergone major structural changes during the past 10 years. Like other departments, planning has felt the downsizing crunch. Beyond that, planning has a new focus, and with the emphasis on strategy execution and line management involvement, the staffing requirements have changed. In addition, some planning officers, along with some public relations specialists, have been given the added responsibility of a marketing function, and others are responsible for such functions as public relations, pricing, joint ventures, technology planning, and development of health maintenance organizations and preferred provider organizations.

According to national studies by the American Hospital Association's Society for Healthcare Planning and Marketing, full-time-equivalent planning positions dropped from an average of 3.2 per hospital in 1982 to 1.9 in 1985, 2.0 in 1987, and 1.8 in 1989 (in 1989, the average

Figure 15. Strategic Business Planning Framework

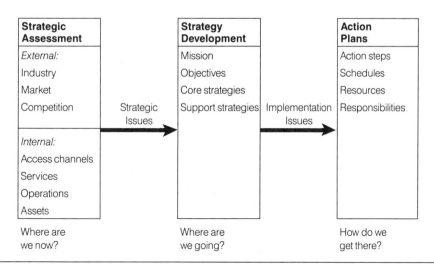

Strategic Assessment		Strategy Development		Action Plans
External:		Mission		Action steps
Industry		Objectives		Schedules
Market		Core strategies		Resources
Competition	Strategic Issues	Support strategies	Implementation Issues	Responsibilities
Internal:				
Access channels				
Services				
Operations				
Assets				
Where are we now?		Where are we going?		How do we get there?

From J. Abendshien, *A Guide to the Board's Role in Strategic Business Planning.* American Hospital Publishing, 1988, p. 13.

was 1.7 for small- and medium-size hospitals and 2.1 for hospitals with more than 450 beds). However, averages can be very misleading because planning staffs vary by the organization's size and complexity. A multihospital system's headquarters or a large tertiary care institution could need a very large staff. Organizational arrangements also vary widely. Some hospitals have a separate, distinct planning department; others combine planning with marketing or corporate development. Because planning departments function in so many different ways, there is no one right way for a department to be organized.

Generally, the planning department reports to the CEO and is a vice-presidential-level position. In very small institutions, the CEO is often the planning officer or, alternatively, a single person is responsible for planning, marketing, public relations, development, and other related tasks. At other organizations, a single vice-president or director may oversee all of these areas but supervise several people who actually perform the tasks. Common titles for the highest-ranking planning executive include vice-president of planning; vice-president of planning and marketing; vice-president of business development, corporate development, or corporate strategy; and even chief operating officer (COO). By and large, although many progressive organizations have oriented planning and marketing toward line management positions, other organizations prefer to have planning and marketing function as staff positions.

Occasionally, planning officers have risen through the ranks to become COOs and CEOs. The outlook remains unchanged for effective planning officers in the 1990s who are willing to expand the scope of their careers. As the planning profession has evolved, however, the skills mix demands have changed as well. The great majority of planning officers hold master's degrees, generally in an area related to health care. In the future, however, a growing number will probably hold master's degrees in business administration as opposed to master's degrees in health care administration or public health. The need for financial acumen has skyrocketed, and computer skills have become essential in order to prepare forecasting models, perform spread-sheet analyses, and create sophisticated tracking mechanisms for monitoring operational activities. Communication skills, political savvy, and facilitating and negotiating abilities have become necessary, too, as planning officers have found themselves increasingly involved in group management, consensus building, and physician relations activities. Overall, the planning officer is functioning in a much more action-oriented role than previously and is a key player in many important operational and managerial tasks.

With larger planning staffs, some of these skills are likely to be more vital to one planning position than another. For example, some planning staffs might have one person assigned to clinical programs and another to facilities. The skills of those two individuals would, of course, be quite different. More difficult is the department that combines several job categories in one position. When one person is responsible for planning, marketing, and public relations — and that does occur in small hospitals — it is a considerable challenge for that person to effectively fulfill all of the requirements of the three areas. To augment staff, as well as to add objectivity and experience, it is common to hire outside consultants to perform some tasks, such as the development of a strategic plan. Other tasks, such as data collection and analysis, might be accomplished within the finance department. The smaller the planning department and the more diffuse its responsibilities, the larger the role of the CEO needs to be.

Models and Systems

Planning officers stand in two worlds: the high-technology world and the high-touch world. The difficulty comes with finding the balance and cultivating the necessary side for each situation. On the high-technology side, planning officers need to master computers. Some of the most interesting and telling information that a hospital needs to make its decisions is already available within the hospital's walls. The trick is in figuring out how to uncover the information when many of the systems are not presently compatible. For example, it is not uncommon for hospitals with computerized referral systems or senior membership programs to have difficulty tracking utilization or identifying related revenue. One system can easily track the membership enrollment of a senior membership program, but the hospital's back-office system that tracks admissions and billing and physicians may be totally incompatible with the system tracking membership. Software programs that can perform such integrative tasks do exist, but there are often many obstacles to effective implementation, and ample time must be devoted to making these programs produce the needed data.

For the most part, most large hospitals already have extensive data bases that house data on demographics, competitors, market share, service mixes, physician profiles, and other necessary information. Federal and state departments of health and local agencies supply additional resources. Even when sophisticated data bases do not exist, however, the most basic and necessary information is available within the hospital walls, although not necessarily in an accessible or obvious place or in a usable form.

What specific functions does the planning officer perform? This varies widely, based on whether the planning is a top–down (from the CEO) or bottom–up (from the unit managers) process, whether the planning officer is assigned additional responsibilities (for example, marketing), and whether planning is viewed as a line management or a staff function. Similarly, planning tasks vary dramatically depending on the size of the organization (for example, whether it is a multiunit or single-facility institution), the size of the staff, and the changing needs of the organization. The responsibilities of a planning officer at a sole-provider, rural hospital vary greatly from those of a planning officer at the headquarters of a 25-hospital system. However, in the most generic sense and with recognition that any list cannot cover all of the possibilities, planning officers are engaged in the following tasks:

- *Managing the assessment and analysis process*
  - Environmental assessment — external assessment: Review national, regional, and local trends related to economics, business and industry, governmental issues, public and private payers and insurance, technology, diseases and medical occurrences, population (demographics and life-style), human resources, and other relevant variables.
  - Environmental assessment — internal assessment: Analyze the hospital's strengths and weaknesses and overall areas of operations, mission's effectiveness, market share and position, patient mix, payer mix, services, financial situation, and staffing including physicians.
  - Environmental assessment — competitive assessment: Profile variables examined in the internal assessment (including planned and expected new services and products) for competitor institutions.
  - Data collection and management: Develop intelligence gathering and reporting systems; create and manage data bases; manage network arrangements, hardware and software decisions, market research and analysis, demand forecasting and measurement, financial systems, and other information systems.
- *Orchestrating the strategic planning process*
  - Plan development: Oversee the development of strategic, business, and marketing plans with clear goals, objectives, strategies, and actions outlined; integrate the external, internal, and competitive assessments with the entire planning process; coordinate physician and manpower planning, business unit and/or product planning, community service and mission effectiveness monitoring, financial planning and analysis, and tracking and evaluation activities.
  - Strategy development
  - Training personnel: Guide personnel through the planning process; help them develop better, more effective plans and share assessment information with them; act as internal consultant.
- *Business development and implementation:* Manage new business and product development activities including merger, acquisition, and affiliation evaluation; examine diversification and/or integrative growth opportunities as well as service line development

or discontinuation; implement planned activities; and handle special projects such as managed care, pricing, and quality measurement.

- *Monitoring and evaluating hospital services and projects:* Develop and implement tracking mechanisms to chart the progress and success of ongoing activities, establish financial safeguards to guard hospital resources, and create criteria for project expansion and contraction.
- *Developing linkages to external organizations:* Act as liaison consultants with external agencies, including health systems agencies, state departments of health, metropolitan hospital councils, and other agencies. As required, develop any required documents for these agencies (certificates of need, testimony, and special reports).

Not every planning officer will be involved in all of these activities, but generally these tasks fall within the realm of the planning department.

Productivity

Measuring the productivity of planning departments is very difficult. The planning officer's control over the execution of the strategic plan may be very limited. For example, it is unreasonable to hold the planning officer responsible for improving returns on investments when that improvement is tied directly to the actions of an operational executive. Some may also find it unreasonable to measure the planning officer's batting average in predicting events (noting that even well-known futurists tend to be wrong more often than they are right), while others expect a level of accountability (suggesting that planning officers are paid to anticipate changes and prepare their organizations to deal with them).

However, it is not unreasonable to evaluate the volume and quality of output, the meeting of deadlines, and the general timeliness of projects. The adequacy of the planning system itself can be measured, and the output and appropriateness of data produced by the planning officer are certainly under that person's control. Similarly, planning can be measured by its success in fostering the planning process, generating options for organizational growth, and providing valued internal consulting services to the hospital's CEO and management staff.

Situations and Problems

One of the most fundamental challenges faced by the planning officer is guiding managers to think with a market-driven, long-term focus. A one-year time horizon is adequate for some projects, but others need a much longer time. Similarly, it is difficult to foster strategic thinking when most line managers by necessity focus on day-to-day operational issues. However, thinking longer term (that is, thinking strategically) is an absolute requirement for the planning process, and the planning officer must facilitate this and assist the hospital and its staff in this area.

Planning officers may also be challenged to be the voice of reason when hospital managers examine programs and services that may only be short-term fads. For example, if top management learns that a rival hospital is building a women's pavilion, management may decide to embark on a similar project without considering the marketplace or the consequences of failure. Similarly, a hospital executive may read that innovative hospitals are delivering more services for the elderly and then decide to create an adult day-care center without a full understanding of the demographics of the hospital's area. It is the planning officer's job to maintain the type of information that can help a hospital make informed decisions. If proper resources and data bases are maintained, the planning officer should be able to produce appropriate information before lemminglike management decisions for new projects lead the hospital astray.

Another difficulty is the complexity of gathering information from many different management groups within the hospital as well as from sources external to the hospital. The planning officer must collect and integrate input from the board of trustees, the CEO, physicians, operational executives, vice-presidents of various areas, the chief financial officer, and the managers of hospital units. Developing a participative process that links these disparate groups, many with special interests, can be quite demanding. Beyond that, the planning officer is faced with the classic problem of needing to collect information and motivate people to contribute without having any real control over these people. For example, the planning officer may need to work closely with the vice-president of nursing and the recruitment manager to devise a comprehensive nursing recruitment and retention plan, but the planning officer has no real control over the nursing or human relations personnel. Similarly, the planning officer often must surrender some control as alliances, networks, and corporate offices take over or augment some of the planning officer's tasks. For example, a planning executive at the corporate office of a hospital system may develop a data base and select hardware and software for the system's hospitals' planning departments. The planning officers at the individual facilities may or may not report to the corporate planning executive, and if they do not, they may even resent having another planning specialist making such decisions even if it is accomplished through a participative process.

The politics of the planning officer's position cannot be underestimated. Because planning officers often deliver the CEO's edicts about which projects go forward, which continue at their current level, and which receive no funds or reduced funds, planning officers may face some difficult sessions. This is especially true when physicians are involved because it is so important to develop and maintain strong relations with them. How can the planning officer tactfully explain why a physician's pet project will not be undertaken? How can the planning officer assess the very real threat of that physician then shifting loyalties to another hospital? Sometimes trade-offs and compromises need to be made, and the planning officer needs to have excellent negotiating skills. The planning officer may not always be the person involved in such discussions, but some vice-presidents of planning have found themselves facing just such a challenge.

Some of the tensions of the planning process can be dissipated through the creation of useful criteria for screening project ideas. In *Health Care Marketing Plans: From Strategy to Action* (Homewood, IL: Dow Jones-Irwin, 1984), Steven G. Hillestad and Eric Berkowitz suggest the following screening criteria for project selection:

1. Is the return on the investment adequate?
2. Does it enhance political power?
3. Are estimated revenues sufficient and profitable?
4. Does it require capital? To what extent?
5. Does it require research time?
6. Is a certificate of need required?
7. Does it have a competitive advantage in the marketplace?
8. Does it have a solid market segment?
9. Is it easy for a competitor to duplicate?
10. Is it a process with which the organization is familiar?
11. Does it enhance the stability of the other products offered by the organization?
12. Does it promote product competition?
13. Does it provide for long-range growth?
14. Does it provide for adequate market share?

Setting up such objectives in advance of creating a plan can help line managers and business unit managers to assess their ideas before bringing them to the attention of top management.

Finally, planning is by definition cyclical and iterative. At peak times of the year, the planning department may be understaffed. With the tough economics facing today's hospitals, it is not uncommon for understaffing to be a chronic condition, and as planning officers take on additional responsibilities such as marketing, the expectations can become overwhelming. When one staff person has three or four different responsibilities, one or more projects are bound to receive inadequate attention.

Because of all of these common problems, external consultants are often used for special projects. When funding permits, many hospitals hire market research firms to collect some of the necessary baseline information. Alternatively, a consultant may work with the medical staff or develop the strategic plan. In other cases, departments can be reconfigured to maximize the use of existing personnel. It has proved effective for some organizations to link their planning and marketing departments, for example, or for staff with a special expertise in areas such as physician relations to be hired for long-term staffing needs.

Departmental Analysis

The planning department can be one of the most difficult to analyze. Because planning is organized and practiced in so many different ways at hospitals, a standardized national norm of behavior and expected results does not exist. As noted earlier, planning officers cannot be evaluated on outcomes when they have no control over them, but planning officers can be evaluated on the basis of such *structural* aspects as the degree of focus of the strategic plan, the appropriateness of strategies to market conditions, and the accuracy of predictions and projections, as well as on *process* (including the extent of familiarity with, and acceptance in, the organization). For example, the planning department can be assessed on the basis of the effectiveness of the planning process itself, the comprehensiveness of the strategic plan, the adequacy of the information systems, the coordination of the budget, the coordination of departmental and/or business units' plans, the quality of the internal consulting assistance in developing these plans, the adequacy of the financial analysis and risk–return assessment of projects, and the political sensitivity of the staff. In cases in which planning officers have direct control over implementation and outcome, it certainly makes sense to evaluate those contributions as well.

Public Relations

Overview

Public relations as it is practiced within a given hospital depends on the objectives hospital management sets for the function and the understanding management has of the value of the range of potential activities as well as the budget and staff available to support them. In "Public Relations as a Senior Management Function" (Chicago: American Society for Hospital Marketing and Public Relations of the American Hospital Association, 1989), Robert Ristino defines public relations as:

> a communication function of senior management through which organizations adapt to, alter, or maintain their environment for the purpose of achieving organizational goals. . . . As open systems, hospitals must continuously interact with their environments. Public relations assists this interaction by managing corporate public discourse, monitoring and managing the environment, and managing internal and external relations. . . . Through corporate public discourse, public relations practitioners attempt to control how organizational identity, image, issues and values are perceived and discussed in the public arena. . . . As monitors and managers of the environment, public relations staff scan and span the organization's boundaries—the points at which the consumer and the hospital make contact. As boundary scanners, they collect information useful to many organizational functions, such as planning and marketing. As boundary spanners, they interpret and represent the organization to its publics and its publics to the organization.

The range of public relations activities can best be understood by looking at the kinds of publics with whom the hospital must relate. The *Basic Guide to Hospital Public Relations* (Chicago: American Hospital Publishing, 1984) suggests the following typical publics:

- Patients and former patients, classified as inpatients or outpatients
- Employees, classified as full-time or part-time, salaried or hourly, week or weekend, and so forth
- Hospital visitors, perhaps divided into family and friends
- Physicians, divided by specialty and type of privileges
- Government officials
- Auxilians and volunteers
- Trustees
- Hospital donors, divided by personal and corporate givers
- Potential patient populations, such as senior citizens, young children, women of childbearing age, and so forth

- Hospital suppliers
- Insurance officials
- Students and school guidance counselors
- The media

One goal of public relations is the structuring of a two-way communication system between hospital management and the hospital's publics. A dimension of that system must involve a counseling role for the public relations practitioner:

- Interpreting viewpoints of publics to management with recommendations for appropriate actions and programs
- Reporting trends in attitudes of publics to prepare management to meet changes
- Reporting the findings of public opinion and customer satisfaction research
- Apprising management of the impact that proposed actions and activities may have on the public's perceptions of the hospital
- Counseling management on strategies to avoid public relations pitfalls as well as to capitalize on unrecognized advantages and opportunities

A second dimension of the two-way communications system is targeting communications to reach specific publics with a message designed to elicit specific behaviors and to enhance the credibility of the hospital. The communications activities may include:

- Media relations
- Advertising
- Patient relations, including publications targeted to patients
- Community relations
- Board relations
- Employee relations, including involvement in employee orientation and in-service education
- Physician relations
- Legislative affairs, although specific lobbying activities may be done by the planning department, top-level management, or a public affairs department

The communications capabilities of the hospital may be most sorely tested when the hospital is called on to respond to a disaster, and the public relations practitioner may therefore be a key member in the development and implementation of the hospital's disaster plan.

In establishing good relations with the hospital's publics, the public relations professional may become involved in conducting special events such as health fairs, setting up a speaker's bureau to get hospital representatives in front of public meetings, structuring fund-raising campaigns, operating telephone hot lines for complaints or information, assisting in the recruitment and training of volunteers, and designing sales literature and sales campaigns for health promotion programs and special audience programs (senior services, cancer care services, and so on).

Of increasing importance to the hospital and the public relations practitioner is *image management,* which Robert Ristino (in the article referenced earlier) defines as "controlling how actors in the environment perceive an organization." As Ristino suggests:

A primary function of public relations is managing image, in contrast to marketing whose function is managing product. However, as is evident to most practitioners of health care public relations and marketing, these functions are not mutually exclusive. In fact, establishing an organizational image is normally a marketing function primarily because image plays such an important role in positioning an organization, just as it does with a product or service. But once established, image is, to a large extent, refined and managed through public relations activities.

Organization

The structure of the public relations department depends on whether the hospital is seeking a vice-president who will include management counseling functions in the hospital's approach to public relations and who may also assume responsibility for marketing or is seeking a middle manager responsible principally for publications and handling news and special events. When the public relations function is viewed primarily as a communications function, the practitioner may have a degree in journalism or English and some health care experience. The more highly placed the individual is to be, the more importance should be placed on management experience in health care.

Models and Systems

The processes by which public relations functions are carried out flow from the definition of the hospital's mission and goals, which in turn are translated into definitions of specific strategies. When the hospital's mission statement clearly defines the purpose of the organization, the scope of its activities, and its future direction, public relations and marketing communications activities can be structured to support and refine these definitions.

Underlying the planning process for public relations is research. Depending on the internal capabilities of hospital staff, the objectives and complexity of the research effort, and the availability of staff time and budget, market research might be undertaken by a qualified external consultant under the direction and supervision of the person responsible for public relations functions.

The public relations process generally follows five steps:

1. Identifying the relevant publics and stakeholders for the organization and refining the list to target public relations efforts to those who have the greatest influence over the organization's initiatives (different lists might be constructed for different categories of initiatives)
2. Conducting appropriate research-oriented activities to measure the current attitudes of the relevant publics toward the organization and to gauge likely reactions to possible organizational initiatives
3. Establishing public relations goals in terms of effecting desired changes in public attitude and public perception of organizational image as well as eliciting support for organizational initiatives or reducing the negative influence of opposing groups (for example, addressing the presence of a vocal right-to-life group in the community)
4. Developing cost-effective strategies to achieve public relations goals
5. Implementing actions, evaluating results, and assessing the need for changes in goals or strategies

The publics that might be identified include those highlighted in the overview section of this profile. The measurement of the hospital's current image and the attitudes the public holds can come from qualitative studies (such as focus groups with consumer or employee groups) or quantitative market research (such as patient satisfaction surveys). The structuring of the research tasks as well as the interpretation of the results and the translation into statements of hospital goals and objectives are most effective when not done solely by the public relations practitioner. Without administrative and medical staff support, and perhaps governing board support as well, the results of research may not be translated into effective shared objectives and strategies, and the public relations practitioner may be placed in a position of recognizing problems but having no authority to take actions to resolve them.

The *Basic Guide to Hospital Public Relations* highlights six problem areas for which the public relations practitioner might find strategy development most critical:

- Satisfactorily explaining rising costs and their causes to increasingly skeptical internal and external publics
- Recruiting employees, especially key groups, such as nurses
- Attracting volunteers and auxilians to the hospital
- Defusing press criticism and building strong, positive relationships with the press based on professionalism and mutual respect
- Building community and specific public appreciation for the hospital and its programs, including health education, emergency services, obstetrics, and others. This problem often translates into a need to increase the census by using goal-oriented communication techniques aimed at both potential patients and physicians
- Developing employee and other internal public support for the institution and raising morale and productivity while combating rumors, inclinations to organize, and so forth

Of the activities listed in the overview section of this profile, media relations (including news releases, copy for radio and television public service announcements, and placement of hospital representatives in radio and television interviews) is most likely to be accomplished solely within a public relations department. Other activities are more likely to be conducted in cooperation with other areas of the hospital. For example, patient relations is likely to involve the nursing service and the medical staff and, depending on the structure of the hospital, the education department and the manager of the patient representative program.

Public relations practitioners have traditionally been involved in the development of brochures, booklets, newsletters, fact sheets, and other written materials for a variety of public relations activities. In recent years, video and audio productions have been added to the communications tools of public relations. The nature and frequency with which such tools are used will lead to the need to make make-or-buy decisions about production capabilities. The introduction of affordable desktop publishing hardware and software has made decisions to "make" promotional materials in-house more realistic even for smaller institutions. Given the availability of desktop publishing capabilities in many departments within the hospital and the consequent production of a wide variety of print materials (newsletters, brochures, and so on) within these departments, the public relations professional has often been called on to manage the institution's visual image through the provision of design standards.

Departmental Analysis

Management engineering studies of public relations are seldom undertaken. Because of the administrative nature of public relations, no nationally recognized productivity standards or measures have been developed or accepted. The size and personnel composition of these functions is a largely discretionary issue from institution to institution. The scope of activities and responsibilities also varies significantly among facilities, which also effectively prevents the development of a standard activity profile on which productivity measurement can be based.

In some cases, clerical or administrative work load may be measured to determine the utilization of clerical time. Such studies might be performed by audit (yielding generalizations) or by work sampling (yielding more exact data). However, the management of the qualitative aspects of public relations is difficult to quantify and is generally dealt with by a subjective evaluation of performance and staffing needs.

In the absence of any nationally recognized standards or any consistency in the organizational structure and range of activities, one is left with performing an audit against self-determined and institution-specific objectives. A public relations audit might begin with the list of publics presented in the overview and seek to ascertain how, by whom, and how well communication with these publics is accomplished.

Quality Assurance

Overview

Quality assurance (QA) programs in hospitals, guided by standards set forth in the *Accreditation Manual for Hospitals* published by the Joint Commission on Accreditation of Healthcare Organizations (JCAHO), are designed to be systematic, objective, ongoing, and integrated efforts that focus on the following topics:

- The competence of people providing patient care services (through credentialing, peer review, and other performance evaluation processes)
- The accuracy and completeness of clinical information (through review of medical records and QA reports)
- The physical safety of patients, staff, and visitors (through an infection control program; review of accidents, injuries, and safety hazards; and a risk management program)
- Compliance with professionally established standards of medical care (through the self-monitoring activities of the medical staff and review of utilization management data)
- An organized process to monitor, evaluate, and improve the quality and appropriateness of care provided to patients

Since its founding in 1951, the JCAHO has been a major influence in the evolution of QA programs in hospitals. The consensus-building process through which JCAHO standards are developed has yielded modifications in the standards over the years, moving the focus of the QA program from the hospital's *retrospective* rendering of a professional judgment of the hospital's capability of providing good care to *concurrent* and ongoing evaluation against predetermined, clinically relevant, and valid criteria. These criteria, referred to as *indicators,* may focus on the structures, processes, or outcomes of care (a three-part definition of quality first advanced by Avedis Donabedian and published in *Explorations in Quality Assessment and Monitoring,* Ann Arbor, MI: Health Administration Press, 1980):

- *Structures* are inputs into care, such as resources, equipment, and the qualifications or number of staff members.
- *Processes* of care are those functions carried out by practitioners, including assessment of treatment, planning of treatment, indications for procedures and treatments, technical aspects of treatments, and management of complications.
- *Outcomes* include complications, adverse events, short-term results of specific procedures and treatments, and patients' long-term health and functional status.

The emphasis on concurrent review enables the hospital to identify and correct problems while the patient is still in the hospital or at least still under treatment if he or she has been discharged from the hospital. At this point, problems in care can be quickly addressed and resolved, and the chances of averting potential harm and reducing costs are also greatly improved.

Hospitals have found quality assurance to be an important and yet increasingly more complicated activity. It has become especially important in providing information on the appropriateness and cost-effectiveness of patient care services to regulatory bodies, third-party payers, private industry, and patients. However, the perception of what constitutes quality care tends to be institution specific, and definitions vary widely among providers and consumers. As a result, no definitive method for QA activities has gained universal acceptance in the industry, and hospitals have used a variety of approaches to fit their particular situations, revising and adapting these approaches in response to ongoing changes in the health care environment and advances in QA technology.

There are a number of major efforts under way to advance the state of the art of quality assurance and quality management. For example, under its Agenda for Change, the JCAHO is working toward definitions of appropriate indicators for selected clinical services that can be reflected in its accreditation standards in the 1990s. Ultimately, hospitals will report data on these indicators to the JCAHO, thus yielding a national data base of performance norms against which hospitals will be able to analyze and compare results.

Perhaps the greatest pressure for refining the process of measuring and reporting data on quality of care has been generated by the actions of third-party payers. The Health Care Financing Administration (HCFA) of the U.S. Department of Health and Human Services, for example, releases annual reports to the public on hospital-specific mortality data for Medicare patients. Because the data do not reflect adjustments for age and severity of illness and do not differentiate causes of death unrelated to the admission diagnosis (for example, a patient admitted for cataract surgery who dies subsequent to a myocardial infarction), the public may easily misinterpret high mortality rates as indicative of a hospital that does not render high-quality care. Hospitals therefore must capture appropriate data and be able to report objectively their own assessments of performance. This task is made all the more difficult given that there are a number of systems designed to capture severity-of-illness data (and states such as Pennsylvania have mandated the use of designated systems) but there is no widespread support for any individual system.

Organization

The governing body of each health care facility bears the ultimate responsibility for the quality of patient care and customarily delegates to the medical and hospital staff the responsibility for monitoring and evaluation activities. The approach selected by a hospital to administer, coordinate, and integrate its QA activities should be uniquely suited to the philosophy and clinical mission of the facility. The size and complexity of the organization may also influence the approach taken. Within the hospital structure, the locus of control for quality assurance may be based in administration (usually through a QA coordinator who reports to a senior-level administrator), in the medical staff, or in a joint conference committee of hospital staff, physicians, and trustees. The overriding principle is that quality must be viewed as everyone's business in the organization, and however the program is structured, it must have the active support and involvement of the hospital's administration, the governing board, and medical staff leadership to meet institutional goals for quality assurance.

The manager or physician director of each hospital department and service is responsible for ensuring that required patient care evaluation activities are carried out in his or her area of responsibility. The manager may decide how this will be done but is expected to incorporate a problem-solving process into the routine activities of the department and to focus evaluation and monitoring efforts on those activities that will result in the greatest opportunity for improvements in patient care. In emergency departments, special care units, and hospital-sponsored ambulatory care and home care agencies, evaluation should include the care provided by physicians as well as nursing and other health professionals playing a significant role in services to patients. Whenever patient care problems involve more than one service or department or group of practitioners, all involved are expected to work together to resolve the problems. In so doing, systemic problems in the process of care can be identified, addressed, and resolved.

Delineation of Responsibility

The JCAHO requires the hospital to establish a written plan that delineates the scope of its QA program. Within the major services provided to patients, the plan identifies what is to be evaluated, who among the practitioners providing the service is to identify opportunities to improve care, and how improvement is to be monitored. The plan should also clearly define who holds the responsibility and authority for each QA function. The JCAHO does not require a written plan for each clinical department or support service, but many hospitals find it useful to document QA activities and staff responsibilities specific to their areas.

Lines of communication should also be specified to establish how pertinent information is to be shared across the departments to support integration of the problem-finding and problem-solving components of the system. The plan is usually developed by a dedicated hospitalwide QA staff, reviewed and approved by all appropriate medical and hospital committees, and approved by the hospital's chief executive officer, the president of the medical staff, and the governing board before implementation. The JCAHO requires that the plan be evaluated annually and revised as necessary.

Role of the Medical Staff

Officers of the medical staff in each facility are accountable for ensuring the clinical competence of all physicians and allied health practitioners who receive clinical privileges through its credentialing mechanism. This is usually accomplished through established peer review activities in each department of the medical staff that include the following:

- Determining what clinical privileges each physician will hold
- Recommending governing board approval of appointments and reappointments to the staff
- Setting criteria for evaluating the quality and appropriateness of care
- Monitoring physician performance
- Providing continuing education and appropriate corrective strategies (with objective definitions of events that require corrective action and consistent application of the required corrective strategy)
- Establishing the mechanism by which membership on the medical staff may be terminated

Oversight of these activities may be vested in an appointed director of the medical staff, the chief of staff, the executive committee or the credentials committee of the medical staff, or the joint conference committee of the governing board. The heads of clinical departments usually assume the responsibility for credentials review and recommendations for appointment or reappointment based on this review. The department heads also bear the direct responsibility for ensuring systematic review of physician performance through clinical case review focused on the following factors:

- *Volume indicators:* Monitors of the frequency and scope of services, such as the number of admissions and the number of specific procedures or clinical tests. The data on volume enable the staff to calculate rates of incidence of adverse outcomes or complications as a percentage of the total number of similar procedures, to identify the practice patterns of individual practitioners and the hospital as a whole, and to identify trends important to hospital resource allocation and strategic planning.

- *Occurrence screens:* Predetermined and objective indicators used to signal the need for review. Screens may describe the processes in the delivery of care, clinical events, complications, or outcomes for which data can be collected in order to compare actual results with criteria related to the screen. Events such as unexpected deaths, returns to the operating room, or adverse drug reactions should prompt for investigation to determine whether the events could be traced to structural problems (for example, availability of resources for accurate diagnosis) or process problems (for example, accuracy, timeliness, and technical skill in applying diagnostic protocols).
- *Clinical indicators:* Indicators that screen the care provided by each clinical specialty but that are generally confined to those related to high volume, high risk, or likely problems unique to the clinical specialty. Each clinical department uses such indicators to aid in the identification of opportunities to improve care practices or the performance of individuals or groups of practitioners. These opportunities are identified when collected data elements cross an established threshold set by the clinical department or service. Once the threshold has been reached or crossed, those cases are then examined thoroughly, perhaps by using focused review methodology, to determine the reasons for variation.
- *Focused reviews:* Concentrated reviews of key areas in a department or service determined by their high volume, high risk, or history of identified problems. Focused reviews might target a representative sample of high-volume diagnoses or procedures, all cases over a finite time period, or all cases of low-volume but high-risk care.

Following the standards of the JCAHO, the medical staff must have in place monitoring and evaluation functions for the following five basic types of review:

- *Surgical case review:* Review that addresses the indications and justifications for all invasive surgical procedures, tissue, nontissue, and invasive diagnostic procedures performed in both inpatient and ambulatory care settings. This review uses established occurrence screens and clinical indicators, with data reviewed as part of monthly meetings of clinical departments. Each department's review committee includes a pathologist, when appropriate, as well as members of the clinical department.
- *Blood usage review:* Review that consists of five major tasks: justification/indication for transfusion episodes for all blood products, review of all confirmed transfusion reactions, approval of transfusion policies and procedures, monitoring of adequacy of transfusion services, and review of blood product ordering practices. Reviews are conducted for each transfusion episode, and results are reported at least quarterly. In addition to members from the relevant clinical department, the review committee may include a pathologist, a blood bank/transfusion service chief technologist, a surgeon, and a hematologist.
- *Drug usage review:* Review that examines selected high-volume or high-risk drugs from the major classes of drugs used in the hospital for all uses (empirical, therapeutic, and prophylactic) and for the parameters of appropriateness, safety, and effectiveness. The selection of drugs to be reviewed, decisions about the frequency of review, and the reviews themselves are generally best done at the departmental level.
- *Pharmacy and therapeutics review:* Review that embraces approval of pharmacy policies and procedures; development, maintenance, and modification of the hospital formulary; evaluation/approval of experimental or investigational drugs; and review of serious, untoward drug reactions. Reports should be made quarterly, and the review committee is required to include participation of pharmacy, nursing, and hospital administration personnel, as well as the medical staff.
- *Medical records review:* Review that focuses on the timeliness of completion of the record and the clinical pertinence of documentation. Reviews should be performed

in conjunction with the nursing service, the hospital's administration, the range of clinical services groups, and the medical record department. The reviews for timeliness can be done on an ongoing basis within the medical record department, and medical staff can be asked to review random samples of records against predetermined criteria on at least a quarterly basis.

Depending on the size, complexity, and organization of the hospital, these five review functions may not necessarily be performed by five separate committees; the functions may be accomplished by the medical staff executive committee or a practice monitoring committee, by committees that combine functions (for example, combining surgical case review with blood usage evaluation and combining drug usage evaluation with pharmacy and therapeutics review), or at the departmental level.

Role of Nursing

The nursing service provides services that have a major impact on the quality of patient care; therefore, the department places a high value on quality assurance. Indeed, quality assurance in nursing has had a long and distinguished history of its own. It has evolved separately from, but along the same direction as, QA efforts in medicine, beginning as a retrospective peer review of care provided by nurses assessed largely by examining documentation in the medical record and progressing to evaluation of predetermined clinically relevant and valid criteria to measure outcomes of care. Today, nursing QA activities focus on two areas: checking the achievement of standards and solving patient care problems.

These functions are addressed through a unit-based or divisional structure. At the unit level, staff nurse committees identify opportunities to improve care and develop solutions to resolve patient care problems. Results are summarized on a regular basis and reported through a departmental coordinating committee to nursing administration and to the hospitalwide QA committee. In large departments with clinical divisions, QA activities may be addressed by divisional committees for each specialty.

The responsibility for nursing quality assurance rests with the nurse executive, who customarily delegates the coordination of this function to a member of the nursing administrative staff. Over the years, nursing quality assurance has been assigned to those responsible for staff development, nursing education and research, or patient acuity systems, to an assistant or associate director of nursing, or to a coordinating committee. With recent cost-containment cuts in administrative staffs, quality assurance is frequently combined with other responsibilities. Wherever the position is based, the nursing QA coordinator is responsible for designing, implementing, and maintaining all aspects of the program, as well as for serving as a quality information clearinghouse and interdepartmental liaison for QA issues.

Unit-level committees meet monthly or more often. The nursing department QA committee meets quarterly to review unit activities and to refer or resolve broad issues identified by unit committees. Many hospitals require that the nursing QA coordinator report to the hospitalwide QA department quarterly, and in some hospitals, this individual may also serve as a member of the medical staff QA committee.

Program structure within nursing must be congruent with the department's structure. To be effective, the coordinator must be placed at a level where he or she has direct access to top managers in other departments to ensure prompt communication of significant patient care problems and of difficulties arising within the QA program.

Role of the QA Department

The hospital's administration is responsible for ensuring that qualified staff and other required resources (space, equipment, and technology) are available to implement and maintain an effective monitoring and evaluation system. Most hospitals have a designated QA department or director to provide internal consultation to all medical and hospital staff involved in QA activities, to give technical assistance as needed, and to coordinate the dissemination of all quality assurance, risk management, and utilization data across departments. To be effective, members of the QA staff increasingly need strong data-analysis skills.

The staff structure of the hospitalwide QA department varies widely depending on the size and type of hospital, its overall structure, the extent to which support personnel are already available within the clinical and other patient care services departments, and the hospital's use of computers. Staff size is also determined by the amount of information the department collects, whether it performs concurrent or retrospective review, whether it does 100 percent review on all patients or a random sample, and how integrated it is with such quality-related functions as utilization review, risk management, and infection control. In small hospitals, the QA department may be a one-person operation. In large hospitals, the department may include a QA director, a secretary, and two or more data abstractors. In very large hospitals or medical centers, especially those that centralize all quality-related functions, the QA department may include a staff of as many as 16 to 20 people.

The QA coordinator or QA director is usually a registered nurse or registered medical record administrator. Thus, in small hospitals, the QA coordinator may add QA activities to other responsibilities such as those of director of medical records. In large facilities, the data abstractors are also registered nurses or medical record professionals.

Each department within the hospital (whether clinical, ancillary, or other service) is expected to report its QA activities to the hospitalwide QA department on a planned and systematic basis. The frequency of reporting is based on the scope and volume of service provided and on the impact of the service on direct patient care. Most clinical departments must report monthly or quarterly, depending on their JCAHO and/or local and state requirements. In addition, the overall assessment of the hospitalwide QA plan must take place annually, taking into account the results of these periodic departmental reviews.

The hospital's QA staff reviews and concisely summarizes all reports and ensures that data are reviewed in a timely manner by other appropriate parties. Many hospitals establish a hospitalwide QA committee for this review. Selected members of this committee typically sit on a joint QA committee responsible for overseeing both hospitalwide and medical staff quality assurance.

Integration of Quality-Related Functions

To enhance information exchange and problem resolution, many large hospitals are moving toward an organizational integration of several quality-related functions, including quality assurance, utilization management, risk management, infection control and in some cases, medical records and medical staff affairs. Generally, specific areas of professional expertise are retained, but activities are coordinated so that duplicative effort is minimized.

Relationship of Utilization Management to Quality Assurance

Utilization management in hospitals is the review of the appropriateness of all admissions, tests and procedures ordered, length of stay, and discharge planning practices. The overall utilization management (UM) plan embraces prospective (preadmission), concurrent (at point of admission and during course of stay), and retrospective (postdischarge) review activities. The primary purpose of these reviews is to control health care costs by minimizing unnecessary and inefficient uses of hospital services.

Preadmission review has recently taken on increased significance as a means of identifying opportunities to improve care through the use of alternatives or more effective treatment modalities. Hospitals may flag certain practitioners, procedures, or diagnoses—preselected based on the need to control frequency, intensity, or costs—for routine preadmission review by designated physician advisors. The selection of practitioners, procedures, and diagnoses for review may best be done in concert with the medical staff as an additional aspect of the development of clinical indicators for peer review. In addition to one-on-one counseling between the physician advisor and the admitting physician regarding possible alternative treatment plans, large-scale in-service education programs can be developed on the basis of aggregate data on recurring utilization problems. Preadmission review may also be used to identify early on patient discharge planning needs and to ensure compliance with any preprocedure certification requirements of third-party payers (for example, mandatory second opinions).

Concurrent and retrospective reviews involve the examination of data from the medical record to determine whether patients are receiving treatment that is both necessary and appropriate and data from the patient billing system to determine such factors as average cost per stay for patients with a given diagnosis. Reviews may also be used to compile profiles of the practice patterns of individual physicians and profiles of hospital resource allocation. This evaluative activity is a form of quality assessment and should be clearly connected to the QA program.

Relationship of Risk Management to Quality Assurance

Risk management is an umbrella term that embraces activities designed to protect the hospital from incurring liability in the course of caring for its patients and to reduce the hospital's financial burden through risk financing and claims control. In view of the legal implications and the financial components of risk financing and claims control, hospitals usually maintain the risk management function under a risk manager who is organizationally distinct from the QA program. The risk manager also needs to ensure that policies and procedures incorporate the various requirements set forth by the JCAHO, state agencies and departments of health, and insurance carriers.

Because there are quality-related activities in the risk management program that overlap with the objectives of the QA program, there should be clear lines of communication and data sharing. In the areas of identification and assessment of loss potential and loss prevention and reduction, there is potential for coordination between the risk management and quality assurance programs. For example, the development of occurrence screens in medical staff monitoring described earlier in this chapter is clearly parallel to the following definitions of the Chicago Hospital Risk Pooling Program (*Risk Management Manual,* 1982) of occurrences that need to be reported in a risk management program:

- Occurrences of missed diagnosis or misdiagnosis that result in patient injury, such as failure to diagnose acute myocardial infarction, fracture, serious head trauma, or appendicitis
- Surgically related occurrences such as operations on the wrong patient, wrong procedures performed, incorrect instrument or sponge counts, or unplanned returns to the operating room
- Treatment or procedure-related occurrences such as reactions to contrast material used in a diagnostic procedure, inappropriate exposure to X rays, or burns resulting from improper use of hot packs
- Blood-related occurrences such as wrong blood given to the patient, transmission of disease via infected blood, or inappropriate use of blood
- Intravenous-related occurrences such as administration of the wrong solution, infiltration of solution, or inappropriate infusion rate
- Medication-related occurrences such as administration of the wrong medication or dosage or administration of medication to the wrong patient
- Falls
- Other occurrences that result or may result in injuries to patients or visitors

Clear definitions of reportable occurrences, hospital management support for the importance of occurrence reporting that extends beyond the customary reliance on nursing reports, and physician involvement in the development of criteria and commitment to the program enhance both the risk management and the quality assurance programs. Patterns of risk management problems should lead to appropriate in-service education, development of, or changes in, policies and procedures, or one-on-one counseling.

Relationship of Infection Control to Quality Assurance

Hospital infection control programs are geared toward the identification, prevention, and control of nosocomial (hospital-acquired) infections. Estimates from the Centers for Disease Control [R. W. Haley and others, The financial incentive for hospitals to prevent nosocomial infections under the prospective payment system, *Journal of the American Medical Association* 257(12):1611–14, March 1987] indicate that 5 percent of all patients admitted to a general hospital in the United States develop a nosocomial infection and that the incidence of infection nationally adds four days to the average hospital stay at an annual cost of $4 billion. An effective infection control program that prevents development of nosocomial infections and promotes early identification and treatment can therefore make a direct and measurable contribution—both to the quality of patient care and to a hospital's financial status.

The hospital's intensive surveillance and control activities are generally focused on the types of infections and the types of environmental or clinical factors over which the hospital has the greatest control. The four most common types of nosocomial infections, and therefore those most frequently targeted for intensive surveillance, are surgical wound infections, urinary tract infections, bloodstream infections, and pneumonias. Especially with surgical wound infections, the hospital's achievement of infection control objectives depends on the existence of mechanisms for providing feedback to the responsible parties so that appropriate corrective measures can be implemented. Inasmuch as the surgeon's operating technique is the most significant cause of surgical wound infections, the surgeon's regular and consistent knowledge of the incidence rate of such infections is critical to taking corrective action before the rate escalates to the level of a major problem.

Responsibility for monitoring the program is vested in the hospital's infection control committee, and each hospital designates an infection control specialist (ideally but rarely a trained epidemiologist). Depending on the hospital's size, the infection control coordinator may also act as the QA coordinator; however, it is critical not to limit the effectiveness of the infection control program by compounding too many duties in a single person without giving adequate staff support.

Models and Systems

In structuring the QA program, hospitals generally follow the JCAHO's 10-step model. The nature of the system used to implement the program depends on the institution's size and clinical mission.

The JCAHO's 10-Step Model

Within Standard QA.3 in the *Accreditation Manual for Hospitals, 1990 Edition,* the JCAHO recommends a 10-step monitoring and evaluation process to assist chief executive officers, medical staff officers, and governing boards to meet all requirements for hospital-based QA programs. The overall characteristics required of this process, as stated in Standard QA.3.1, are the following:

- The process is designed to effectively utilize QA resources to identify and take opportunities to make important improvements in patient care and identify and correct problems that have the greatest (or an important) effect on patient care.
- The monitoring process is designed to identify patterns or trends in care that warrant evaluation and/or important single clinical events in the process or outcome of care that also warrant evaluation.

- The evaluation is designed to determine the presence or absence of an opportunity to improve or a problem in the quality and/or appropriateness of care and determine how to improve care or correct the problem.

This model can also be used to evaluate existing hospital and medical staff QA functions on a step-by-step basis as follows:

- *Step 1: Assign responsibility for monitoring and evaluation activities.*
- *Step 2: Delineate the scope of care provided by the organization.* This step is an ongoing process in each department and includes all major services provided, all types of patients served, all types of practitioners providing these services, and all settings in which care is provided. This complete inventory becomes the basis for the selection of targets of review made in subsequent steps.
- *Step 3: Identify the most important aspects of care provided by the organization.* According to Standard QA3.2.1, "These important aspects of care are those that (1) occur frequently or affect large numbers of patients; (2) place patients at risk of serious consequences or of deprivation of substantial benefit when the care is not provided correctly, or the care is not provided when indicated, or the care is provided when not indicated; and/or (3) tend to produce problems for patients or staff."
- *Step 4: Identify indicators (and appropriate clinical criteria) for monitoring the important aspects of care.* The indicators are related to the quality and/or appropriateness of care and may include clinical criteria (sometimes called "standards, guidelines, or parameters of care or practice"). The indicators must be objective and measurable, and they must be based on current knowledge and clinical experience. They may reflect structures, processes, or outcomes of care (as described in the overview at the beginning of this profile).
- *Step 5: Establish thresholds (levels, patterns, or trends) for the indicators that trigger evaluation of care.* Qualified practitioners assign each indicator a predetermined threshold or level of performance against which realistic goals for quality improvement are set.
- *Step 6: Monitor the important aspects of care by collecting and organizing the data for each indicator.* There is ongoing data collection from a variety of sources to adequately monitor and evaluate each indicator and to provide for aggregation of data on a predetermined schedule to detect trends and patterns of practice. All data elements required for internal and external review are identified in advance to minimize duplication of effort in data collection.
- *Step 7: Evaluate care when thresholds are reached in order to identify either opportunities to improve care or problems.* Qualified staff from the department or service involved evaluate care provided when indicator thresholds are reached or exceeded. Physicians proficient in the specific area review any variations in care. According to Standard QA3.2.5, "When initiated, the evaluation of an important aspect of care (1) includes analysis of trends and patterns in the data collected on the indicators; (2) includes review by peers when analysis of the care provided by a practitioner is undertaken; and (3) identifies opportunities to improve, or problems in, the quality and/or appropriateness of care."
- *Step 8: Take actions to improve care or to correct identified problems.* Corrective action must be appropriate to the cause of the problem (changing attitudes and behavior remains the most difficult corrective action to implement).
- *Step 9: Assess the effectiveness of the actions and document the improvement in care.* Through continued monitoring of the important aspects of care, the effectiveness of the action in correcting a problem or achieving a desired improvement is evaluated.
- *Step 10: Communicate the results of the monitoring and evaluation process to relevant individuals, departments, or services and to the organizationwide quality assurance program.*

At a point specified in the written QA plan, all data received and analyzed come together for scrutiny by those in authority. Overall, there should be evidence of integration and coordination of all QA activities, evidence that people in the organization are working together toward a common goal of high-quality care, and evidence that, however organized, the job gets done. Finally, there must be evidence of an annual evaluation of the program's effectiveness.

System Design

There are many ways in which the process described in the preceding section may be implemented, although the ultimate responsibility lies with the hospital's governing board. In large medical centers, physicians may be employed as managers of multidivision clinical departments. These physician managers coordinate the identification and resolution of issues and problems concerning patient care in each respective area through a team effort within each department. In this type of setting, the reviews for which the medical staff is responsible may be accomplished through a network of quality assurance–related standing committees and subcommittees of the medical staff, including, for example:

- Departmental QA committees for large departments such as medicine, surgery, and pediatrics
- A quality of care committee whose members include physician representatives from each of the medical center's clinical departments
- A surgical case, blood usage, and hospital mortality review committee
- A drug usage and pharmacy and therapeutics review committee
- A utilization management committee
- An infection control committee
- A risk management committee
- A QA executive committee whose members include all the chairpersons of all the QA committees

Members of the medical staff provide direction with respect to medical care, and a QA program staff employed by the medical center performs all the support activities for the respective committees. A QA manager, also employed by the hospital, coordinates all QA activities. The QA executive committee, which includes key representatives from the hospital's administration, coordinates the medical center's overall QA program and reports program activities to the medical staff executive committee and the governing board of the hospital.

An alternative approach taken by a community hospital with no medical school affiliation and no chief of staff or medical director employed by the hospital features parallel tracks for hospital department and medical staff QA activities that converge in a joint QA committee (or joint conference committee) established by the governing body to maintain and support an ongoing QA program. Membership on this joint committee often includes the medical director of the QA program, officers of the medical staff, representatives from the governing board and the hospital's administration, the chairman of the credentialing committee, the QA/UM systems director, the nursing QA coordinator (or director of nursing), and the hospital's risk manager.

The medical staff track ensures that all requirements are met for review of physician practice and clinical care; and in its track, the hospital has established mechanisms for departmental evaluation of all patient care services, including such overarching programs as those for utilization management, risk management, and infection control. The hospital also provides personnel and resources to direct and support the total QA effort. The program is evaluated on an annual basis by the joint QA committee with input and assistance from other committees, clinical departments, and hospital departments.

Under this two-track model, the governing board appoints a physician recommended by the medical staff and the hospital to serve as the medical director of the QA program.

This physician oversees all QA monitoring activities carried out by the medical staff department committees, reviews all reports, represents the medical staff on the hospital QA committee, and reports on the status of the program to the medical staff executive committee and the joint QA committee.

The director for QA/UM systems is the key coordinator and integrator of all aspects of the QA program. The QA/UM director provides resources, direction, and support to department managers and physicians involved in quality assurance, reviews all QA activity reports from hospital departments, and determines appropriate disposition. The director attends related hospital and medical staff committee meetings, meets regularly with the physician director to ensure the integration of interdisciplinary QA activities, sits on the hospital QA committee, and is a member of the joint QA committee.

In small, nondepartmentalized hospitals, the responsibility for QA activities may be delegated to two committees: a medical staff committee and a hospital departments committee. Members of these committees provide initial review of quality indicators in assigned areas of responsibility and report findings to a coordinating committee. Quality assurance staff employed by the hospital provides support to each committee. Out of necessity, small hospitals tend to coordinate quality assurance, utilization management, risk management, and infection control functions within these same three committees.

In small hospitals in which the size of the medical staff may not permit objective review by peers of like specialty, coordination with the medical staffs of other hospitals in the region may provide a viable alternative.

Problems and Challenges

Health care organizations and QA professionals for the foreseeable future will continue to work toward consensus on the meaning of quality care and how it can best be measured and improved. Attempts will also continue to be made to measure the cost-effectiveness of QA activities and to answer the question in everyone's mind, "What, if any, impact do QA activities have on the quality of patient care?"

Within specific organizations, QA efforts have encountered long-standing problems in gaining physician acceptance of the need for, or the value of, required QA activities. The involvement of physicians in defining QA program objectives, analyzing data, and designing clinically useful follow-up strategies has improved the success of QA programs.

Another difficult area for many programs is moving QA activities away from identifying the "problem of the month" to continuous monitoring and implementing actions designed to resolve the problem, particularly when this involves changing thought patterns and behavior, as well as actions that seize opportunities to improve care *before* problems occur. Again, the extent to which clinicians and managers are involved in planning, implementing, and assessing the effectiveness of QA activities encourages ownership in the program and increases commitment to the resolution of patient care quality problems and to the achievement of excellence.

Quality assurance is also struggling to enter the computer age. The need is compelling; basic manual and spread-sheet tracking systems are no longer adequate to deal with current mandates to collect, synthesize, analyze, and report ever-increasing amounts of data to a variety of groups in myriad formats.

Hospitals must assess their current data management capabilities and look for more efficient methods to capture and exchange quality, utilization management, and risk management information across departments. To be effective and efficient, a QA/UM data management system must be part of the mainstream of a comprehensive, interrelated, clinical information management system. In some organizations, this may mean purchasing a microcomputer with appropriate applications software. In other facilities, it may mean designing and developing a comprehensive mainframe program.

An example of a cross-referenced data base in such a system would include the following information:

- Patient admissions and discharges
- Credentialing and privileging of physicians and professional staff
- Incident and occurrence monitoring
- Aspect of care and indicator monitoring
- Procedure monitoring (for example, blood utilization and drug usage evaluations)
- Infection control monitoring

The ability of computers to analyze and quantify massive amounts of information will prove invaluable to providers in future debates over the quality of health care.

Radiation Therapy Department

Overview

The radiation therapy department's principal function is the treatment of oncological diseases (cancer) through the use of ionizing radiation, which shrinks or destroys cancer cells and other abnormal tissue growths by breaking down the cells at the atomic level. Radiation oncology works in concert with medical oncology, which provides diagnostic and clinical treatment services to cancer patients, including chemotherapy. Surgical oncology, another subspecialty within oncology, treats malignant tumors by surgically removing them. Approximately 40 to 50 percent of the cancer patients treated in the United States each year receive some form of radiation therapy, either alone or in combination with other forms of treatment, including surgery and chemotherapy. Although the hospital's radiation therapy department treats both inpatients and outpatients, the trend in cancer care in the United States is to administer radiation therapy, as well as chemotherapy, on an outpatient basis.

Three kinds of basic equipment are used in most radiation therapy departments: cobalt units, linear accelerators, and superficial X-ray machines. Larger departments may also use orthovoltage machines, phototherapy machines, brachytherapy machines, and stereotactic radiosurgery machines. All radiation therapy equipment requires shielding of some kind to keep dangerous radiation from escaping the treatment area.

The cobalt unit usually is used for deep-radiation therapy; it uses a radioactive isotope to generate the therapeutic radiation beam. Electricity rather than a separate radiation source is used to generate the therapeutic ionizing radiation in the linear accelerator and superficial X-ray units, which have applicability in the treatment of a wide range of oncological diseases. The linear accelerator is much more powerful than the cobalt unit, and its beam is much more concentrated. Therefore, treatment by a linear accelerator is very precise. A computerized treatment simulator is used to determine the amount and location of radiation treatment to be delivered by the linear accelerator.

The radiation therapy department relies on the expertise of several different groups of professionals and technologists, including radiation oncologists (physicians, usually radiologists, specializing in radiation oncology), radiation physicists, physicist assistants (known as dosimetrists), radiation therapy technologists, radiation therapy nurses, and dietitians.

Organization

In most hospitals, the radiation therapy department reports to the associate administrator or vice-president of professional services. In many small hospitals, radiation therapy may be a subdepartment of the radiology department and report to the associate administrator or vice-president of ancillary services.

In a stand-alone radiation therapy department, the department head is usually a radiation oncologist, and the day-to-day management of the department is often the responsibility of the chief radiation physicist. In such organizational structures, all the professional and technical staff report to the chief physicist, with the exception of the physicians. In large hospitals, the physics support staff might report to the chief physicist, the technical staff might report to the chief radiation therapy technologist, and the nursing staff might report to the department's nursing coordinator.

A radiation physicist, with or without the assistance of a dosimetrist or physicist's assistant, is responsible for developing the details of the individual treatment plan prepared for every patient who is referred by a medical oncologist to the department for treatment. As part of treatment preparation, a radiation physicist (or a mold-room technician in a large hospital) is also responsible for preparing the individualized blocks and molds made out of a leadlike substance that protect the patient's vital organs from unwanted radiation damage during therapy.

Radiation therapy technologists are responsible for the actual delivery of the treatment: calibrating therapy unit equipment, verifying all doses according to the treatment plan, positioning the patients during treatment, and delivering the prescribed doses. In most hospitals, a senior radiation therapy technologist is also responsible for maintaining the supplies used by the department. The department's equipment is usually maintained under contracts with outside maintenance firms.

In many hospitals, a dietitian may be available to provide nutritional counseling to radiation therapy patients. Registered nurses experienced in cancer treatment provide nursing assistance and follow-up care for patients receiving radiation therapy. The department may also use nonprofessional employees to transport inpatients between the nursing floors and the department, or transporters from the radiology department or a centralized patient transportation service may perform this function.

The radiation therapy department is often linked by computer with the radiation therapy departments of other medical centers for the purpose of sharing information. On-line computer capabilities also help medical and radiation oncologists to develop the best possible treatment plan for each patient.

The department's hours of operation usually begin around 7 a.m. and end in the late afternoon. The workweek is usually five days, although some outpatient cancer centers schedule therapy on Saturdays as well.

A number of institutions have created oncology or cancer centers. Under this concept, inpatient and outpatient cancer treatment services are coordinated with both the medical and radiation oncology professionals working within the same organization. In most cases, such centers are housed within the hospital or in a separate wing of the hospital. One of the main advantages of the oncology center is that all patient scheduling, reception, and record keeping can be fully coordinated by the same staff. From a clinical standpoint, this concept also provides a better environment for the interaction of medical and radiation oncologists. Under the oncology center model, the center is managed by a professional manager who is concerned not only with the day-to-day coordination and functioning of the center, but also concerned with marketing the center to the community. The physician contracts with both medical and radiation oncologists are generally managed by someone from senior management within the hospital.

Models and Systems

The models and systems of the department revolve around one primary goal: the successful treatment of patients suffering from oncological diseases. Although the course of radiation therapy can last up to 22 weeks, depending on the severity of the patient's condition, individual treatments usually last only a matter of minutes, and so the radiation therapy staff must be able to respond effectively to fast turnaround times.

The operations of the department can be divided into three principal areas: initial evaluation of the patient and development of the patient's treatment plan, determination of the specific treatment regimen needed to carry out the treatment plan, and provision of the radiation therapy modalities prescribed in the treatment plan.

A radiation oncologist from the department works with the patient's medical oncologist to evaluate the potential benefit of radiation therapy and develop a treatment plan specific to the patient's condition. The patient's overall treatment plan may include chemotherapy, radiation therapy, or a combination of both. Many times, radiation and chemotherapy are undertaken after the patient has undergone surgery for the removal of malignant tissue. The plan may also include implanting radioisotopes or other materials during surgery to deliver a constant dosage of radiation therapy to specific tissues.

After the patient has been evaluated by his or her physician and the department's radiation oncologist and the treatment plan has been agreed on, the radiation physicist determines the best method of applying radiation therapy for that particular patient. The duties of the physicist include the following (in large hospitals, some or all of the duties might be performed by a dosimetrist or a mold-room technician under the supervision of the physicist):

- Determining the dosage of exposure to radioisotopes or other sources of ionizing radiation. The dosage plans indicate the appropriate penetration angles and the axis referencing for the radiation beam. The plans usually are determined with the aid of an on-line computer, and small departments with limited computer capability are often linked to a larger medical center's computer system for this purpose. The computer helps generate possible dose applications to minimize the possibility of damaging the healthy tissues surrounding the target areas.
- Constructing special shielding to minimize damage to surrounding tissues.
- Performing calculations to verify the dose levels prescribed for the duration of each treatment.
- Calculating doses needed for surgical radiation implant therapy.

After the physicist or dosimetrist has formulated the dosage regimen and calculated the dosages necessary to implement the treatment plan, a radiation therapy technologist carries out the actual therapy by positioning the patient and operating the therapy equipment.

Situations and Problems

The following situations might indicate the need for an efficiency study in the department:

- Inefficient scheduling whereby patients are scheduled in 30-minute time slots, although most therapy applications take less than 15 minutes.
- Full-time patient transporters assigned to a department. This may or may not be justified given that the majority of a department's patient caseload is often walk-in outpatients. Also, inpatients scheduled for therapy might be scheduled at various times of the day, not together, thus making transportation systems inefficient. A management engineer should investigate sharing transportation staff with other departments if this is not already being done (see the Transportation Department profile).
- Suspected high percentage of lost charges.
- Two or more technologists assigned to each piece of equipment when cross-training might eliminate the need to assign two technologists to each therapy unit every day.
- A lack of patients scheduled between 11:00 a.m. and 1:00 p.m. (lunch) and in the late afternoon (after 3:00 p.m.), which results in lost revenue for the department. Radiation therapy equipment is expensive, and it should be fully utilized to offset capital costs.
- Radiation therapy units that have a high percentage of downtime. Machine downtime often creates havoc in patient scheduling and shortfalls in revenue. Traditionally, depart-

ments have signed outside maintenance contracts for servicing their equipment. However, large departments should consider the feasibility of recruiting and hiring their own staff for machine maintenance.

Departmental Analysis

A review or study of a radiation therapy department might include the following areas:

- *Staffing:* Time standards should be established for all procedures in the department, such as cobalt treatment or linear therapy procedures. The end result should be to establish a productivity management report for the department.
- *Patient scheduling:* Two questions should be asked: Does the present schedule optimize staff and equipment time? Is the scheduling system manual or automated? An automated system using a microcomputer may be more efficient than a manual system for a large department.
- *Cost:* The actual cost for all procedures should be determined.
- *Departmental layout:* The physical layout of the department may lead to inefficient patient flow.
- *Word processing:* There should be up-to-date systems to handle clerical functions in the department.
- *Future growth:* The monitoring of growth, the marketing of the service, and the acquisition of new equipment should be given priority.
- *Clinical coordination:* The feasibility of a consolidated medical and radiation oncology center should be considered.

Recent MONITREND data for the radiology-therapeutic functional reporting center are provided in table 20.

Table 20. HAS/MONITREND Data for Radiology-Therapeutic: Six-Month Medians for Period Ending December 1988

	National Bed Size Groups							
Indicator	Under 50	50–74	75–99	100–149	150–199	200–299	300–399	400 and Over
Procedures per adjusted discharge[a]	0.0	0.0	0.06	0.05	0.10	0.10	0.11	0.10
Paid hours per procedure[b]	0.0	0.0	1.34	1.44	1.07	1.27	1.17	1.29

[a]Procedures per adjusted discharge = radiology-therapeutic procedures/(total discharges/radiology-therapeutic RCC). The radiology-therapeutic RCC (ratio of charges to charges) is an adjustment factor that is computed as follows: Radiology-therapeutic RCC = radiology-therapeutic inpatient revenue/(radiology-therapeutic inpatient revenue + radiology-therapeutic outpatient revenue).

[b]Paid hours per procedure = radiology-therapeutic paid hours/radiology-therapeutic procedures.

Source: HAS/MONITREND, 1988. Please refer to page x for more information about the data presented in this table.

Radiology Department

Overview

The radiology department is basically responsible for the recording on film of images produced by X rays as well as for the development and interpretation of X-ray film. These responsibilities are generally referred to as diagnostic radiology. However, rapid technological advances in radiological specialty areas have broadened the focus of most hospital radiology departments to include separate subdepartments or cost centers for diagnostic radiology as well as for ultrasound, nuclear medicine, computerized axial tomography, and magnetic resonance imaging. In fact, it is now common to find radiology departments changing their name to the diagnostic imaging department or the medical imaging department. The structure of the department is determined by the volume of work performed in each specialty.

In addition to performing the various kinds of diagnostic imaging, the radiology department maintains several operational systems: scheduling, reception, registration, indexing, filing, report transcription, patient escort or transportation, and transmission of the final report. The department receives its casework by means of requisitions and referrals from attending physicians. Examination scheduling used to be performed only for fluoroscopies or special procedures, but now it has been expanded to include almost all examinations (particularly outpatient examinations) to provide greater control of work load by hour of the day.

Radiology departments offer 24-hour service. In small hospitals, the 11 p.m. to 7 a.m. shift is staffed by on-call personnel. In general, the majority of examinations are performed during the morning hours, mostly because fluoroscopies, which require that the patient fasts before the testing, are scheduled for the morning.

Most of the work is performed in the main radiology department or in freestanding ambulatory care centers, surgicenters, or diagnostic imaging centers. However, some examinations such as cystoscopies are also performed in the surgical suite with portable machines. The cardiology department usually performs certain diagnostic studies as well, most commonly, ultrasound. Some large hospitals also use satellite X-ray stations, which may be located in the emergency department or other areas of the hospital.

As mentioned earlier, the imaging specialty areas of nuclear medicine, ultrasound, computerized axial tomography, and magnetic resonance imaging are most commonly part of, or very closely related to, the radiology department. Nuclear medicine is the employment of radioisotopes injected into the body to detect abnormal tissue. Usually, nuclear medicine

NOTE: *The authors of this profile acknowledge the source of the descriptions of nuclear medicine, ultrasound, computerized axial tomography, and magnetic resonance imaging to* The Complete Book of Medical Tests *by Mark A. Moskowitz, M.D., and Michael E. Osband, M.D. (New York: Norton, 1984). Readers in need of more in-depth information are urged to consult the full original text.*

193

is part of the radiology department or the pathology department and laboratory. Sometimes it is a separate department altogether.

Ultrasound is an imaging technology that employs sound waves and echos to produce an image. It is steadily gaining in popularity, particularly because it does not utilize radiation.

Computerized axial tomography (often referred to as CT or CAT scanning) is a complex technique that utilizes X rays for studying cross sections of various body parts at different angles. It is particularly well suited for the detection of neurological problems. This technology, introduced in the early 1970s, is now widely available and is fast becoming a primary examination. Hospitals as small as 100 beds may provide CT scanning on-site, and smaller hospitals may share CT scanning services and frequently provide such services through a mobile vendor.

Magnetic resonance imaging (MRI) is the use of radio signals and powerful magnets rather than radiation or sound waves to create an image. It is more expensive than X rays or CT scanning and is relatively new. However, many hospitals have entered into joint ventures to cost-effectively share the use of MRI units on a regularly scheduled basis. Small hospitals frequently provide MRI services through a mobile vendor.

Organization

The radiology department in medium- to large-size hospitals usually includes a radiology administrator and a medical director. The radiology administrator reports to a vice-president or associate administrator. The medical director is a radiologist (a physician who specializes in radiology) who is usually not salaried but rather is paid a professional fee for the interpretation of examinations. Board certification may not be required, but it is preferred because of the complexity of the new imaging procedures. There is increasing specialization and training of radiologists in such areas as echocardiography (ultrasound of the heart), CT scanning, and MRI. Some hospitals are served by a physician radiologist group, which may provide expertise to several hospitals.

Among the other personnel in the department are radiology technologists, who mix contrast media, position the patient, and perform the examination or exposure of film. They are generally trained in two-year or three-year programs, but bachelor's degree programs are also available. Many training programs are hospital based. Certification is given by the American Registry of Radiologic Technologists. A chief technologist usually has managerial as well as technical responsibilities in a small hospital.

Radiology aides and darkroom technicians are usually trained on the job. The aides' function is to provide support for the technologists in positioning patients and carrying out the examinations. The radiology aide may also escort the patients to and from their rooms. Darkroom technicians develop the exposed film and provide the film to the radiologist for interpretation.

Radiology clerks, who act as receptionists and do filing and other clerical tasks, are not required to have special credentials. The typing of the radiologist's report is performed by a transcriber. A radiology transcriber who has been trained in a medical transcription training program is preferred. Some transcribers complete two-year medical secretary programs in which they study radiological terminology.

Models and Systems

The diagnostic imaging process consists of three basic steps: (1) examination, (2) development of film or processing of digital study data, and (3) reading and interpretation of the film or study.

Diagnostic Radiology

There are many types of diagnostic radiographic examinations, each requiring different procedures. These procedures are generally divided into four classifications, as follows:

- *Routine (nonextended) procedures:* Routine procedures usually involve the spine, neck, chest, and extremities (legs, arms, hands, feet) and follow the three basic diagnostic imaging steps. The examination (film exposure) is usually performed by a radiology technologist.
- *Fluoroscopic procedures:* Fluoroscopies (commonly called fluoros) are usually used to study the digestive tract or the urinary tract. Patients receive an injection or enema or are required to swallow a medium before the film is exposed. A specialized machine allows continuous radiographic display of the body area. Film exposures are made by the radiologist, who is viewing the area that is examined. Common fluoroscopic examinations are the gastrointestinal (GI) series (upper and lower), the barium enema, the barium swallow, the gallbladder examination, and the intravenous pyelogram. Unlike routine procedures, fluoroscopies are performed by a radiologist, with assistance from the technologist.

    There are several steps in a fluoroscopic examination. A routine exposure of the abdomen (or scout film) is made before the fluoroscopic examination begins. Next, the patient receives the injection, enema, or medium for swallowing, followed by film exposure and the radiologist's examination. Finally, a routine exposure of the abdomen (or postprocedure film) is made after the fluoroscopic examination. This last exposure is sometimes referred to as one-hour film, post, or overhead. A series of postprocedure films may be taken.
- *Special procedures:* Special procedures are complex fluoroscopies that may require minor surgical procedures. A radiologist performs the examination with assistance from one or more technologists. Such procedures are usually scheduled in advance because they require special preparation.
- *Mammography:* Mammography is the radiographic examination of the breast. Either unilateral or bilateral examinations are performed, but most are bilateral. X-ray film for mammographies is developed to show a positive rather than negative image. The process is called xeroradiography, which utilizes a special developer.

Film exposures are taken from different views, the most common of which are posterior–anterior (PA), lateral, and oblique. Patient visits to the radiology department may require multiple radiographic procedures, and statistics must clearly distinguish between visits and examinations when used for analysis.

A common work-flow model used in radiology is batch processing for fluoroscopies. The actual fluoroscopic examination is performed by a radiologist, but the other films (scout and post) are not. Therefore, patients are guided through the following procedure: (1) all scout films are taken in room A by the technologist only, (2) all fluoroscopies are taken in room B by the radiologist and technologist, and (3) any required post films are taken in room A by the technologist only. The advantage of this flow process is that it reduces the setup time for scout, fluoroscopic, and post films and minimizes the amount of idle time for the radiologist, the technologists, and the equipment. The main disadvantages are to the patient: increased waiting time, additional movement from room to room, and the possibility for feeling lost in the system.

The departmental operations for diagnostic radiology can be summarized through the use of a flow diagram (figure 16) and include the following activities:

- *Reception and registration:* Greet patients, log and schedule appointments, answer telephone, complete registration forms, and process charging and billing data; usually performed by a clerk.

Figure 16. Departmental Operations for Diagnostic Radiology

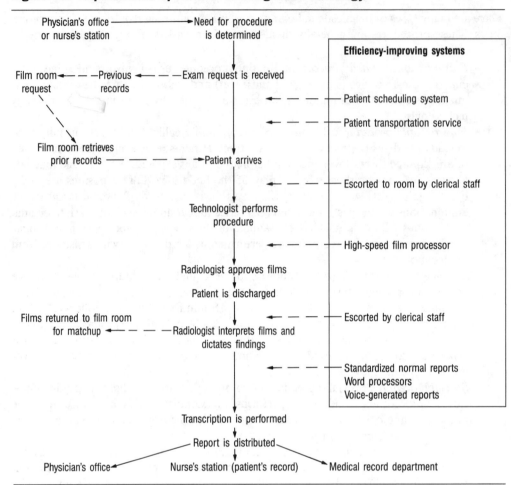

- *Radiographic examination:* X rays are taken as described previously.
- *Development of film:* Generally, the exposed film is fed manually through the film processor and checked for quality. Some radiographic equipment has an automatic developer as part of the camera.
- *Reading and interpretation of film:* The radiologist examines the film, makes a professional interpretation, and usually dictates the report into either a central or local dictating system. Telephone reports to physicians for nonemergency examinations are generally available within 24 hours after the complete procedure.
- *Radiology report transcription:* A medical transcriber or secretary transcribes the report. Transcription may be a centralized or decentralized (departmental) function in a hospital. Contract services are also available. Typically, the report is distributed to the department's file, the medical record department, and the referring physician. In most departments, reports are transcribed on the same day that the examination is performed. Written reports are generally available within two days after the complete procedure. Technological advances in word processing have improved the efficiency of the transcription process. A technology in its developmental stages is the voice-generated report, a typed report that is generated from the electronic interpretation of the user's voice.
- *Indexing and filing:* The indexing system used is similar to the patient record index in the medical record department, but it may also serve as a combination index

and radiographic report file. The radiologist's reading of films is usually dictated, transcribed to a report, and filed in the report file. Films are also retained on file. Retention of the report file and the film file are required to meet applicable statute-of-limitations requirements, which may vary from state to state; however, the contents of the department's record is subject to interpretation and definition on the part of the department.

- *Patient escort or transportation:* Patient escort may be performed by an aide or escorter from the radiology department. Hospitals with a centrally pooled escort service may transport radiology patients by using a call system or by following the examination schedule. The escorting or walking of patients to the dressing room prior to examination time increases the efficiency of the technologist.

Nuclear Medicine

Nuclear medicine consists of a number of tests in which internal tissues and organs can be studied by means of radioisotopes, or materials that give off radiation that can be detected by scanning devices. The type of radioisotope that is chosen for a given test depends on which organ or tissue needs to be evaluated.

The test begins when the patient ingests the radioisotope orally or receives a veinal injection. After a period of time, the radioisotope becomes concentrated in abnormal tissue to a different degree than in normal tissue. A scanning device, called a rectilinear or gamma camera, is positioned over the tissue being studied, and measurements are taken to determine how much radiation is being given off by the various tissues. The camera converts these measurements into a permanent image for interpretation by a radiologist. A written report states the findings for the referring physician.

Nuclear medicine is commonly employed to evaluate the effects of strokes and to detect tumors and inflammation, heart damage, blood clots, and abnormal tissue of the bone, liver, spleen, thyroid, and kidney. Parts of organs can be seen by these means that would not be seen on X-ray film.

Ultrasound

Ultrasound is a technique that enables physicians to see internal tissues by means of sound waves and their echos. The operating principle is that sound waves reflect in different ways depending on the density of the tissue.

The equipment for this technique includes a transducer and an oscilloscope/computer. The transducer is like a microphone except that it both emits sound waves and detects their echos. The area under study is lubricated with mineral oil or some other lubricant to enhance the conductivity of the sound waves, and the technician moves the transducer back and forth over the skin. The oscilloscope/computer converts the echos into a picture on a screen, which can be recorded on special paper. Ultrasound is especially valuable for examining soft tissues, such as the fetus during pregnancy, the heart, the abdomen, and the veins and arteries.

CT Scanning

Computerized axial tomography, or CT scanning, is the use of X rays to study specific planes of the body, that is, cross sections of the chest or of specific organs. It is much more effective than standard X-ray procedures, and it enables physicians to examine parts of the body from many different angles.

To begin the test, the patient is asked to lie down on a special table that constitutes part of the CT scanner. The scanning unit itself looks like a giant ring that encompasses both the table and the patient. Once moved into the appropriate position for a particular study, the scanning unit rotates in a complete circle around the patient, all the while sending an X-ray beam through the patient's body as well as detecting it once it leaves the body. Contrast dyes injected into the patient improve the scanner's ability to detect abnormalities. The resulting beam is analyzed by a computer and converted into an image on a CRT screen. The image displays tissues in various shades of gray, depending on the density or abnormality of the tissue. Permanent pictures are made for review by a radiologist, who conveys his or her findings in a written report.

Generally, CT scanning is of two types: the brain scan and the body scan. In the brain scan, physicians can look for the presence of cancerous tissue or study the effects of a stroke. In the body scan, physicians can detect an enlarged aorta or cancer of the kidney, pancreas, liver, or lung.

Magnetic Resonance Imaging

Magnetic resonance imaging (also called nuclear magnetic resonance) produces an image that is similar to that of a CT scan, but the technique utilizes radio signals and magnetism rather than radiation. The equipment includes a huge magnet so powerful that it can align some of the hydrogen atoms of the body into one direction. This forced alignment is used to detect various densities of body tissue.

To begin the test, the patient is positioned inside the magnet. The magnet is turned on and the atoms become aligned. Seconds later, a radio signal is trained on the body part being studied, which disrupts and energizes the aligned atoms until the signal is cut off. With the signal gone, the atoms again align but at different rates. These rates depend on the type of tissue—bone, fat, liquid—to which the atoms belong.

A computer analyzes the different rates of realignment and translates the data into picture form. As with other types of diagnostic imaging, the radiologist studies the picture and writes his or her report.

Staffing and Productivity

Due to the extensive training required to perform many of the specialty procedures, each specialty area may be staffed separately. However, because of increasing shortages of technologists, administrators are looking for personnel with competency in more than one specialty and are encouraging cross-training of staff.

Normative staffing data are based on paid hours per procedure and, according to recent MONITREND data, may range from 1.3 hours for diagnostic radiology in a hospital of 100 to 149 beds to 1.8 hours for CT procedures in the same size hospital. Other data of this type are provided in tables 21 through 23.

A standardized work-load measurement system for radiology was not available until recently. Radworks, developed by American Healthcare Radiology Administrators, is the beginning of such a system and may help departments to study productivity and determine appropriate levels of staffing.

Departmental Analysis

An analysis of the radiology department might include all functions of the department, or it might focus on such specific problems as upcoming construction, budgeting, new billing systems, and establishing cost-effective mobile unit services.

The performance and productivity of the department can be measured by quantifying such factors as volume and mix of examination procedures, room utilization, and staff utilization. Such a study may include determining actual start and stop times for activities while taking into account such differentiations as the type of patient, the room, the number of staff, the type of examination, the waiting time, the number of people in the waiting room, simultaneous examinations, the hour of day, the day of week, and delays in patient processing. The institution of a management reporting system can help ensure ongoing monitoring of productivity in these ways.

Staffing can be determined on the basis of quantitative data plus other factors such as vacation, sickness, holiday, indirect activities, idle time inherent in the system (equipment breakdown or scheduled maintenance, for example), and nonproductive time. The skill level required for departmental activities should also be analyzed.

Most radiology department managers have utilized time standards by type of examination to implement a case mix–sensitive, labor-based relative value system to monitor productivity and establish optimum staffing levels. The professional organization for radiology managers has actively supported this relative value system. In addition, many managers have performed product costing and cost-based charging analyses, which are particularly useful as hospitals establish relationships with managed care systems.

Table 21. HAS/MONITREND Data for Radiology-Diagnostic: Six-Month Medians for Period Ending December 1988

Indicator	National Bed Size Groups							
	Under 50	50–74	75–99	100–149	150–199	200–299	300–399	400 and Over
Procedures per adjusted discharge[a]	1.63	1.98	1.90	2.10	2.09	2.33	2.49	2.50
Paid hours per procedure[b]	1.19	1.15	1.22	1.32	1.34	1.43	1.48	1.60

[a]Procedures per adjusted discharge = radiology-diagnostic procedures/(total discharges/radiology-diagnostic RCC). The radiology-diagnostic RCC (ratio of charges to charges) is an adjustment factor that is computed as follows: Radiology-diagnostic RCC = radiology-diagnostic inpatient revenue/(radiology-diagnostic inpatient revenue + radiology-diagnostic outpatient revenue).

[b]Paid hours per procedure = radiology-diagnostic paid hours/radiology-diagnostic procedures.

Source: HAS/MONITREND, 1988. Please refer to page x for more information about the data presented in this table.

Table 22. HAS/MONITREND Data for CT Scanner: Six-Month Medians for Period Ending December 1988

Indicator	National Bed Size Groups							
	Under 50	50–74	75–99	100–149	150–199	200–299	300–399	400 and Over
Procedures per calendar day[a]	0.82	1.63	2.54	4.40	7.30	10.99	14.51	23.02
Paid hours per procedure[b]	0.83	1.38	1.74	1.84	1.71	1.62	1.77	1.87

[a]Procedures per calendar day = CT scanner procedures/days in period.

[b]Paid hours per procedure = CT scanner paid hours/CT scanner procedures.

Source: HAS/MONITREND, 1988. Please refer to page x for more information about the data presented in this table.

Table 23. HAS/MONITREND Data for Nuclear Medicine: Six-Month Medians for Period Ending December 1988

Indicator	National Bed Size Groups							
	Under 50	50–74	75–99	100–149	150–199	200–299	300–399	400 and Over
Paid hours per adjusted patient day[a]	0.02	0.04	0.04	0.05	0.05	0.05	0.05	0.06

[a]Paid hours per adjusted patient day = nuclear medicine paid hours/(total patient days/nuclear medicine RCC). The nuclear medicine RCC (ratio of charges to charges) is an adjustment factor that is computed as follows: Nuclear medicine RCC = nuclear medicine inpatient revenue/(nuclear medicine inpatient revenue + nuclear medicine outpatient revenue).

Source: HAS/MONITREND, 1988. Please refer to page x for more information about the data presented in this table.

Improvements in departmental systems might be gained from a study of the following factors:

- The scheduling of patients and the feasibility of scheduling staff based on work load by hour of the day
- The transportation of patients to and from radiology appointments
- The efficacy of clerical systems (this includes reviewing the filing system, including access, retrieval, merging, registration, logging, and transcription; file retention policies should also be analyzed; and the radiology record system should be compatible with the medical record system)
- The physical layout of the department
- Forms use and design
- Systems for effective and efficient communication

Other topics for study include preventive maintenance contracts, equipment costs, purchasing policies and procedures, the charging structure, and the possibility for silver recovery from film processors.

Renal Dialysis Department

Overview

Although there is no known cure for chronic renal failure, there are currently three treatment options: hemodialysis, peritoneal dialysis, and transplantation. Renal disease is estimated to occur in 151 people per million population per year. Nationally, there are about 98,000 patients currently undergoing dialysis, with about 80,000 in hospitals and 18,000 at home. Approximately 9,000 kidney transplants are performed annually.

Hemodialysis involves the removal of waste products from a patient's blood through the use of a dialysis machine, a process that takes an average of three to four hours, three times per week. Peritoneal dialysis does not involve a dialysis machine, but instead involves the instillation of an electrolyte solution (dialysate) into the peritoneal cavity via an indwelling catheter. Electrolyte balance is accomplished by the movement of ions from the blood across the peritoneum and into the dialysate solution, which is then drained from the peritoneal cavity. This method uses an average of four to five exchanges per day. Peritoneal dialysis in the inpatient setting is usually performed by staff nurses from the medical/surgical nursing unit rather than by the renal dialysis unit or its nurses. However, peritoneal dialysis is no longer limited to the inpatient setting. Many institutions have taught end-stage renal disease (ESRD) patients all the skills needed to enable them to perform continuous ambulatory peritoneal dialysis (CAPD) at home. Nationally, approximately 17 percent of dialysis patients are on CAPD. This program has been extremely satisfying for those patients who are capable of controlling their treatment and who value being independent from a fixed hemodialysis treatment schedule. Transplants are the third treatment option, but this option is not always available or appropriate for all patients.

Organization

The organizational structure of the renal dialysis department depends on the range of services offered, but a typical reporting structure for an institution offering a full range of acute and chronic inpatient and outpatient renal dialysis services is illustrated in figure 17.

Inpatient dialysis may consist of peritoneal dialysis at the patient's bedside or hemodialysis in the inpatient hemodialysis unit. The inpatient unit also serves as the emergency backup for CAPD patients who develop complications and require hemodialysis.

Chronic hemodialysis units customarily are open six days per week, Monday through Saturday, and the hours of operation depend on the number of stations and the volume of patients. Patients are customarily scheduled for treatments on a Monday–Wednesday–Friday or a Tuesday–Thursday–Saturday calendar.

Figure 17. Typical Reporting Structure for a Renal Dialysis Department

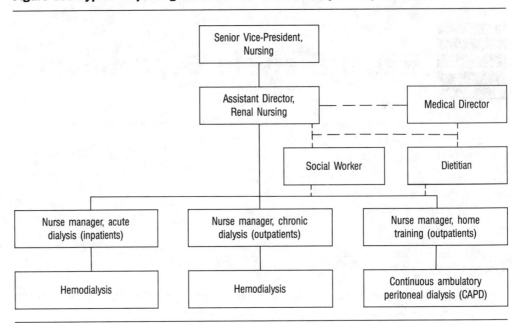

Hemodialysis units have a medical director who oversees the quality of medical care provided to the facility's patients. The medical director typically participates in administrative decisions regarding policies, supplies, and equipment. The medical director is also the principal liaison between the nephrologists who admit patients and the hemodialysis unit.

Patient care is customarily managed through the use of an interdisciplinary treatment team made up of a physician, a nurse, a social worker, and a dietitian. The registered nurse assumes the responsibility for all the professional issues related to the patient's care. These duties include patient assessments, care planning, administering intravenous medications, and supervising all the technical aspects of direct patient care. Licensed practical nurses and technicians work under the supervision of registered nurses to provide most of the direct patient care. These duties include putting patients on machines, taking vital signs, monitoring the dialysis machines, and taking the patients off the machines.

As required by federal regulations, the social worker on the treatment team addresses the psychosocial needs of the patients. The social worker customarily helps the patients to arrange transportation and to cope with the stress, depression, or changes in life-style that accompany chronic disease.

A dietitian is also required by federal regulations. Dialysis treatment alone is not sufficient to maintain the patient's long-term health. Dietary restrictions must be followed, and patients must be instructed, consulted, and monitored regarding needed dietary adjustments and compliance. Federal regulations also require that a transplant surgeon participate in managing each patient's care, and an agreement must exist between the dialysis facility and a transplant center. Interdisciplinary patient care conferences are required to review and update each patient's needs and prescription for therapy.

Hemodialysis units also typically have one or more supply aides. These personnel are responsible for ordering and storing all inventory and outside purchase supplies as well as any sterile instruments, kits, or supplies.

Home dialysis (CAPD) training units are customarily open Monday through Friday during daytime working hours. A nurse is available by pager to cover the hours that the home training unit is closed. The CAPD client is customarily taught that treatment of renal failure includes diet and fluid modification, medication therapy, and dialysis. A renal dietitian is actively involved in the diet and fluid modification training. The clients in CAPD training are taught the principles of continuous ambulatory peritoneal dialysis, normal kidney function, and what happens to the body when the kidneys fail to function properly. They are taught about their particular renal disease—symptoms, significance of blood chemistry values, measurement of weight, blood pressure, vital signs, and sterile and aseptic techniques. Most important, the clients are taught to assume responsibility for planning their care and treatment along with members of the home training team. During CAPD training, the client is taught how to perform solution exchanges and catheter care and what to do if spike or solution set contamination should occur. They are also taught to recognize the signs and symptoms of peritonitis, the major complication of CAPD. A CAPD nurse is on call 24 hours a day if contamination should occur and the client needs to come to the hospital for a solution transfer set change.

Operational Systems

This section describes operational systems for both hemodialysis and home dialysis.

Hemodialysis

Operational systems in chronic hemodialysis units are customarily designed to ensure the smooth flow of patients and a steady but optimum work load for staff. To this end, patient appointment times are customarily staggered because a large proportion of the work load is concentrated at the start and end of a dialysis run (getting the patient on and off the dialysis machine). Daily schedules must provide time for staff breaks and time to clean and set up the dialysis machine for the next patient. During the three- to four-hour run, dialysis nurses monitor the patient's vital signs and provide patient education and emotional support while monitoring fluid balance and watching for signs and symptoms of uremia or hypotension.

Many disposable supplies are utilized during a patient's hemodialysis treatment, for example, dialysate, blood lines, intravenous saline bags, artificial kidneys, needles, syringes, and so forth. Storage areas for these supplies should be an integral part of space planning. Planning considerations should also include the availability of backup machines, an isolation station for hepatitis B and human immunodeficiency virus-positive patients, and separate patient and staff bathrooms and eating areas. Ancillary equipment includes centrifuges, activated clotting machines, conductivity meters, and scales to weigh patients before and after each treatment. Current regulations require 110 square feet of space per treatment station, and each station is typically equipped with a dialysis machine, a reclining chair, an individual television, a blood pressure cuff, an airway, and a bite stick. Recent treatment trends include the more common and accepted reuse of the artificial kidney. Better equipment and standards have made reuse of the artificial kidney a safe and beneficial practice, both financially and with respect to patient care. For example, better equipment and standards have decreased the frequency of first-use syndrome, an immune response affecting approximately 10 to 20 percent of patients when an artificial kidney is used for the first time.

Hemodialysis facilities usually find it necessary to provide water treatment as an integral part of making dialysis machines operational. Water treatment can be accomplished through a variety of methods such as reverse osmosis, deionization, and carbon filters.

Professional staff in hemodialysis units customarily undergo an extensive orientation period (six to eight weeks of training is not uncommon), which consists of both classroom and clinical experience. This program describes equipment operation, the disease process, medications, diet, and psychosocial issues.

Reimbursement for outpatient hemodialysis is provided through the federal government (Medicare) under the end-stage renal disease (ESRD) program. A composite rate is established for each facility, and care must be provided within the established rate. Medicare reimburses 80 percent; secondary insurers pay the remaining 20 percent. It is estimated that it costs $25,000 per year to hemodialyze one patient. Hemodialysis facilities are inspected for compliance with ESRD regulations through the U.S. Department of Public Health. Hospital-based dialysis facilities are also regulated by Joint Commission on Accreditation of Healthcare Organizations requirements.

Home Dialysis

Although the government favors home dialysis, it is not always a feasible treatment option for every patient. The patient's potential as a home training candidate depends on his or her medical condition, emotional stability, home situation, and desire and ability to learn.

Home dialysis training units are responsible 24 hours a day for all the patients at home plus patients in training. The ESRD program allows 12 training sessions for each patient on how to perform self-dialysis. Certain laboratory tests are routinely performed monthly or at specified intervals. Any training over 12 sessions or tests in addition to these covered must be justified by the provider in writing. They are then either paid for or denied by the Medicare intermediary. Following the training period, patients are seen by appointment for monthly follow-up care.

The hospital receives prospective reimbursement from Medicare for providing home dialysis training, supplies, emergency backup, and monthly follow-up. The reimbursement rate is based on the wage index of fixed geographical areas. The cost of CAPD supplies ranges from $8,000 to $12,000 per year, depending on the equipment used. The cost of dialysis training and supplies used during training and thereafter at home are paid for from day one as follows: 80 percent by the primary insurer and 20 percent by Medicare for the first 12 months and 80 percent by Medicare and 20 percent by the primary insurer thereafter.

Extensive CAPD orientation and certification in patient CAPD procedures is ongoing for the registered nurses and licensed practical nurses who staff home training units, intensive care units, and inpatient units.

Situations and Problems

Departments providing chronic or home training dialysis services must deal with professional issues as well as operational problems. The major professional issue is keeping current with the latest technological changes. Active literature reviews and extensive in-service education are both important parts of a successful program. The major operational problems are scheduling patients and coordinating each patient's care. Scheduling patients can be difficult when patients are delayed while receiving diagnostic care in other departments (for example, radiology). Coordinating each patient's care can be extremely difficult when multiple dietary revisions must be made while medications are being adjusted.

Staffing and Productivity

Staffing levels for hemodialysis units primarily depend on patient volume and the effectiveness of the schedule in stabilizing work load and work flow. Staffing systems based on patient acuity have also been developed and published. At the very least, a licensed nurse is required whenever a patient is being dialyzed. Staggered patient schedules permit nurses to care for multiple patients. Typical units plan a staffing ratio of one nurse for two and one-half patients going up to a maximum of one nurse to three patients when necessary due to sick calls and other factors. In the course of each eight-hour shift, each nurse might see five or six patients but would not complete five or six treatments because two or three patients would carry over to the next nursing shift.

Staffing levels for home training units are much lower than for hemodialysis units. An average nurse-to-patient ratio for staffing in dialysis home training units is one nurse to twelve patients, but this ratio ranges from one to five to one to twenty, depending on the size and growth potential of the unit.

Recent MONITREND data for the hemodialysis functional reporting center are provided in table 24.

Traditional productivity-monitoring systems include variable standards for patient-related activities and constant standards for support functions. An example of a variable standard is: 2.30 variable required hours per chronic dialysis unit patient. An example of a constant standard is: 6.14 hours of clerical support per day of unit operation.

Productivity-monitoring systems are well suited to the structured setting of a hemodialysis unit. This is particularly true when standards can be accurately developed and reliably applied using a validated patient acuity system. The variability of supporting CAPD patients operationally and emotionally in individual home settings makes establishing variable standards much more difficult.

Departmental Analysis

Topics of study for analyzing the renal dialysis department might include the following:

- *Staffing and scheduling:* Matching staff hours to the patient schedule and patient volumes. Staggering patient arrivals to reduce work-load peaks and to make it easier for one nurse to care for more than one patient at a time.
- *Patient flow/patient delay analysis:* Analyzing the types and magnitudes of delays and recommending operational or scheduling alternatives.
- *Productivity-monitoring systems:* Developing variable and constant work-load standards to provide routine comparisons between the amount of work performed and the labor resources required to handle that work load.
- *Patient acuity systems:* Implementing a system for quantitatively assessing the care required by each patient through the use of patient care indicators. Although widely implemented for most nursing inpatient units, such a system has not yet been developed or published for renal nursing patients.
- *Quality assurance systems:* Implementing nursing quality assurance programs, which commonly focus on professional practice issues, such as patient teaching, documentation, and ensuring that established standards of care are being delivered. Unitwide quality assurance programs commonly focus on problem-solving issues and discussion of current advances and innovations described in the literature.
- *Purchasing and stocking procedures:* Implementing sound materials management practices such as minimum order points, economic order quantities, and inventory turnover targets.

Table 24. HAS/MONITREND Data for Hemodialysis: Six-Month Medians for Period Ending December 1988

Indicator	National Bed Size Groups							
	Under 50	50–74	75–99	100–149	150–199	200–299	300–399	400 and Over
Treatments per calendar day[a]	0.0	0.0	0.88	0.85	6.00	6.29	4.50	6.13
Paid hours per treatment[b]	0.0	0.0	4.54	5.02	4.01	4.16	5.14	5.10

[a]Treatments per calendar day = hemodialysis treatments/days in period.

[b]Paid hours per treatment = hemodialysis paid hours/hemodialysis treatments.

Source: HAS/MONITREND, 1988. Please refer to page x for more information about the data presented in this table.

Respiratory Care Department

Overview

Respiratory care is a relatively new specialty; it was first practiced in the mid-1950s and early 1960s. Although some institutions organized formal departments during this period, many hospitals simply employed "oxygen orderlies." Today, most departments are less than 20 years old.

There are two types of services provided by respiratory care departments: diagnostic and therapeutic. The diagnostic services section most commonly performs pulmonary function testing, arterial blood gas analysis, and monitoring and analysis of exhaled gases. Pulmonary function testing is the assessment of the effectiveness of a patient's lung function. Most pulmonary function testing is done by having the patient exhale and measuring the exhaled volume over a period of time. This may also include studies of gas exchange and may be repeated as needed to follow the patient's progress or regress. In addition to pulmonary function testing, the diagnostic services section may assist with stress testing, bronchoscopies, electrocardiograms, and echocardiograms.

Therapeutic services include a large number of treatment modalities that represent the majority of the department's work load. Common forms of therapy include incentive spirometry, postural drainage, chest physiotherapy, oxygen therapy, aerosol therapy, intermittent positive pressure breathing (IPPB), metered dose inhalers, and ventilator care. These forms of therapy can be described as follows:

- *Incentive spirometry:* For patients who may have a condition that hinders them from taking a deep breath, incentive spirometry is an inspiratory maneuver that encourages patients to take a deep breath. Deeper breathing reduces the likelihood of pulmonary complications. Different devices measure the inspiratory volume and provide an indicator to encourage a patient to reach a higher volume. The goal is to have the patient repeatedly take slow, deep breaths and hold those breaths for three to five seconds.
- *Postural drainage:* Postural drainage is a therapy used to encourage the drainage of mucus or foreign matter out of the lung. The patient is placed on an adjustable table or bed in various positions in order to drain the mucus or foreign matter from the 10 segments of the right lung and 8 segments of the left. Each segment empties into the main airway at a different angle.
- *Chest physiotherapy:* Chest physiotherapy is the rhythmic application of the hands or a pneumatic percusser to the chest to facilitate the removal of secretions from the segments of the lung. Vibration of the chest may also be applied by hands or vibrator. Chest physiotherapy is used with postural drainage. Deep breathing exercises may also be done between periods of chest physiotherapy.

- *Oxygen therapy:* Oxygen therapy is the administration of oxygen to a patient to prevent or relieve a low blood oxygen condition. Oxygen can be administered via a wide variety of devices including cannulas, simple masks, partial rebreather masks, nonrebreather masks, aerosol therapy (water/saline particles suspended in a gas), and ventilator therapy. Levels of oxygen can be monitored noninvasively by pulse oximetry or invasively by drawing arterial blood specimens.

- *Aerosol therapy:* Aerosol therapy is the treatment of an illness or condition by the inhalation of aerosol particles, which may include medication, water, or saline. The most commonly used tool for aerosol therapy is the hand-held nebulizer with medications. In another type of therapy, heated aerosols are given to patients through artificial airways that bypass the nose and mouth. The heated aerosols replace the function of the nose by warming and humidifying the inspired air. Aerosol generators may be disposable or permanent. Permanent aerosol generators commonly include cool mist tents and ultrasonic nebulizers.

- *Intermittent positive pressure breathing (IPPB):* Treatment by IPPB involves the administration of deep breaths to a patient by using a device that administers measured quantities of air and/or oxygen under pressure. Positive pressure is the indicated treatment when patients need to take bigger breaths than they can generate on their own or when patients have become psychologically attached to the positive pressure breath. This treatment may not be effective when too much or not enough pressure is used. The volume of breath must be monitored to ensure that a larger than normal breath is being administered.

- *Metered dose inhalers:* Metered dose inhalers are small aerosol cannisters that give medications at a precisely metered dose. Patients must be taught the proper way to use metered dose inhalers or the inhalers are of no value. Patients unable to manipulate the device or take a deep breath on their own are not candidates for metered dose inhalers. Although metered dose inhalers are not new, many hospitals are showing renewed interest in them as a less expensive form of medication delivery than handheld nebulizers.

- *Ventilator care:* Patients are placed on ventilators (sometimes inappropriately called respirators) because of respiratory failure or impending respiratory failure. The basic ventilator provides three features: the oxygen percentage, the breaths per minute, and the breath. Various other mechanical, diagnostic, or pneumatic devices may be available on different makes and models. The respiratory practitioner is responsible for knowing which type of ventilator would be most appropriate for each type of patient. The respiratory practitioner is also responsible for ensuring that all alarms, parameters, and other diagnostic equipment are set up, operational, and appropriate for the patient's illness or condition. The physician must order each item and parameter, but the practitioner should be qualified and prepared to recommend and explain how the equipment can best be utilized. Ventilator care also includes the suctioning of the artificial airway, stabilization of the artificial airway, ventilator parameter checks, medication delivery, and diagnostic monitoring or tests.

Inpatients, outpatients, and emergency patients receive therapy for a variety of conditions, but inpatient care usually represents at least 90 percent of the department's work load. The inpatient population therefore determines the work load of the respiratory department to a much greater extent than it might in other departments. However, the implementation of reimbursement based on diagnosis-related groups has greatly decreased the work load of many respiratory therapy departments because some treatments (IPPB in particular) have come under sharp attack by a number of groups that question the treatments' efficacy and value.

Historically, IPPB made up a large portion of the department work load. As the use of IPPB therapy has decreased, the growth of departmental work load has leveled off because the use of other therapies has not filled the gap. Reimbursement for other treatment modalities has also declined, making the respiratory care department less of a revenue-generating department than it once was.

The home care of patients represents a potentially significant market for respiratory care departments. Legislation is pending that would, depending on licensure, approve Medicare home care reimbursement certification for respiratory therapy practitioners. At present, the reimbursement structure encourages patients to rent equipment. Even in this setting, hospitals have the opportunity to subcontract with rental companies to provide therapists' services for instruction and follow-up.

Organization

The respiratory care department generally consists of a manager or technical director, supervisors of functional areas (depending on the size of the department), and therapists and technicians. A medical director is required by Joint Commission on Accreditation of Healthcare Organizations (JCAHO) standards to be responsible for medical matters and may work either part-time or full-time, depending on the department's size. The medical director may be an anesthesiologist, a pulmonary specialist, or another type of physician with an interest in respiratory care.

Two types of workers commonly found in the respiratory care department are the certified respiratory therapy technician (CRTT) and the registered respiratory therapist (RRT). A CRTT has 12 to 18 months of training and has passed an examination administered by the National Board for Respiratory Care. An RRT has 2 to 4 years of training and has passed both a CRTT and an RRT examination, also administered by the Board for Respiratory Care. A specialty examination for neonatal/pediatric care is currently being developed.

The RRTs and CRTTs report to supervisors and/or medical directors. The JCAHO recommends that the department manager or technical director be an RRT. Typically, the manager or director needs three to five years of experience, with at least three years of supervisory experience. Supervisors usually need one to three years of experience and usually need to be certified and/or registered. A registered therapist is generally preferred.

Many hospitals do not distinguish job responsibilities for CRTTs and RRTs. The pay scale, however, is different. For those hospitals that do distinguish between CRTT and RRT responsibilities, the RRT is more likely to perform the managerial, supervisory, and teaching functions, with the CRTTs reporting to the RRTs.

In the diagnostic services section of the department, two other types of workers may be employed—the certified pulmonary function technologist (CPFT) and the registered pulmonary function technologist (RPFT). The technologists have completed specialized training in pulmonary function testing and equipment and have passed examinations administered by the National Board for Respiratory Care.

Staffing patterns are designed according to the department's work load, with most staff members scheduled during the day and evening shifts. Night staff may consist of one or two persons, depending on the patient need, the size of the facility, and the department's policy. Most departments provide services 24 hours a day, seven days a week, without varying staff from day to day in spite of potential variances in the work load. However, the hours of operation depend on the size of the hospital, the department's work load, and the patient mix.

Some of the smallest hospitals have explored alternatives to providing night-shift respiratory therapist coverage when there are no patients on ventilators. The option of using on-call staff has proved practical only when nursing services has agreed to cover respiratory functions and when the on-call personnel are close enough to the hospital to satisfy emergency response guidelines.

Many respiratory care departments have been reorganized in combination with electro-cardiology (EKG) and electroencephalography (EEG) departments to form cardiopulmonary service departments. As a result, cardiology and pulmonary diagnostic testing have been integrated into a cardiopulmonary laboratory unit. This merger has provided both improved, integrated cardiopulmonary services and the opportunity for improved staff utilization.

Models and Systems

The respiratory care department is likely to be centralized, although large hospitals may take a decentralized approach in specialty areas. Almost all therapeutic work is performed at the bedside. Diagnostic functions may be performed at the bedside (especially in the intensive care unit), but most diagnostic work is performed in the department. Cross-training between the therapeutic and diagnostic services sections is common, especially in small hospitals and in hospitals where the hours of operation of the therapeutic area are longer than those of the diagnostic area.

Respiratory therapy equipment may be either manual or automated. In the therapeutic area, automated equipment is required for the treatment of severe illnesses. The diagnostic area primarily uses automated equipment, particularly for testing purposes. The clinical computer has recently been introduced to the department and is being used particularly in the pulmonary laboratory.

The department may use a combination of disposable and reusable equipment. The reusable equipment may be cleaned and sterilized either in the respiratory care department or in central supply. Disposable equipment for patient units may be stored and replenished either by the department or by central supply.

The department director is responsible for the selection and purchasing of major pieces of equipment for the department. Daily supplies may be procured, stored, and distributed by any respiratory staff member as assigned and trained by the department director. Some of the routine ordering and stocking can be delegated to clerical support staff.

Paperwork systems are almost always manual. A clerk or secretary may transcribe workload data provided by the respiratory care staff onto charge slips, and charges may be handled manually. The technologist staff may also perform this function.

Situations and Problems

The fact that much of the work is performed away from the department makes it difficult for supervisors to assign appropriate personnel for various tasks. As a result, the proper use of equipment, which must be mobile but accounted for at all times, can be difficult. Breakage of small but expensive equipment is a related problem.

The charging system is another area of concern because most departments use manual rather than automated methods for transcription of therapists' and technicians' data for income purposes. Cash flow can be affected adversely by untimely posting of charges and by lost charges.

A third area of concern is that, in some departments, some of the work ordered may not be performed. In the past, as a result of staffing shortages, treatments were sometimes ordered and not provided. Although this is becoming less a problem as the department's work load decreases, quality control considerations dictate the importance of monitoring and documenting cases when work was ordered but has not been performed. In some cases, however, the respiratory care supervisor may have decided that the ordered therapy was not necessary. It is therefore important that the department director and medical director develop protocols for defining what is appropriate respiratory care.

A fourth concern is that respiratory therapists tend to become managers on the basis of technical rather than administrative skills. This may result in a poorly run or inefficient department. More respiratory schools are now offering management classes and/or a clinical rotation with managers.

A major political concern relates to the control of the department. Administratively and medically, the department manager may report to a physician who is seldom present in the department. A difficult working environment as well as supervisory problems may result.

Financial conflicts between the hospital and the medical director may occur because the medical director may receive a percentage of the department's income. Because the physician may also be a primary source of orders for services to be rendered by the department, this presents a potential conflict of interest.

Utilization of the department's services is often directly related to the amount of time devoted by the medical director to the education of the medical staff. This is part of the reason for the leveling off of the department's work load. Saturation of the market is the other major factor. The number of physicians who have become more knowledgeable about respiratory care has grown so that it is no longer a novelty.

Departmental Analysis

Because the work load of the department is determined by the inpatient population and the seasonal nature of some respiratory diseases (for example, influenza and asthma), fluctuating work loads throughout the year require analysis. The use of respiratory program students as part-time employees has been successful in some hospitals for providing greater flexibility during seasonal variations. Also, cross-training personnel and combining respiratory care with EKG and EEG increase the flexibility of the department in small hospitals.

In addition to analyzing work load, evaluations should address staffing, equipment, and systems. With regard to staffing, consideration should be given to hiring staff with appropriate levels of skills. For example, clerical or cleaning tasks performed by therapists might be handled by less-skilled and lower-paid personnel instead.

Among the many topics for analysis are the following:

- All positions and functions; task assignments, balance of work load, and documentation of individual performance of task assignments; appropriateness of task allocation in relation to the type of employee. One difficulty of such an analysis is that, although the typical department is centralized, the work performed by staff is decentralized. For comparisons of work-load units and paid hours in hospitals of various sizes, see the recent MONITREND data provided in table 25 for the respiratory therapy functional reporting center.
- Systems and information processing; charge system; flow patterns; reduction of duplication of effort; maximization of income; reduction of work not completed; timeliness of departmental processes.

Table 25. HAS/MONITREND Data for Respiratory Therapy: Six-Month Medians for Period Ending December 1988

Indicator	National Bed Size Groups							
	Under 50	50–74	75–99	100–149	150–199	200–299	300–399	400 and Over
Work-load units per adjusted patient day[a]	1.97	2.36	1.45	1.75	1.25	1.13	1.31	1.63
Treatments per adjusted patient day[b]	1.19	1.25	1.30	1.27	1.31	1.21	1.31	1.40
Paid hours per adjusted patient day[c]	0.66	0.84	0.81	0.64	0.64	0.58	0.60	0.67
Work-load units per treatment[d]	0.90	1.28	1.01	0.78	0.92	1.05	0.70	1.31
Paid hours per 100 work-load units[e]	30.67	25.00	36.76	60.91	46.97	51.16	51.72	50.23

[a]Work-load units per adjusted patient day = respiratory work-load units/(total patient days/respiratory therapy RCC). The respiratory therapy RCC (ratio of charges to charges) is an adjustment factor that is computed as follows: Respiratory therapy RCC = respiratory therapy inpatient revenue/(respiratory therapy inpatient revenue + respiratory therapy outpatient revenue).

[b]Treatments per adjusted patient day = respiratory treatments/(total patient days/respiratory therapy RCC).

[c]Paid hours per adjusted patient day = respiratory paid hours/(total patient days/respiratory therapy RCC).

[d]Work-load units per treatment = respiratory work-load units/respiratory treatments.

[e]Paid hours per 100 work-load units = respiratory paid hours/(respiratory work-load units/100).

Source: HAS/MONITREND, 1988. Please refer to page x for more information about the data presented in this table.

- Equipment use; capital equipment needs; reduction of delay factors; use of disposables versus reusable supplies.
- Department's size and location; storage requirements; work sites; systems for disbursement of equipment; procedures for start/stop notification of therapy orders; procedures for equipment cleaning, turnover, and supply stock levels.
- Compliance with JCAHO standards.

Other projects for departmental analysis include the following:

- Development of a quality control and monitoring program
- Cost analysis of disposable versus reusable items, space requirements, and supplies
- Implementation planning for such new systems as a computerized order-entry/charge-entry system
- Cost analysis of services or equipment
- Layout analysis of department to accommodate basic flow
- Improvement of the department's policies and procedures

Although respiratory care departments are not as large or as profitable as they were years ago, they still perform an important role in patient care and patient safety. Much of the department's recognition within the hospital comes from its knowledge of ventilator care. However, the outpatient community knows it best for its treatment of chronic respiratory conditions.

Risk Management Department

Overview

Risk management in health care is a function that strives to reduce or control potential financial loss from clinical activities (professional liability), loss of property, and/or employee activities. This function traces its origins to the so-called malpractice insurance crisis of the mid-1970s. Before that time, the functions now conducted by hospital risk management were usually performed by commercial insurers and their brokers. However, as commercial liability insurance became difficult and expensive to obtain, hospitals saw the need to manage their own exposure to risk. The profession of health care risk management was born out of this need.

Activities and Responsibilities

Risk management is a process that requires the identification of potential risks, the evaluation or measurement of those risks, the choice of methods to handle the risks (either by risk control, risk financing, or more likely, a combination of methods), the implementation of a plan, and finally, the constant evaluation of the method(s) employed. The person charged with identifying potential risk exposures is the risk manager. He or she gets information from a number of sources, including but not limited to the following:

- Incident reports (reports that document the particular facts of an accident or misadventure such as an employee's injury or a patient's ingesting the wrong medication)
- Patient complaints
- Committee reports, including quality assurance, tissue review, and safety
- Reports of legal actions
- Security reports
- Requests for medical records
- Third-party reports (for example, those of the Joint Commission on Accreditation of Healthcare Organizations, state agencies, and the peer review organization)

The risk manager must evaluate, in terms of severity, individual occurrences requiring specific and immediate actions as well as the trends or frequency of occurrence of certain events that may indicate the potential for a severe loss. In gathering and evaluating this information, risk managers rely on an effective data base or risk management information system (RMIS) to abstract information so that trends can be monitored. Sometimes, hospitals may choose to have data tabulated or interpreted by an external data service. The data obtained, although useful to the risk manager, also serve as an information source for the quality assurance function and may also be required by the commercial liability insurer of the facility. In addition, many facilities have an interdisciplinary committee that is concerned with the function of risk management, and such information obtained and maintained by the risk manager is reviewed by that committee.

In identifying and evaluating risk situations, the risk manager helps to enable the hospital's administration to know of situations and conditions in which specific corrective action may be needed. Meetings involving the administration, departmental managers, and/or senior managers may formalize specific changes to policies, procedures, and practices for eliminating or minimizing the exposure to risk. A task force or working group may be created, or a specific department may be assigned the responsibility for addressing specific problems.

Organization and Staffing

The organization, size, and reporting relationships of the risk management function in a hospital depend on its defined role and mission, both of which are determined by several factors:

- The size of the facility
- The management and organization of the facility
- The setting or mission of the facility
- The administration's perception of the function of risk management
- The type or method of risk financing employed by the facility (for example, self-insurance, commercial insurance, pooled insurance, or a combination of these)

Large facilities may have one to three full-time persons dedicated to the risk management function. An effective risk management program requires well-trained personnel not only to review incident reports, but also to carry out the other duties now associated with risk management. For example, in many hospitals the risk management function also includes claims investigation and claims evaluation and management, which require specialized training and skills beyond the clinical aspects of risk management.

Risk financing requires personnel who are knowledgeable about the operation of the insurance market, insurance contracts, and the underwriting requirements of insurance companies. Such personnel have specific knowledge about hospital professional liability insurance, automobile and aircraft liability insurance, director's and officer's liability insurance, general liability insurance, and the various property insurance and worker's compensation insurance coverages.

In small facilities, risk management may be performed by a person who has other administrative responsibilities, for example, safety, patient representation, or quality assurance. The emphasis in small programs may be more on the clinical aspects of risk management than on the broader range of functions performed by risk managers of large institutions. Nevertheless, with the growing interest in all exposures to loss as well as in government regulation and the JCAHO's recent mandate for risk management, the duties of risk management are expanding even in small facilities.

As the duties and depth of responsibilities of the risk management function increase, this function will most likely report to higher and higher levels of authority, even to the chief executive officer or to the hospital's board of trustees. The more successful and complete risk management programs have the unqualified support of the highest levels of management and governance.

Situations and Problems

An effective risk management program requires the participation and cooperation of all departments within the facility, including the medical staff. Effective lines of communication are essential. Nevertheless, the natural reluctance on the part of individuals to draw attention to their potential faults often creates a problem for the risk manager in obtaining prompt and current information about potential risk situations. The reporting of occurrences or incidents by those persons involved must be encouraged and should not be seen as a method to institute punitive or disciplinary action. For example, the medical staff should be urged to report situations in which the manner of patient care may have produced a potentially compensable event. Employees of the facility should be provided the opportunity to report hazardous conditions that might expose patients, property, or other employees to loss, without fear of reprisal and with a level of anonymity.

Because risk management relates to the operation of many departments of the facility, its involvement can be construed as interference with the authority of those departments. Therefore, care must be exercised in the communication of risk management's role and its potential benefits. For example, the early involvement of the risk management function in the review of contracts, affiliation agreements, and hospital and nursing policy formulation can often provide a perspective not otherwise available.

Departmental Analysis

Measurement of planned activities—such as the number of incident reports received, claims reported, or lawsuits investigated or the risk manager's participation on various hospital committees—often defy a good evaluation. However, a lowered loss frequency, improved loss ratios, and reduced cost of loss (insurance premiums and/or self-insurance contributions) are calculable and can partially serve to evaluate the performance of a facility's risk management program from both a risk control and risk financing standpoint.

Social Services Department

Overview

The origin of hospital-based medical social services dates back to 1905, when the value of having a professionally trained individual working with patient and family problems created by social conditions was observed by Richard C. Cabot, M.D., chief of medicine at Massachusetts General Hospital in Boston. Since then, the roles, services, and functions of social workers in hospitals have continued to expand.

Today's social worker is a member of a professional team concerned with the social welfare of the patient. Typically, the social worker is able to improve the effectiveness of hospital care by helping the patient solve social problems such as those related to family relationships, employment, finances, legal issues, and other areas that may contribute to the illness itself or that may interfere with treatment, such as physical discomfort, isolation, fear, and anxiety.

The services provided by the social services department can be divided into three broad categories: services to patients and their families, services to the hospital, and services to the community. The most significant of these categories is services to patients and their families, which can include:

- Discharge planning
- Screening and case finding for at-risk populations (screening and case finding involve the review of admissions to identify cases that would benefit from the assistance of social services in the discharge planning processes)
- Providing psychosocial assessments (the provision of psychosocial assessments involves the assessment of how well a patient and/or family will be able to manage the patient's care and/or financial needs after discharge)
- Counseling patients and family members
- Assisting patients with financial arrangements
- Providing information about community services and benefits
- Making referrals to other resources

The social services department is usually responsible for the coordination of discharge planning, either to the home or to another institution. With the advent of prospective payment systems and the emphasis on shorter lengths of stay, the social worker has assumed a greater role in managing the patient's length of stay. In this role, the social worker may assist the patient and family in effecting a timely discharge to the patient's home with the appropriate level of home health care assistance. Alternatively, when a discharge to home is not feasible, the social worker assists in the transfer of the patient to another facility such as a nursing home or a rehabilitation facility. In this role of managing the length of stay, the social worker may assist in making arrangements for home health care, nursing home placement, or referral to community resources for financial, emotional, and social needs; the social worker may also coordinate transportation to ensure the patient's access to continuing medical services.

Organization

The organization of the social services department may vary depending on the size of the hospital and the administrative relationships that exist within the institution. The typical department includes a director of social services, who reports to the senior administrative level. Depending on the size of the department, there also may be an associate or assistant director, as well as a supervisor of social services staff assigned to various units within the hospital, such as the medical, surgical, obstetrical, or gynecological services. The social services staff includes social workers (with either master's or bachelor's degrees in social work) as well as clerical staff. The size of the institution is not as important in determining the department's size as the commitment of the hospital's administration to provide social services is.

Most social services departments maintain a Monday-through-Friday daytime schedule. Scheduled hours may be extended in departments with special needs such as emergency services or alcohol detoxification; alternatively, these needs may be covered by staff on an on-call basis.

Social services may be either centralized or decentralized. The primary advantages of a centralized department are that the caseload can be handled more efficiently, supervision of staff is easier, and peer interaction is facilitated. A decentralized department may be more effective because it allows specialized staff to be dedicated to particular units, thus making staff more readily accessible to individual units. However, the social worker dedicated to a particular department or unit may not be able to work with the caseload as efficiently and may lack peer interaction.

Many hospitals also have social services and projects (such as substance abuse, child abuse, and meals-on-wheels programs) that are supported by the government or private foundations. Even though these programs are externally funded, from the department's perspective, the staff members should be considered hospital employees and report to the director of social services.

Models and Systems

The number of sessions a social worker has with a patient or family depends on the nature of the problem. The sessions vary in length from 10 to 15 minutes to perhaps 45 minutes and may be held daily or weekly. For example, the social worker might need to see a young, severely ill child frequently, while the social worker might not need to see another patient at all but instead works exclusively with the family in weekly meetings. In other cases, family meetings might include the patient.

It is estimated that for every 60 to 90 minutes spent directly with a patient or family member, social workers spend another 30 minutes in related work such as meeting with community agency representatives, making telephone calls, attending to paperwork, recording supervisory conferences, attending educational conferences, and performing other indirect activities.

The social services department typically maintains extensive statistics concerning contacts with patients, family members, and other individuals, as well as related activities. These statistics should be kept in a uniform and systematic manner and should be documented in a manner that satisfies the requirements of local, state, and federal regulations. The statistics generally should include the number and duration of interviews with patients and family members, contacts with community agencies, and collateral interviews with significant persons in the patient's personal environment, such as employers. This documentation of time spent is important as a component of case management and productivity measurement and should be maintained on a daily basis.

Although many social services departments still manage their case information manually, there is a growing trend toward using computerized social services information systems because of the detailed nature of the case statistics kept and because of the usefulness of such records in case management and productivity improvement programs. The Society of the Hospital Social Work Directors (SHSWD) of the American Hospital Association has developed a minimum data set for use by social services departments and has endorsed a particular computerized social services information system. This combination should yield an interesting comparative data base for use in evaluating the social services department's performance in the future. Several other case management information systems are also on the market, and some departments have developed their own information systems.

Situations and Problems

The hospital social services department faces many challenges and problems in its attempt to have a positive impact on the patient during his or her hospital stay. The depth of the department's involvement often depends on the level of the administration's commitment to the program. Some administrators place less value on the social services function and opt for a narrowly defined role for the social services department limited to discharge planning, work with patients referred to the department, and other related activities. At the opposite end of the spectrum is an administration that is willing to go beyond the limited definitions of social services and encourage screening and case finding for at-risk populations. This generally provides the department with a much larger percentage of the hospital's patients to serve. Because social services generally are not directly reimbursable, social services departments are often faced with the challenge of justifying the benefits of their services.

Because the social services department is concerned primarily with the patient's welfare, conflicts may occur with other hospital personnel whose duties overlap or possibly oppose those of the social workers. For example, nurses, who are important to the discharge planning function, may feel resentment when the social worker deems it necessary to intervene on the patient's behalf. In another area, problems might develop if the social worker assisted a patient in setting up a payment structure for the hospital bill while the accounting department wanted immediate payment through normal channels. These types of situations can make adversaries of social workers and other hospital personnel and should be handled carefully to minimize conflict. The best way to minimize conflict is for the administration to outline clearly its goals and expectations for the social services department and to communicate those goals and expectations to the hospital staff and the medical staff.

Other problems faced by the social services department include pressure to discharge patients, either to make hospital resources available for other patients or to shorten lengths of stay, which is to the financial advantage of the hospital under prospective payment systems. This pressure to discharge can be aggravated by shortages of nursing home beds and home health resources. Staff recruitment can also be a problem, as can be keeping abreast of constantly changing Medicare and Medicaid regulations.

The social worker in today's environment is often confronted with the need to assist the patient and family in arranging for appropriate care once the patient is discharged or transferred while at the same time helping the hospital to keep the patient's length of stay within expectations and departmental expenses at a minimum.

Departmental Analysis

Social services departments, because of their function and because of their relatively small size in the institution, have not been studied extensively by management engineers. The SHSWD attempted to establish national productivity measures (units of time needed to perform specific functions) several years ago, but the society was unsuccessful because of regional differences in procedures.

The SHSWD was able to establish and publish a relative value system in the late 1970s. However, the assessment of staffing needs is still a subjective rather than an objective activity. This is an important factor under prospective payment systems. The social services department may need to justify its staff and services to the institution at the bottom line. To do so, it must demonstrate its ability if not to generate revenue at least to save the hospital money through shorter stays and improved patient satisfaction and care.

In assessments of staffing requirements, the department's role in assisting patients in traditional social services functions must be combined with expectations concerning the role of the department in the discharge planning process. Hospitals should assess overall strategies for coordinating the management of patient care and length of stay. The management engineering study is one way to demonstrate the cost-effectiveness of the department.

The role of the hospital social services department varies significantly from hospital to hospital, as do the definitions of various social services procedures. Therefore, it is difficult to cite national norms for social services staffing levels. Although gross norms currently exist through sources such as MONITREND, these norms do not take into account the wide variation in activities in social services departments. The presentation of a standardized data set by the SHSWD along with the widespread use of its endorsed computerized social services information system hold great promise for the development of meaningful comparative information and standards. This could enable the tailoring of standards to the characteristics of individual social services departments and greatly facilitate productivity analyses.

A detailed departmental statistical system, whether manual or automated, also provides an opportunity for productivity monitoring at the department level, as well as by individual social worker. From a management engineering perspective, care must be taken to describe required staffing in terms of the time needed to perform various activities as compared to the time actually taken to perform activities because most of these systems record actual, not required, time.

In studies of the department's staffing needs, the following situations generally indicate the need for fewer staff:

- A centralized department
- No system for case finding and screening for at-risk patients
- No specialized programs such as child abuse, alcohol detoxification, or meals-on-wheels programs
- A narrow role for social services as defined by the hospital's administration
- A focus limited to discharge planning
- A work schedule limited to the weekday day shift

The following characteristics generally indicate the need for higher levels of staffing:

- A decentralized department
- A system for extensive case finding and screening for at-risk patients
- Many specialized programs requiring dedicated social services staff or staff with special qualifications and skills
- A broad role for the social services department as defined by the hospital's administration
- A work schedule that includes coverage of specialty areas such as the emergency department on nights and weekends

There are many areas in a typical social services department in which management engineering can become involved. Some of these project areas might include the following:

- Development of departmental and individual productivity-monitoring systems that use the department's statistical systems
- Analysis of the costs and benefits of a manual versus a computerized social services information system
- Assistance in the development and implementation of a computerized social services information system
- Analysis of the staffing requirements and costs of a centralized versus a decentralized staffing approach
- Analysis of the staffing requirements, costs, and benefits of case finding versus referrals as a source of social services caseload
- Review and analysis of the discharge process to determine whether the process can be streamlined to facilitate earlier discharges

Recent MONITREND data for the social work services functional reporting center are provided in table 26.

Table 26. HAS/MONITREND Data for Social Work Services: Six-Month Medians for Period Ending December 1988

Indicator	National Bed Size Groups							
	Under 50	50–74	75–99	100–149	150–199	200–299	300–399	400 and Over
Discharge units per calendar day[a]	7.41	13.92	18.13	28.20	38.06	54.16	70.05	106.33
Discharges per social work FTE[b]	151.90	143.42	163.39	157.20	157.41	138.00	132.50	138.63
Paid hours per adjusted patient day[c]	0.15	0.15	0.13	0.14	0.13	0.14	0.15	0.14
Paid hours per discharge unit[d]	0.36	0.48	0.39	0.43	0.47	0.51	0.59	0.58

[a]Discharge units per calendar day = discharge units/days in period.

[b]Discharges per social work FTE = total discharges/social work FTEs.

[c]Paid hours per adjusted patient day = social services paid hours/(total patient days/overall RCC). The overall RCC (ratio of charges to charges) is an adjustment factor that is computed as follows: Overall RCC=gross inpatient revenue/gross operating revenue.

[d]Paid hours per discharge unit = social services paid hours/discharge units.

Source: HAS/MONITREND, 1988. Please refer to page x for more information about the data presented in this table.

Surgical Suite

Overview

Surgery is a type of medical practice in which disease is cured, injuries are repaired, and deformities are corrected by means of manual operative procedures. The surgical suite is composed of general-purpose operating rooms in addition to specialty rooms for cardiac surgery, cystoscopy, and other services. Many hospitals have also constructed separate ambulatory surgical units for the hospital's outpatient surgical caseload. A recovery room or postanesthesia recovery unit is also part of the surgical suite.

The surgical suites in community and teaching hospitals perform the same basic functions, and yet there is a substantially different environment in teaching hospitals. Complex procedures may be performed more frequently in teaching hospitals with several surgeons participating on one case and some acting as physician's assistants. Procedures in teaching hospitals also tend to take longer because of additional teaching support and cases being performed by residents. Consequently, more nursing and technical support is needed in a teaching hospital.

Typically, the surgical suite is available between 7:00 a.m. and 3:30 p.m., Monday through Friday, for scheduled surgery. Generally, hospitals with fewer than 300 beds place the surgical nursing staff on call to cover weekday evening and night shifts and all weekend shifts for emergency cases. In larger hospitals and teaching hospitals, these shifts may be staffed.

Surgical patients may represent up to 60 percent of total admissions in many hospitals. The surgical suite contributes heavily to the utilization of other hospital ancillary services. The success of this utilization depends on good communication among surgical personnel and personnel in other departments. Some of the departments directly involved are admissions/registration, laboratory, radiology, pharmacy, environmental services, laundry, and nursing.

Organization

Surgeons from all specialties, usually private physicians, are granted privileges to operate at the hospital. The chief of surgery is a medical doctor who is elected to the position by the peer group of surgeons. The position usually does not command an additional salary, but it is considered a prestigious one. In large teaching hospitals, however, it may be a salaried position reporting to the medical director or an administrator.

The major surgical specialties or services are the following:

- General surgery
- Plastic and reconstructive surgery

- Orthopedic surgery
- Ophthalmology
- Neurosurgery
- Otolaryngology
- Vascular surgery
- Gynecology
- Thoracic surgery
- Urology

The surgical group usually has a formal relationship with the medical staff of the hospital, but not a direct relationship with the hospital's administration.

Anesthesiologists are medical doctors who administer anesthesia during surgical procedures and provide medical direction for the recovery room. Anesthetists are generally certified registered nurse anesthetists (CRNAs) and act as assistants under the direction of anesthesiologists. The same group of anesthesiologists and anesthetists may serve several community hospitals. This service may be provided by a hospital-based department of anesthesia, or it may be provided by a private group of anesthesiologists under contract with the hospital.

The typical operating room nursing team consists of one circulating nurse and one scrub nurse. The circulating nurse is a registered nurse who functions outside the sterile field surrounding the operating table. The functions of this nurse are to coordinate activities, record events, and obtain supplies. The scrub nurse may be a licensed practical nurse or a surgical technologist who functions within the sterile field. The functions of the scrub nurse are to assist the surgeon and organize and pass instruments. More complex surgical procedures may require additional scrub nurses, circulating nurses, and physician's assistants.

A physician's assistant may be another physician or an individual specially trained as a physician's assistant. Some surgeons employ a scrub nurse as a personal assistant. Certain procedures require a medical doctor to be the physician's assistant, who may be called a first assistant. The assistant retracts the surgical opening and assists the surgeon with the surgical procedure. Surgical house officers (residents) often serve as physician's assistants in teaching hospitals.

Aides and orderlies are generally used for patient transportation, patient positioning, and cleanup work. Aides may clean, check, and wrap instrument kits. Orderlies are responsible for patient transportation and cleanup (discarding trash, mopping floors, and so on).

The operating room and recovery room nursing staff reports to a nurse manager. Each nurse manager is responsible for the day-to-day work of his or her assigned unit, whether it is an operating room or a recovery room. Nurse managers report to either a surgical suite supervisor or director. The supervisor or director oversees the entire department and is involved with planning, budgeting, and developing policies and procedures, as well as with maintaining intradepartmental relationships.

The surgical suite's management structure and the interrelationships of the structural elements are unique and may be quite complex. There is a hierarchical arrangement in which multiple disciplines (nurses, surgeons, anesthesiologists, and administrators) must interact and in which a variety of mechanisms are utilized to ensure the orderly conduct of business. This hierarchy is characterized by at least four separate vertical lines of authority that must be integrated at some level within the system. These include nursing, administration, anesthesiology, and medical staff. The integration of these lines of authority can be accomplished by instituting and enforcing well-defined policies and procedures and by implementing a surgical suite committee. The surgical suite committee allows representative input from each of the areas. This committee traditionally participates in the governance of the surgical suite.

Operational Systems

The terms *surgical case* and *surgical procedure* are often but erroneously used interchangeably. A case refers to the patient, and a procedure is a specific surgical activity performed, such as an appendectomy. A patient may have many procedures performed as part of his or her case.

Surgical patients generally fall into one of the following three categories:

- *Inpatients:* Patients who are usually admitted to the hospital one day before surgery and emergency room patients who have been admitted through the emergency department
- *Morning admits:* Elective surgery patients who arrive at the hospital on the morning of surgery and who are admitted to a hospital bed (due to changes in reimbursement, most patients having elective surgery are admitted the morning of surgery)
- *Same-day ambulatory surgery patients:* Outpatients who come to the hospital the morning of the procedure and return home the same day
- *Minor outpatients:* Patients who are scheduled for minor surgical procedures requiring local anesthesia (these patients typically return home the same day; often, the surgery is performed in an area adjacent to the surgical suite and may or may not be performed by surgical staff)

With the emphasis on cost containment, there has been a transition in recent years from inpatient surgery to ambulatory and outpatient surgery. Ambulatory surgery patients typically represent 50 to 60 percent of a hospital's surgical caseload.

Ambulatory surgery is arranged for extensive outpatient surgical procedures that often require general or spinal anesthesia. Ambulatory patients are usually instructed to arrive two to three hours before the scheduled case start time in the ambulatory surgery unit. The patient is then transported to the operating room, where the procedure is completed. After surgery, the patient recovers in the postanesthesia care unit (recovery room) and then typically is transferred back to the ambulatory surgical care unit for observation before being discharged the same day.

An ambulatory surgical care unit consists of a bed and recliner chair and may be in a clinic area. The advantage of this type of service is that it reduces patient and hospital expense for less intensive surgical procedures.

Preadmission testing (PAT) is usually arranged for ambulatory surgery patients and requires that the patient come to the hospital one to three days before surgery as an outpatient so that preoperative tests (for example, X rays, laboratory tests, electrocardiograms) can be completed. Some hospitals also arrange for the anesthesiologist to evaluate the patient during the preadmission testing process.

The two essential elements in the functioning of the operating room are the case scheduling system and the materials management system.

Case Scheduling

The surgical case scheduling system is an organized approach for scheduling surgical procedures. An effective scheduling system is complex, consisting of numerous interrelated elements. Designing an effective scheduling system demands comprehensive analysis, creativity, careful attention to facts, and sensitivity to the needs of those affected by the system, particularly the surgeons. Controversy surrounds the question of what the time on the operating room schedule represents. The problem is not whether the scheduled time represents incision, induction, or in the room time but that all parties interpret the schedule the same way.

There are two types of case scheduling systems: conventional (or first-come, first-serve) scheduling and block scheduling. Well-defined scheduling policies and procedures should include information on operating hours, scheduling procedures, preoperative requirements, block allocations (including a mechanism for revisions, if applicable), emergencies, on-call surgery, assistants, distribution of the operating room schedule, starting time for surgery, monitoring delays, and closing the schedule.

A conventional case scheduling system is essentially a first-come, first-serve system in which cases are scheduled in the order in which they are requested. The advantages and disadvantages of conventional scheduling are listed in figure 18.

A block scheduling system incorporates specific blocks of surgery time, in specific operating rooms to be available for a particular surgical service, group of surgeons, or individual surgeons. Block scheduling holds the reserved period for the specified use until a designated time before the day of surgery (for example, 48 hours or 72 hours in advance). When the block of time is not booked with cases at that point, the reservation is lifted and the block becomes available for use by other surgeons. The advantages and disadvantages of block scheduling are listed in figure 19.

Computer support for the scheduling function, including microcomputer-based systems, is available and can help simplify the scheduling process. Automated scheduling packages provide case volume and case length information.

Significant warning signs of scheduling inefficiencies and problems in the surgical suite include the following:

- Increased complaints from surgeons, anesthesiologists, and patients
- Large and frequent variances in the number of scheduled versus actual case starts
- Case turnover times over 30 minutes (case turnover time is the time needed to clean up from one case and prepare for the next)
- Increased case cancellations

Figure 18. Advantages and Disadvantages of a Conventional Case Scheduling System

Advantages	Disadvantages
• Slack time in schedule is reduced. • Surgeons with longer scheduling lead times who wish to perform several procedures, one after another, can be accommodated. • System is easy to set up.	• Surgeons who perform procedures with shorter scheduling lead times often must accept less desirable surgical times. • A starting time may not be assigned until the day before surgery. • Inefficient case flow for unrelated specialty procedures may result. • A surgeon often must accept starting times for cases spread throughout the day. • It is harder to book urgent cases on short notice. • "Phantom" booking can often occur in order to reserve prime operating room time in advance. • System is difficult to manage.

Figure 19. Advantages and Disadvantages of a Block Scheduling System

Advantages	Disadvantages
• Surgeon can plan on established time for surgery. • Competition among surgeons for desirable times is reduced. • Afternoon operating room utilization can be improved. • Continuity of case flow for staff and equipment requirements is improved. • Surgeons or specialists with short lead times have easier access to the schedule. • The hospital can attract or market new surgeons or services. • The system distributes surgical demands more evenly.	• It is difficult to perform more procedures than planned in the established time block. • Accommodation of special situations, such as a visiting surgeon, is difficult. • Blocks must be updated periodically and adjusted for surgeon usage.

To avoid such problems, departments should institute a case scheduling system that achieves desired levels of staff and facility utilization.

Materials Management

The second essential element in the functioning of the surgical suite is the materials management system. Its objective is to provide the right supplies, instruments, and equipment to the right location, at the right time, and in the right condition for use. An operating room is a unique environment because of the quantity of supplies, and the sterile conditions that are required as well as the high costs and time constraints involved. The materials management system must coordinate a variety of single-use products, special-order supplies, reprocessed instruments, and delicate equipment. Errors may cause case delay, jeopardize patient safety, or create unnecessary expenses.

The traditional approach to materials management in the surgical suite involves support from the central service department for instrument processing and selected supplies. In some hospitals, this function is performed by surgical suite personnel. Supplies are maintained in the surgery department and in individual operating rooms. Special-order supplies are ordered by nursing personnel. Items needed for a particular case are selected or picked by the surgical team (circulating and scrub nurses) between cases.

Hospitals following centralized materials management principles typically rely on the case cart system, which delivers fully prepared carts to the surgical suite the evening or morning of surgery. Typically, carts are prepared by support staff in an adjacent central service department. The carts are filled with instruments, equipment, and supplies as documented on surgeon case preference cards. These cards specify all the items the surgeon needs for the scheduled procedure. Carts are delivered via a closed container route in advance of the scheduled surgery. Some carts also function as the scrub nurse's back table. At the completion of the case, instruments and equipment are returned in the cart for reprocessing. Emergency procedure carts are kept ready in the surgical suite. The case cart system offers opportunities to control expensive supplies and equipment, consolidate inventories, use support personnel in preparing cases, and reduce case delay.

Some automated surgical suite management systems allow for the automation of the surgeons' preference listing and case cart requisitions. Such systems automatically generate the specific case cart requisition in the central processing department whenever a particular surgeon and procedure are scheduled.

Efficient surgical suites utilize inventory par (average usage) levels for inventory within the operating room. The establishment of par levels helps streamline the ordering of supplies on a daily or weekly basis. The use of par levels also serves to control excessive supply ordering since what is ordered on a par-level system is essentially what has been used for the day or week.

Many hospitals have transferred the daily supply inventorying, ordering, and replenishment function for the surgical suite to the materials management department. The establishment of appropriate par levels by surgical suite personnel makes this transition possible.

Staffing and Productivity

The surgical suite is usually an expensive area to operate because of equipment cost, instrument cost and high instrument inventories, the relatively large staff required, and other items such as utility costs. To go along with this high cost, a relatively low level of utilization of available facilities is sometimes experienced. This utilization is related to demand for service. The resources of the hospital, such as the availability of nursing personnel, beds, and anesthesiologists as well as the surgeon's personal schedules can be, but often are not, related to this demand.

Percentage average operating room utilization is a sensitive and meaningful measure of surgical suite facility utilization. Percentage average operating room utilization is calculated by the following formula:

$$\text{Percentage average operating room utilization} = \frac{\text{Average room use during the scheduled surgery period}}{\text{Room time available for scheduled surgery}}$$

Average room use includes the inpatient room time plus the amount of time needed for room preparation and cleanup.

Utilization of 75 to 85 percent is considered to represent a potentially attainable utilization level. At this level, the surgical suite's facilities are being used at capacity. When the utilization rate is above 85 percent, management should consider expanding scheduled surgical time. Below 60 percent facility utilization, management should consider decreasing the hours available for scheduled surgery.

There has been a good deal of work done to improve the facility utilization of operating rooms. Because the surgical procedure itself is considered a medical procedure that should be left to the discretion of the surgeon, the most recent attempts to improve operating room utilization are based on improving factors other than the surgeon's time. Some of these factors are reduced cleanup and setup times for the rooms, improved scheduling systems, more functional surgical suite layouts, improved patient transportation systems, and better utilization of the holding area. Improvements in these areas allow additional surgical cases to be processed. The desired results are improved operating room utilization (for example, larger caseload) and increased hospital revenue.

The surgical suite usually requires an average of two staff nurses (circulating and scrub) per case. Support staff includes a charge nurse, aides, orderlies, and secretaries. Depending on the degree to which supply, instrument, and housekeeping functions are the responsibility of the surgical suite, 4.8 to 6.5 staffing hours per case are required, with a target utilization of 75 to 80 percent. Recent MONITREND data for the surgical service functional reporting center are provided in table 27.

Table 27. HAS/MONITREND Data for Surgical Service: Six-Month Medians for Period Ending December 1988

	National Bed Size Groups							
Indicator	Under 50	50–74	75–99	100–149	150–199	200–299	300–399	400 and Over
Surgical visits per 100 medical and surgical and pediatric adjusted discharges[a]	33.66	44.65	49.65	53.83	55.48	58.06	64.90	65.14
Minutes per visit[b]	64.75	63.48	70.37	75.83	74.27	79.50	85.21	94.82
Paid hours per visit[c]	8.38	10.60	10.98	10.92	11.69	12.66	13.93	15.69
Paid minutes per surgical minute[d]	8.16	9.41	9.55	9.05	9.61	9.99	10.59	10.67
Surgical visits per calendar day	1.50	3.88	5.09	9.06	12.23	17.35	23.83	35.57

[a]Surgical visits per 100 medical and surgical and pediatric adjusted discharges = surgical visits/([medical and surgical + pediatric discharges]/[surgical RCC/100]). The surgical RCC (ratio of charges to charges) is an adjustment factor that is computed as follows: Surgical RCC = surgery inpatient revenue/(surgery inpatient revenue + surgery outpatient revenue).

[b]Minutes per visit = surgical minutes/surgical visits.

[c]Paid hours per visit = surgery paid hours/surgical visits.

[d]Paid minutes per surgical minute = (surgery paid hours × 60)/surgical minutes.

Source: HAS/MONITREND, 1988. Please refer to page x for more information about the data presented in this table.

The recovery room is usually staffed exclusively by registered nurses, but in larger hospitals aides may work in the recovery room. A registered nurse usually handles two or three patients, depending on the condition of the patients. Expected lengths of stay in the recovery room are 1.5 to 2.5 hours for patients under general anesthesia and 1.0 to 1.5 hours for outpatients or patients under local anesthesia. Discharge of the patient from the recovery room is at the discretion of the anesthesiologist.

Departmental Analysis

In conducting a departmental analysis, the following methodologies are typically utilized in obtaining information:

- Interviews
- Questionnaires (nursing, anesthesia, and physicians)
- Calculation of facility utilization
- Documentation and analysis of existing systems—patient flow, materials handling, case scheduling
- Direct observation of daily activity
- Case-delay data collection

Improvements resulting from a system analysis could include the following:

- Improved scheduling systems might increase accessibility and increase the number of surgical procedures performed.
- An improved scheduling system would even out the surgical caseload, eliminating unnecessary peaks and demands on operating room and recovery room staff, anesthesia staff, and ancillary departments.
- Cost savings might result through elimination of unneeded extended hour coverage, use of part-time staff, and identification of overstaffing.
- An improved charge system design might increase revenue and reduce lost charges.
- Reductions in supply costs might be gained through stock control.
- Reductions in case delay might be gained through improved work flow.

To successfully manage and promote change within the surgical suite, one must understand the functioning of the operating room, its relationship with other areas of the hospital, its perceived importance among physicians, and its place within the health care delivery system.

Telecommunications Department

Overview

Instantaneous and reliable communication is vital to every health care facility. Communications systems in hospitals may include administrative, patient, and public telephones; electronic paging; and emergency dispatch, including ambulance and helicopter two-way radios. In many hospitals, these systems are maintained by a telecommunications department. In addition, the department may be responsible for various alarm systems, including both fire and security alarms; the intercom system, which may include Muzak entertainment; and a facilitywide local area paging network that can transmit on either its baseband (local in-house paging system) or broadband (long-range paging system) channels. Some departments have also branched out to provide answering service coverage for private physicians' offices. The extent to which a department will be responsible for some or all of the named areas depends largely on the facility's size.

In addition to the more obvious requirements, it is important for the telecommunications department to be responsive to external demands because the public's first contact with the facility is often the switchboard operator. A slow response or an unfriendly attitude creates a negative impression and lowers the caller's confidence in the hospital.

The management engineer must realize the potential problems associated with poor or missed communications. Poor communications can lead to overall organizational inefficiencies, higher costs because of the introduction of temporary and shortsighted solutions to problems, and poor public image. Also, missed communications can sometimes be life threatening. For example, a delay in issuing cardiac codes or the inability to reach on-call specialists in a timely fashion could possibly endanger patients.

Organization

Because a facility's size is often the factor that determines the overall responsibilities of the telecommunications department, institutions with fewer than 200 beds may not have a formal department. In such institutions, there is usually a telephone switchboard operated by clerical staff or receptionists under the supervision of an assistant administrator.

In larger institutions, there might be a more formal structure supervised by a director of telecommunications, who performs all budgeting, staffing, and planning functions for the department. Responsibilities include overseeing any telephone installations, moves, or changes of equipment as well as planning future modifications to the hospital's telecommunications services and equipment. The director of telecommunications usually reports to an assistant administrator or director of support services, although in more and more hospitals this position is reporting to a chief information officer.

The director may be assisted by a chief operator, who supervises daily telephone and paging operations at the switchboard. This function may include implementing the director's staffing schedule, solving problems for patients and physicians, billing for answering service customers, and supervising the response to alarms.

Operating Systems

The major function of the telecommunications department is to provide telephone services throughout the facility. Before January 1984, the provision of such communications services was relatively easy in that the component parts of the overall system could be purchased from a single vendor. When the federal government completed its divestiture proceedings against American Telephone and Telegraph (AT&T) in January 1984, the number of options multiplied, as did the complexity of the selection process. The telecommunications director now deals with all vendors and makes all decisions on equipment, features, and networking.

In small institutions, the phone system usually consists of either a central office (CO) service (Centrex) or a small private branch exchange (PBX). Central office services allow direct dialing to all extensions; PBX services require all incoming calls to go through a switchboard. Central office services are usually provided by the local phone company, and PBX services usually are obtained from one of the many vendors now in the market.

Large facilities combine the benefits of CO and PBX services by having certain direct inward-dialed (DID) calls bypass the switchboard and go directly to the departments' extensions. This reduces switchboard traffic volume and therefore reduces staffing requirements.

Other new telecommunication technologies are also being marketed as productivity aids. Among the features that are usually desired are:

- Touchtone dialing
- Call pickup (a feature that enables everyone in a department to input a code on their telephone sets to answer any other telephone extensions in their department)
- Call forwarding
- Conferencing capability
- Consultation hold features (a user with a single line set—that is, without a hold button—can put a call on hold)
- Transferability of incoming calls
- Transferability of outgoing calls
- Restriction capabilities on individual phone units (restricting phone use to in-house calls or to in-house and local calls—that is, disallowing long distance calls unless they go through the operator)
- Direct outward dialing
- Direct inward dialing
- Remote access (a feature that allows a caller from outside the hospital to call a predetermined number, dial in a security code, and access the calling features of the hospital's telephone system)
- Speed dialing
- Data transmission capabilities
- Expansion capabilities (the ability to add stations and/or extensions or to add features)
- Energy management and monitoring (thorough investigation should be conducted to ensure that this feature will be cost-effective for the institution)

It should be noted that telephone instruments are sometimes selected for image rather than functional utility. For example, multiple push-button sets, electronic speaker phones, CRT display units, automatic-dial features, and memory devices can add significant cost for a questionable return on investment. Because of recent technological innovations, today's decisions may appear less than optimum within a short time. It is therefore important to institute a planning process for telecommunications that attempts to define functional requirements, technical capacities, and organizational considerations over intermediate- and long-range periods.

Another major responsibility of the telecommunications department is to notify physicians when they are needed to handle an emergency. This is often done by means of a paging system. Long-range or local paging systems (often called beepers) can transmit and receive tone, voice, or digital signals. Signal transmitters can be located either within the facility itself or at remote sites. Local transmission from the facility is usually adequate for short-range signals. Remotely located transmitters often belong to vendors who specialize in long-range transmitting capability.

Some of the largest hospitals maintain their own emergency dispatch system. Such hospitals typically operate their own fleet of ambulances and/or operate their own medical airlift service, either helicopter or fixed wing. The emergency dispatch system is used to dispatch ambulances or aircraft to transport patients to or from other hospitals and to transport critically ill persons to the hospital from remote locations.

A recent development expected to have a major impact on telecommunications is the car telephone, which is made possible by cellular technology. Large institutions in major population centers will be the first to see this service introduced. Where it is already in use, this feature has proved effective in reducing response times.

The major difficulty facing the telecommunications department is choosing a new telephone switch for the hospital. When the director does not have the up-to-date expertise to configure a new telephone switch in regard to trunking, networks, and so forth, the use of a telecommunications consultant may be necessary. Other but less major departmental difficulties typically include covering unplanned operator absences, ensuring satisfactory operator response time, maintaining up-to-date on-call schedules for medical and hospital staff, negotiating needed versus requested telephone extensions and features, and controlling long distance expenses.

Staffing and Productivity

Staffing guidelines depend directly on the range of services provided by the hospital's telecommunications department and the resulting work load by hour of day and day of week. Staffing and scheduling considerations most commonly start with a telecommunications traffic survey to document types and volumes of both incoming and outgoing calls. Management engineering analysis most commonly includes the use of the Poisson distribution to quantify the impact of random demand and alternative staffing levels on average caller waiting times by hour of day and day of week. Staffing levels are customarily determined by the administration on the basis of these projected average waiting periods. Staffing schedules are then developed to schedule staffing working hours to best fit the hourly needs for console coverage.

The department's ability to monitor its productivity depends directly on its ability to obtain viable statistical data on the range of services offered by each institution. In most telecommunication areas, statistics should be collected on incoming and outgoing calls (by trunk line if possible), long distance calls, long distance call duration, frequency of paging requests, frequency and duration of emergency code actuation, and other similar factors. Unfortunately, obtaining this base of data is rarely cost-effective without the aid of a traffic management software system or a similar device that is capable of generating these types of statistics automatically. Some of these computer-assisted system functions are available only by special request for finite sample time periods and still require extensive manual analysis and tabulation. For optimum application to productivity reporting, statistical volumes are needed on a cost-effective, ongoing basis.

Departmental Analysis

Systems engineers might consider the following areas for more detailed evaluation:

- A detailed evaluation of long-distance calls, including both their destinations and frequencies, could be undertaken. Long distance expenses can account for up to half of the total operating expenses for the telecommunications area. Once reliable data have been collected, cost reduction alternatives can be explored. These might include using different vendors, restricting long distance access by phone or by individual, and using direct charge-back mechanisms.
- A long-range planning process could be initiated by the systems engineer. The goal of the planning process should be to define current and future requirements and to investigate the cost and benefits of the many available alternatives.
- Data communications requirements could be evaluated by a team, including the engineer, the telecommunications director, and the information systems and data processing director. The feasibility of local area networks, relative to future needs and in consideration of current capabilities, should be determined.
- An evaluation of an electronic mail system, relative to cost and benefits, could be done by a similar team.
- An evaluation of written policies and procedures for the telecommunications department could be undertaken. The department's policies and procedures should include such items as physician paging procedures, emergency code procedures, alarm actuation procedures, disaster procedures, and procedures for establishing remote communication capabilities.
- The method and policy for providing patients with telephone service should be evaluated. It should be recognized that patient telephone service is a possible revenue-generating function for the medical facility. However, it is suggested that consideration be given to the potentially adverse public relations impact of large surcharges for long distance calls.
- Different scheduling alternatives for operators could be analyzed. The switchboard must be staffed 24 hours a day, seven days a week, with special consideration for ensuring weekend and holiday coverage. Different scheduling possibilities, including four-day workweeks, might be advantageous in facilitating vacation scheduling and covering sickness and incidental time off without excessive use of overtime hours.
- The cost of moves and changes of telephone instruments could be investigated. The cost of moves and changes can be substantial; however, such costs are often overlooked when renovation costs are estimated. Newer digital technology can lessen this expense in the case of moves with no wiring changes (location of jacks, and so on). Records of work orders for changes and moves should be retained for future reference and planning purposes. A potential method of controlling the cost of moves and changes is through a contract with the telephone vendor for moves, changes, or installations at a flat rate.
- A study could be done to determine whether the given features of a system are utilized. It is sometimes true that features are available but are not used by staff because of poor preparation and education or lack of confidence. Orientation programs should be conducted for new employees, and review sessions should be conducted on an ongoing basis for current staff.
- The feasibility of establishing an in-house or community physicians' answering service could be examined. This evaluation should include operator work load, staffing, type of equipment, the billing process, and the required clerical support.
- The controls for ordering and installing various telephone instruments could be evaluated. Each department requiring phone services should be analyzed to determine the optimal amount and type of equipment required for functional efficiency. For example, needs may differ among the medical center's business office and its operating room, clinical laboratory, or physical plant departments. Similar controls should also be established for the periodic reevaluation of the telephone requirements for each department.

Transportation Department

Overview

Transportation is a function performed in every health care facility, regardless of its size or sophistication, and is not limited in scope to patient transport. The methods by which the transportation function is performed, however, vary significantly from one institution to another. Some institutions have a transportation department that is responsible for the movement of patients, supplies, and equipment. Others have separate departments for each of these activities, and the patient transport function is called patient transportation, escort service, or courier service. This profile focuses on the transportation of patients as a separate function.

The transportation department is usually responsible for one or more of the following activities:

- Inpatient escort services after admission and discharge
- Patient transportation to and from ancillary departments for inpatients, emergency department patients, and occasionally outpatients
- Routine maintenance or repair of rolling equipment used for patient transportation

The transportation department may provide services Monday through Friday, 7 a.m. to 3 p.m., or it may operate 24 hours a day, seven days a week.

The transportation function can have a tremendous impact on the productivity of the ancillary departments and nursing units it services. The effective management of the transportation services through communication, dispatching, and scheduling increases the efficiency of the transportation function, thereby minimizing delays in ancillary departments and nursing units while providing a valuable patient service. For this reason, it is essential that the department develop effective systems, procedures, and staffing.

Organization and Operations

The transportation department may be managed by a department director or a supervisor, depending on the size of the institution and the nature and scope of services provided. The department manager may report to the administrator for support services, the director of materials management, or the director of the nursing service.

The department usually consists of a department manager, shift dispatchers, and transporters. The department manager should have a good understanding of hospital operations and should have the skills necessary to be an effective communicator and supervisor of staff.

In addition, he or she needs to be sensitive to the needs and problems of a variety of other hospital departments.

Shift dispatchers, who are responsible for supervising the second and third shifts, may also supervise the first shift in the absence of the department manager. The transporter position is usually considered an entry-level position, with on-the-job training in proper lifting and transportation techniques. Because these are entry-level positions, turnover in the department is usually high, with a number of employees transferring to other positions within the institution.

The department is usually responsible for some or all of the rolling transportation equipment in the institution. Some institutions have developed a centralized department with the primary goal of developing control and responsibility over the condition and availability of wheelchairs and stretchers.

Centralized and Decentralized Systems

Most transportation departments have evolved from decentralized systems. Departments such as radiology, physical therapy, surgery, and nursing traditionally have used aides and attendants to transport patients to and from the departments. In addition, the admissions/registration and emergency departments require patient escort services. As an institution grows, the economies of scale from a centralized transportation service can be realized by pooling resources into one department that satisfies transportation needs throughout the institution.

When there is a shortage of nursing personnel, a centralized transportation service allows nurses to spend less time transporting patients and more time on other activities. Studies have indicated that there is a cost benefit to having lower-paid staff transport patients.

Although many institutions have a centralized transportation function, rarely is true centralization ever achieved. In many instances, individual departments still transport patients, supplies, and equipment independent of the transportation department. Common examples include the transportation of trays by the food service department, mail delivery by the mail room, supply and equipment delivery by materials management, and patient transportation by surgical suite personnel.

A centralized department generally has the advantage of better use of transporters, maintaining a smaller staff than what would be required under decentralization, and improving control of transportation through a central dispatcher. The advantages of a decentralized department include having a staff that is committed to a given area and that understands its specific needs and having a staff available to perform other support tasks in the department.

Communication

The most common form of communicating a request for transportation is the telephone. When requesting departments call the central dispatch office, a dispatcher logs the request and assigns the first available transporter to the request. Once the requested trip has been accomplished, the transporter calls the central office for another assignment prior to returning to the office.

When a hospital has a hospitalwide information system, a message or mailbox feature allows requesting departments to transmit requests via computer. Once the requesting department enters a request into the computer, a request order is printed in the central dispatch office. The dispatcher then assigns the request to a transporter. This method of requesting transportation services eliminates telephone calls and can improve hospital productivity. An additional benefit is the potential for having the computer maintain statistics on the number of trips by area.

Dispatching

To a great extent, dispatchers control transporter productivity. Requests for transportation should be logged according to the time requested, the requesting department, the type of transport, any special equipment needed, the time of dispatch, and the time completed. These detailed logs are very useful in determining required staff by hour of the day, as well as individual transporter productivity. Although most transportation departments keep manual dispatch logs and statistics, the capability does exist for automated logs that significantly reduce the time spent in statistical data manipulation.

Although some transportation activities can be scheduled at regular intervals (for example, mail and supply deliveries, elevator operator schedules, routine equipment maintenance, and so forth), the majority of the department's work load depends on the level of activity in ancillary departments. As a result, it is very important to match transportation staffing with projected ancillary department volumes.

One of the keys to productive transportation services is the procedure whereby transporters call the dispatcher the moment they finish their last call. This system allows the dispatcher to assign the transporter to a request close to his or her current location. Low productivity can be expected when transporters do not call the dispatcher and return to the office to receive their next request.

Scheduling

Scheduling systems in hospitals range from very sophisticated centralized patient scheduling systems to decentralized systems. The predictability of the transportation department's work load is directly related to the number of departments that schedule patient activities. A centralized hospital scheduling system usually provides the transportation department with a schedule of all ancillary department treatments, which allows the dispatcher to assign transporters to ensure that all patients are transported on time. The result produces fewer complaints and higher departmental productivity.

Without centralized patient scheduling, staffing patterns must be established by using historical work-load statistics, and the ability to make daily adjustments in transporter work schedules to accommodate unusual fluctuations in work load are limited at best. This shortcoming usually results in lower productivity levels because the tendency is to staff for peak work-load levels to minimize complaints, which frequently results in overstaffing. Complaints from ancillary departments will be higher when peak periods of work load are not handled.

Staffing

The major problem in any centralized transportation system is the development of staffing patterns that achieve an acceptable level of productivity and minimize complaints from departments serviced. Some level of delay in patient treatments or procedures inevitably occurs whether the transportation function is performed by each department or through a centralized system. The increased staffing flexibility possible with an effectively managed centralized transportation system should minimize such delays.

When economies of scale are to be realized by centralizing the transportation function, a high level of productivity must be maintained to offset the additional expenses for supervisors, dispatchers, and office space not required in a decentralized system. High levels of productivity with minimal complaints can most easily be achieved when patient scheduling systems are in place in the departments to be serviced.

As in any department, efforts to increase productivity often result in an increase in minor delays (and therefore complaints). An administrative decision as to the number of minor delays that are acceptable may be required. Once this desired level of service is identified, appropriate staffing guidelines and target productivity levels can be developed.

Staffing levels for a transportation department are determined by three factors: the number of trips, the distance required for the trips, and the type of trips. A rule of thumb for staffing is 0.50 paid hours per trip. If the hospital is very large, the distance and thus the time required will be greater. The third factor, type of trip, means that staffing levels are affected by the percentage of nonpatient transports. Most hospitals have a certain amount of non-patient transport, which usually does not exceed 20 percent in a traditional service.

Work-load measurement and performance standards should be based on the type, volume, and required time per trip for the variable work-load component. The constant activities include required hours for supervisors, dispatchers, and elevator operators as well as the time required for repairs and maintenance of transportation equipment. Required time per trip depends on the departments serviced (location within facility), the method of transportation (wheelchair versus stretcher), and the time of day.

Departmental Analysis

Departmental analyses generally focus on department staffing, staff scheduling, and additional activities with which the transportation department may be involved. Other topics of analysis may be transportation equipment requirements and an evaluation of centralized versus decentralized transportation systems.

- *Evaluating departmental performance:* Basic departmental performance can be determined by reviewing staff productivity, average response time per each type of call and by area, number of complaints, and average trip time. The department should have an ongoing program of reviewing performance to predetermined goals of response time.
- *Determining staffing requirements:* A management engineering staffing analysis of the transportation function should address work-load requirements by hour of day for each day of the week. Trip times vary by time of the day also, and so average trip time per shift for each department serviced should be identified. The development of staffing guidelines based on weighted work-load standards is preferred.
- *Analyzing scheduling systems:* A detailed review of the hospital scheduling system may indicate that poor scheduling within ancillary departments causes transporter work load to fluctuate and create delays and low productivity. Improved coordination and communication between the ancillary departments and transportation can reduce delays.
- *Determining whether the system should be centralized or decentralized:* A comprehensive review of the transportation needs of the institution can determine whether a centralized or decentralized system is preferred. Items to consider are cost benefit due to lowering the skill mix of transporter, availability of scheduling information, and cooperation from administration, ancillary departments, and nursing.
- *Identifying other activities with which transportation could be involved:* Many institutions expand the role of the transportation department to include transporting mail, supplies, and equipment. Many of these activities can be accomplished without increasing the total need for transporters but rather by increasing productivity. Each activity should be reviewed carefully to determine its appropriateness and cost benefit.

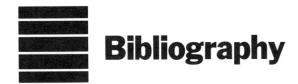

Bibliography

Administration

Aikens, C. *Hospital Management*. Edited by S. Reverby. New York City: Garland Publishing, 1985.

American Hospital Association. *Managing under Medicare Prospective Pricing*. Chicago: AHA, 1983.

Bassett, L., and Metzger, N. *Achieving Excellence: A Prescription for Health Care Managers*. Rockville, MD: Aspen, 1986.

Berman, H. J., and others. *The Financial Management of Hospitals*, 6th ed. Ann Arbor, MI: Health Administration Press, 1986.

Brown, J. H., and Comola, J. *Improving Productivity in Health Care*. Boca Raton, FL: CRC Press, 1988.

Gerber, L. *Hospital Restructuring: Why, When and How*. Chicago: Pluribus Press, 1983.

Goldstein, J., and Spivack, J. Gain-Sharing for Hospitals: Organizational Impacts. AHA report no. MG37. Chicago: American Hospital Association, 1987.

Joint Commission on Accreditation of Healthcare Organizations. *Accreditation Manual for Hospitals*. Chicago: JCAHO, 1987.

Kirk, R. *Healthcare Quality and Productivity: Practical Management Tools*. Rockville, MD: Aspen, 1988.

Malsky, S. J. *Hospital Administration for Middle Management: A Practical Approach*. St. Louis: Warren H. Green, 1988.

McDougall, M. D., Covert, R. P., and Melton, V. B., editors. *Productivity and Performance Management in Health Care Institutions*. Chicago: American Hospital Publishing, 1988.

Moore, T. F., and Simendinger, E. A. *The Effective Health Care Executive: A Guide to a Winning Management Style*. Rockville, MD: Aspen, 1986.

Thomas, A., and Schramm, W. Functional Analysis: An Approach to Hospital Reorganization. AHA report no. AB68. Chicago: American Hospital Association, 1986.

Admissions/Registration Department

Abney, S. Customizing a Turnkey Admission/Discharge/Transfer System to Meet Hospital Goals. AHA report no. AM56. Chicago: American Hospital Association, 1985.

American Hospital Association. *The Hospital Admitting Department*, 2nd ed. Chicago: American Hospital Publishing, 1986.

Blanchet, K. D., and Switlik, M. M., editors. *Handbook of Hospital Admitting Management*. Rockville, MD: Aspen, 1985.

Cochard, R., and Colaberdino, R. Productivity management in the hospital admissions department. *Journal for Hospital Admitting Management* 13(4):5–8, Spring 1988.

Covert, R. P. Management, productivity and admitting departments. *Journal for Hospital Admitting Management* 13(4):3–4, 25, 27, Spring 1988.

Dahlstrom, G. A., Sliwinski, R. T., and Sweetland, K. Integrating Preadmission with Patient Care. AHA report no. AM65. Chicago: American Hospital Association, 1986.

Pehkonen, J., and Chawla, N. Initiating Nursing Assessment, Utilization Review, and Discharge Planning in the Admitting Process. AHA report no. AM55. Chicago: American Hospital Association, 1985.

Rowland, F., and Henne, M. Integration of the Admitting and Outpatient Departments into Patient Registration. AHA report no. AM63. Chicago: American Hospital Association, 1985.

Scott, J., and Jones, D. Centralized Scheduling. AHA report no. AM53. Chicago: American Hospital Association, 1985.

Ambulatory Services

Antle, D. W., and Reid, R. A. Managing service capacity in an ambulatory care clinic. *Hospital and Health Services Administration* 33(2):201–11, Summer 1988.

Berman, S., editor. *Ambulatory Health Care Standards Manual, 1988.* Chicago: Joint Commission on Accreditation of Healthcare Organizations, 1987.

Brislin, J., and Wasvick, J. Same-Day Surgery Center: A Hospital-Based Solution. AHA report no. OU19. Chicago: American Hospital Association, 1986.

Budd, G. B. Productivity: the challenge for ambulatory services. *The Journal of Ambulatory Care Management* 11(1):1–12, Feb. 1988.

Card, W. F., and others. *Sample Indicators for Evaluating Quality in Ambulatory Health Care.* Edited by M. Duffy and K. Hill. Chicago: Joint Commission on Accreditation of Healthcare Organizations, 1987.

Carviez, J. A. Systems for Managing an Ambulatory Care Clinic in a Large County Hospital. AHA report no. OW02. Chicago: American Hospital Association, 1987.

Hardin, S. S., and Altus, G. D. Systems Approach to Outpatient Scheduling. AHA report no. OU62. Chicago: American Hospital Association, 1986.

Hill, K. L., editor. *Quality Assurance in Ambulatory Health Care.* Chicago: Joint Commission on Accreditation of Healthcare Organizations, 1987.

Icading, D. R. Staffing a Satellite Ambulatory Care Clinic. AHA report no. OW07. Chicago: American Hospital Association, 1987.

Joint Commission on Accreditation of Healthcare Organizations. *Monitoring and Evaluation of the Quality and Appropriateness of Care: An Ambulatory Health Care Example.* Chicago: JCAHO, 1988.

Lazenby, T. M., and Kachhal, S. K. Information System for a Multiple Location Ambulatory Care Operation. AHA report no. OU82. Chicago: American Hospital Association, 1987.

Lewellen, G. Consumer Awareness in Outpatient Services. AHA report no. OU23. Chicago: American Hospital Association, 1986.

Moen, R. S., editor. *Accreditation Handbook for Ambulatory Health Care: 1987-88 Edition.* Skokie, IL: Accreditation Association for Ambulatory Health Care, 1987.

Newcomb, C. S., Rupp, L. B., and Townsend, G. L. Staffing Model for a Satellite Ambulatory Care Center. AHA report no. OW09. Chicago: American Hospital Association, 1987.

O'Connor, J. P. Ambulatory Surgery Scheduling. AHA report no. OR28. Chicago: American Hospital Association, 1987.

Page, J. A. Managing in the Ambulatory Area: Successful Operations Analysis of Outpatient Care. AHA report no. OW03. Chicago: American Hospital Association, 1987.

Page, J. A., and Pille, B. L. Ambulatory Care Delivery System Analysis Using an Integrated Systems Approach. AHA report no. OU14. Chicago: American Hospital Association, 1987.

Reichertz, P. L., and Engelbrecht, R., editors. *Present Status of Computer Support in Ambulatory Care.* New York City: Springer-Verlag, 1987.

Rostenberg, B. *Design Planning for Freestanding Ambulatory Care Facilities: A Primer for Health Care Providers and Architects.* Chicago: American Hospital Publishing, 1986.

Skadura, C. M. Computerized Simulation of the Ambulatory Surgery Area. AHA report no. OW08. Chicago: American Hospital Association, 1987.

Thielen, C. M. Determining the Quality of Service and Accessibility for Outpatient Visits. AHA report no. OU21. Chicago: American Hospital Association, 1986.

Waldrop, R. T., and Smith, S. P. Assessment Tool for Patient Classification and Nurse Staffing in Ambulatory Care within a Metropolitan Area Teaching Hospital. AHA report no. OU14. Chicago: American Hospital Association, 1987.

Winston, W. J., editor. *Marketing Ambulatory Care Services.* New York City: Haworth Press, 1985.

Cardiac Catheterization Laboratory

Dougherty, E., and others. The future looks bright for cardiac catheterization. *Health Care Strategic Management* 7(1):1, 14–18, Jan. 1989.

Purcell, J. A. *Cardiac Catheterization,* rev. ed. Atlanta: Pritchett and Hull, 1987.

Ronning, P. L., and others. Developing effective invasive cardiology services. *Hospital Technology Series* [American Hospital Association] 7(23):1–106, 1988.

Sanders, W. J. A cardiology productivity network. *Computers in Healthcare* 7(7):22–24, July 1986.

U.S. General Accounting Office. *Sharing Cardiac Catheterization Services: A Way to Improve Patient Care and Reduce Costs.* Report to the Congress. Washington, DC: General Accounting Office, 1977.

Central Service Department

American Society for Hospital Central Service Personnel. *Ethylene Oxide Use in Hospitals: A Manual for Health Care Personnel.* Chicago: American Hospital Publishing, 1982.

American Society for Hospital Central Service Personnel Staff. *Training Manual for Central Service Technicians.* Chicago: American Hospital Association, 1986.

Anonymous. 1988 survey of salaries, education and organization structure in central service and materiel management. *Journal of Healthcare Materiel Management* 6(7):28–32, Oct. 1988.

Dornette, H. L., editor. *Central Service Technical Manual.* Chicago: International Association of Hospital Central Service Management, 1981.

Imhof, J. L. Managing morale and productivity in central service. *Journal of Healthcare Materials Management* 4(5):64–66, 70, 72, Sept.–Oct. 1986.

Kisro, F., and others. Developing productivity standards for performance in the central processing department. *Hospital Materiel Management Quarterly* 9(4):70–76, May 1988.

Markus, F. E., and Christie, J. Storage in central service. *Hospital Topics* 64(3):42–46, May–June 1986.

Mayworm, D. E. CS resources: vital tools for job performance. *Journal of Healthcare Materiel Management* 5(7):50–51, Oct. 1987.

Messer, T. J. *Simplicity in Management of Productivity and Quality Control.* Chicago: American Hospital Association, 1987.

Reichert, M. *Criteria Based Performance Appraisal for the Central Service Technician.* Chicago: American Hospital Association, 1987.

Clinical Engineering Department

Al-Fadel, H. O. Clinical engineering productivity improvement. *Journal of Clinical Engineering* 11(5):355–59, Sept.–Oct. 1986.

David, Y., and Rohe, D. Clinical engineering program productivity and measurements. *Journal of Clinical Engineering* 11(6):435–43, Nov.–Dec. 1986.

Fennigkoh, L. *Management of the Clinical Engineering Department: How to Convert a "Cost Center" to a "Profit Center."* Brea, CA: Quest Publishing Co., 1987.

Furst, E. Productivity and cost-effectiveness of clinical engineering. *Journal of Clinical Engineering* 11(2):105–13, Mar.–Apr. 1986.

Goodman, G. The profession of clinical engineering. *Journal of Clinical Engineering* 14(1):27–37, Jan.–Feb. 1989.

Johnston, G. I. Are productivity and cost-effectiveness comparisons between in-house clinical engineering departments possible or useful? *Journal of Clinical Engineering* 12(2):147–52, Mar.–Apr. 1987.

Mahachek, A. R. Management and control of clinical engineering productivity: a case study. *Journal of Clinical Engineering* 12(2):127–32, Mar.–Apr. 1987.

Shaffer, M. J., and others. Clinical engineering in a downsizing environment. *Medical Instrumentation* 22(4):201–4, Aug. 1988.

Electroencephalography and Electrocardiology Departments

Devereux, R. B., and others. Cost-effectiveness of echocardiography and electrocardiography for detection of left ventricular hypertrophy in patients with systemic hypertension. *Hypertension* 9(2, Pt. 2):1169–76, Feb. 1987.

Grauer, K., and others. Computerized electrocardiogram interpretations: are they useful for the family physician? *Journal of Family Practice* 24(1):39–43, Jan. 1987.

Mirvis, D. M., and others. Instrumentation and practice standards for electrocardiographic monitoring in special care units. A report for health professionals by a Task Force of the Council on Clinical Cardiology, American Heart Association. *Circulation* 79(2):464–71, Feb. 1989.

Willems, J. L. Common standards for quantitative electrocardiography. *Journal of Medical Engineering and Technology* 9(5):209–17, Sept.–Oct. 1985.

Emergency Department

American College of Emergency Physicians. *Quality Assessment in the Emergency Department: A Practical Handbook.* Des Plaines, IL: ACEP, 1984.

Brooks, D. K., and Harrold, A. J., editors. *Modern Emergency Department Practice.* London: E. Arnold, 1983.

Georgopoulus, B. S. *Organizational Structure, Problem Solving, and Effectiveness: A Comparative Study of Hospital Emergency Services.* San Francisco: Jossey-Bass, 1986.

Helmer, F. T., and others. Determining the required nurse staffing of an emergency department. *Journal of Emergency Nursing* 14(6):352–58, Nov.–Dec. 1988.

Kuypers, M. E. A computerized log and integrated quality assessment program for the small emergency department. *Quality Review Bulletin* 15(5):144–50, May 1989.

Matson, T. A., editor. *The Hospital Emergency Department: Returning to Financial Viability.* Chicago: American Hospital Publishing, 1986.

Mitchell, F. P. Timeliness of care in the accident and emergency department. *Hospital and Health Services Review* 83(3):127–31, May 1987.

Overfelt, F. C., and McCarthy, E. Operations Audit of the Staffing and Pricing Practices of an Emergency Department. AHA report no. ER72. Chicago: American Hospital Association, 1986.

Page, J. A., and Pille, B. Analysis of the Hospital-Based Emergency Department: Measuring the Impact of the Changing Ambulatory Environment. AHA report no. ER44. Chicago: American Hospital Association, 1987.

Page, J. A., and Pille, B. Utilizing a participative analysis approach: the key to implementing a successful productivity monitoring system or cost accounting program – case study: emergency department. *National League for Nursing Publication* 20-2191:455–64, Dec. 1987.

Peisert, M., and others, editors. *The Hospital's Role in Emergency Medical Services Systems.* Chicago: American Hospital Publishing, 1984.

Smeltzer, C. H., and Curtis, L. An analysis of emergency department time: laying the groundwork for efficiency standards. *Quality Review Bulletin* 13(7):240–42, July 1987.

Energy Management and Maintenance

Agnello, S. Cost-saving opportunities for HVAC installations. *Health Facilities Management* 1(4):22–25, Dec. 1988.

American Hospital Association. *Cost Containment through Energy Management: A Guide to Executive Action.* Chicago: AHA, 1984.

American Hospital Association. *Energy Management.* Chicago: AHA, 1984.

Anonymous. Lowering hospital energy costs: a comprehensive approach. *Health Progress* 68(8):72, 74, Oct. 1987.

Hunt, V. D., compiler. *Energy Conservation in Health Care Facilities.* Atlanta: Fairmont Press, 1983.

Sitwell, C. R., and others. Energy management: the returns are worth the investment. *Dimensions in Health Service* 64(4):11–13, May 1987.

Environmental Services

Collins, B. J. The hospital environment: how clean should a hospital be? *Journal of Hospital Infection* 11(suppl. A):53–56, Feb. 1988.

Famularo, D. Automated Approach to Quality Assurance within an Environment Services Department of a Kaiser Permanente Medical Center. AHA report no. HU21. Chicago: American Hospital Association, 1987.

Gillespie, J., and others. Forecasting Staffing Alternatives in the Facility Planning Process: A Turnkey Approach to Developing Housekeeping Staffing Levels. AHA report no. HU37. Chicago: American Hospital Association, 1985.

Kurth, J. M. *Hospital Environmental Services Policy and Procedure Manual.* Rockville, MD: Aspen, 1986.

Miller, C. B. *Policy and Procedures Training Manual for the Environmental Health Service Department,* 2nd ed. St. Louis: Catholic Health Association, 1984.

Printup, B. The hazards of executive housekeeping. *EHT* 10(6):10–12, June 1989.

Fiscal Services

American Hospital Association. *Chart of Accounts for Hospitals.* Chicago: AHA, 1976 [out of print].

Berman, H. J., and others. *The Financial Management of Hospitals,* 6th ed. Ann Arbor, MI: Health Administration Press, 1986.

Bley, C. M., and Shimko, C. T. *A Guide to the Board's Role in Hospital Finance.* Chicago: American Hospital Publishing, 1987.

Bradford, C. K., and Tiscornia, J. F. *Monitoring the Hospital's Financial Health: A Guide for Trustees.* Chicago: American Hospital Publishing, 1987.

Brown, B. J., and Ross, A. *Integration of Clinical and Financial Information Systems in Health Care.* Rockville, MD: Aspen, 1986.

Caruana, R. A. *Organizing a Healthcare Financial Services Division,* 3rd ed. Westchester, IL: Healthcare Financial Management Association, 1989.

Esmond, T. H., Jr. *Budgeting Procedures for Hospitals,* 3rd ed. Chicago: American Hospital Publishing, 1982 [out of print].

Hackett, K. L. An initial look at billing productivity. *Healthcare Financial Management* 40(11):125, Nov. 1986.

Harrison, M., and Kapur, R. Management Systems: We Do Product Costing Right. AHA report no. AE05. Chicago: American Hospital Association, 1986.

Herkimer, A. G., Jr. *Understanding Hospital Financial Management,* 2nd ed. Rockville, MD: Aspen, 1986.

Hofman, M. Systems management: strategies to increase effectiveness. *Healthcare Financial Management* 40(6):44–48, June 1986.

Hutchison, R. L. Operational and Economic Feasibility Analysis: Evaluation of Capital Expenditures Using Discounted Cash-Flow Techniques. AHA report no. AE09. Chicago: American Hospital Association, 1986.

Kading, D. R., and Malstrom, E. M. Manufacturing Cost Recovery Method Adapted for Use in a Health Care Facility. AHA report no. AE02. Chicago: American Hospital Association, 1986.

Kazemek, E. A., and Grauman, D. M. The CFO's role in strategic planning. *Healthcare Financial Management* 41(2):94, 99, Feb. 1987.

Kukla, S. F. *Cost Accounting and Financial Analysis for the Hospital Administrator.* Chicago: American Hospital Publishing, 1986.

Lacusta, M. P. Application of Productivity Information to the Hospital Budgeting Process. AHA report no. AC27. Chicago: American Hospital Association, 1985.

Lewellen, G. L. Cost Analysis to Support Product Information. AHA report no. AE03. Chicago: American Hospital Association, 1986.

Marrapese, R. L., and Titera, W. R. *Internal Control of Hospital Finances: A Guide for Management,* rev. 1989 ed. Chicago: American Hospital Publishing, 1989.

McCall, K. A. Cost Outlier Review Process. AHA report no. AE10. Chicago: American Hospital Association, 1986.

Moncarz, E. S. *Financial Accounting for Hospital Management Instruction Manual.* New York City: Van Nostrand Reinhold, 1986.

Seawell, L. V. *Hospital Financial Accounting Theory and Practice.* Oak Brook, IL: Healthcare Financial Management Association, 1987.

Ventrone, J. M. Productivity in the business office: a practical approach. *Patient Accounts* 9(6):2–3, June 1986.

Food Service Department

Anonymous. Evaluating your dishroom. *Hospital Food and Nutrition Focus* 5(4):5–6, Dec. 1988.

Anonymous. Measuring trayline productivity. *Hospital Food and Nutrition Focus* 3(3):1, 3–4, Nov. 1986.

Macks, G. C., and Brye, P. L. Measurement of Workload and Activities of Clinical Dietitians. AHA report no. DI30. Chicago: American Hospital Association, 1986.

Murray, I. P., and Upton, E. M. Labour productivity in hospital foodservice. *Journal of the Canadian Dietetic Association* 49(3):178–81, Summer 1988.

Pellegrino, T. W. *Selecting a Computer-Assisted System for Volume Food Service.* Chicago: American Hospital Publishing, 1986.

Puckett, R. P., and Miller, B. B. *Food Service Manual for Health Care Institutions,* 1988 ed. Chicago: American Hospital Publishing, 1988.

Soth, D. G. Quality and productivity: food service systems. *Hospital Materiel Management Quarterly* 9(4):11–15, May 1988.

Stokes, J. F. *Cost-Effective Quality Food Service: An Institutional Guide,* 2nd ed. Rockville, MD: Aspen, 1985.

Sullivan, C. F. *Management of Medical Foodservice.* Westport, CT: AVI Publishing Co., 1985.

Human Resources/Personnel Department

American Hospital Association. *Staff Reductions.* Chicago: AHA, 1984.

American Hospital Association. Human Resources Management in Health Care Institutions. Policy and statement. Chicago: AHA, 1986.

American Society for Hospital Personnel Administration. *A Basic Guide to Health Care Personnel Policies and Procedures.* Chicago: American Hospital Association, 1984.

Bartels, B. M., and Gee, K. L. Human resources management: keystone for productivity. *Health Care Supervisor* 5(2):47–53, Jan. 1987.

Carter, C. C. Professional recruitment can save both time and money. *Provider* 13(2):48–49, Feb. 1987.

Erf, S., and Badel, J. *Hospital Restructuring: Employment Law Pitfalls.* Chicago: Pluribus Press, 1985.

Feinberg, W. J. *Directory of Hospital Personnel, 1987.* Deerfield, IL: Whole World Publishing, 1986.

McDougall, M. D., Covert, R. P., and Melton, V. B., editors. *Productivity and Performance Management in Health Care Institutions.* Chicago: American Hospital Publishing, 1988.

Rosenbloom, J. S., editor. *The Handbook of Employee Benefits: Design Funding and Administration,* 2nd ed. Homewood, IL: Dow Jones-Irwin, 1988.

Information Systems Department

American Hospital Association. *Guide to Effective Health Care Information Management and the Role of the Chief Information Officer.* Chicago: AHA, 1988.

Austin, H. The economics of information systems. *Computers in Healthcare* 7(6):43–4, 46, June 1986.

Brown, B. J., and Ross, A. *Integration of Clinical and Financial Information Systems in Health Care.* Rockville, MD: Aspen, 1986.

Deluca, J. F. Cost Benefit/Cost Effectiveness Analysis for Microcomputer Acquisition and Placement in Hospitals. AHA report no. DA38. Chicago: American Hospital Association, 1986.

Denaburg, J. S., and Myers, N. Staff Training: Essential to a Successful Computer System. AHA report no. DA94. Chicago: American Hospital Association, 1985.

Girard, R. E. Productivity and information systems. *Computers in Healthcare* 10(2):26–28, 30, Feb. 1989.

Herser, B. S. Chief Information Officer in an Environment of Dynamic Change. AHA report no. DA79. Chicago: American Hospital Association, 1987.

Kahl, K. L., Markiewicz, G., and Riechert, T. Common Data Base Supports Cost Control and Productivity Management. AHA report no. DA37. Chicago: American Hospital Association, 1986.

McHugh, M. L. Increasing productivity through computer communications. *Dimensions in Critical Care in Nursing* 5(5):294–302, Sept.–Oct. 1986.

Stern, S. K. Microcomputers—becoming hospital-wide productivity tools. *Healthcare Computing and Communications* 3(2):18–19, Feb. 1986.

Walters, R. W., and Lincoln, T. L. Using information tools to improve hospital productivity. *Healthcare Financial Management* 41(8):74–76, 78, Aug. 1987.

Zinn, T. K., and DiGiulio, L. W. Actualizing system benefits. *Computers in Healthcare* 9(8):34–35, 38, Aug. 1988.

Intensive Care Unit

Fein, I. A., and Strosberg, M. A., editors. *Managing the Critical Care Unit.* Rockville, MD: Aspen, 1987.

Hayne, A. N., and Bailey, Z. W. *Nursing Administration of Critical Care.* Rockville, MD: Aspen, 1982.

Mudd, D. L. Monitoring productivity and quality indicators in a critical care setting. *Nursing Management* 19(10):96A–96H, Oct. 1988.

Waisbren, B. A. *Critical Care Manual: A Systems Approach Method.* New Hyde Park, NY: Medical Examination Publishing Co., 1985.

Laboratory

Baumgardner, D. L., and Ryerson, P. J. Standard Costing: A Base for More Effective Laboratory Decision Making. AHA report no. LB18. Chicago: American Hospital Association, 1985.

Fitzgibbon, S. *Laboratory Manager's Problem Solver.* Oradell, NJ: Medical Economics Books, 1985.

Gopaul, D., and Botz, C. K. Determining productivity and unit costs in a bacteriology laboratory. *Canadian Journal of Medical Technology* 48(3):99–103, Sept. 1986.

Hallam, K. Turnaround time. Part II. How labs improve their performance. *Medical Laboratory Observer* 20(8):39–41, 44–46, Aug. 1988.

Howanitz, P. J., and Howanitz, J. H., editors. *Laboratory Quality Assurance.* New York City: McGraw-Hill, 1987.

Rubenstein, N. M. *Handbook of Clinical Laboratory Management.* Rockville, MD: Aspen, 1986.

Shaw, B. W. Development of Computer Based Laboratory Workload Standards. AHA report no. LB53. Chicago: American Hospital Association, 1986.

Taylor, J. K. Participative management lifts lab productivity. *Medical Laboratory Observer* 18(4):46–50, Apr. 1986.

Umiker, W. O., and Yohe, S. M. *Performance Standards for Laboratory Personnel.* Oradell, NJ: Medical Economics Books, 1984.

Westgard, J. O., and Barry, P. L., editors. *Cost-Effective Quality Control: Managing the Quality and Productivity of Analytical Processes.* Washington, DC: American Association for Clinical Chemistry, 1986.

Wilson, F. *Cost Control in the Clinical Laboratory.* Mission Viejo, CA: Scientific Newsletter Enterprises, 1985.

Laundry Department

Abramson, D. Improvements at hospital laundry have increased productivity, services. *Laundry News* 13(1):23, Jan. 1987.

Beermann, B. Fewer pounds per laundry operator hour can improve efficiency, safety and quality. *Laundry News* 13(8):11, Aug. 1987.

Billimoria, N. Development of Standard Times in Hospital Laundry. AHA report no. LD60. Chicago: American Hospital Association, 1986.

Carr, S. Space: a hidden asset. Ten recommendations for reducing laundry space while increasing productivity. *American Laundry Digest* 53(3):18–19, Mar. 15, 1988.

Gardner, J. Laundry streamlines operation to achieve higher productivity. *Laundry News* 12(2):21, Feb. 1986.

Joint Committee on Health Care Laundry Guidelines (U.S.). *Joint Committee Guidelines for Health Care Linen Service.* Hallandale, FL: Textile Rental Services Association of America, 1984.

Maintenance Department

American Society for Hospital Engineering. *Maintenance Management for Health Care Facilities.* Chicago: American Hospital Association, 1984.

Joint Commission on Accreditation of Healthcare Organizations. *Plant, Technology and Safety Management Handbook,* 2nd ed. Chicago: JCAHO, 1989.

Rodenbaugh, P. *Maintenance Management by Computer.* Chicago: American Hospital Association, 1984.

Marketing

Bart, B. D., and others. Getting the most out of your marketing research: guidelines for strategy and policy. *Journal of Hospital Marketing* 2(1):45–60, 1987.

Bullis, R. J., and others. The marketing executive in today's health care environment. *Journal of Hospital Marketing* 1(3–4):19–23, Spring–Summer 1987.

Conway, J., editor. *Hospital Marketing,* rev. ed. Philadelphia: Leonard Davis Institute of Health Economics, 1986.

Costello, M. M. Selecting and training the hospital-based physician services representative. *Hospital Topics* 65(4):18–19, July–Aug. 1987.

Folland, S., and others. Implications of prospective payment under DRGs for hospital marketing. *Journal of Health Care Marketing* 8(4):29–36, Dec. 1988.

Goldsmith, M., and others. Strengthening the hospital's marketing position through training. *Health Care Management Review* 11(2):83–93, Spring 1986.

Hamm, G. L., Weber, J., and Schwartz, R. G. Practical Market Analysis Model. AHA report no. AB84. Chicago: American Hospital Association, 1987.

Keckley, P. H. *Market Research Handbook for Health Care Professionals.* Chicago: American Hospital Publishing, 1988.

Kieffer, M. C., and others. Searching for the marketing leader—straight talk from the headhunters. *Healthmarketing* 6(1):7–9, Jan.–Feb. 1987.

Larkin, D. Developing a marketing function in a multi-hospital system: how to define your job. *Health Marketing Quarterly* 3(2–3):37–45, Winter 1985–Spring 1986.

Lazenby, T. M., and Kachhal, S. K. Customer Satisfaction Survey: Development of the Process Analysis of Results. AHA report no. AB10. Chicago: American Hospital Association, 1987.

McDevitt, P. Learning by doing: strategic marketing management in hospitals. *Health Care Management Review* 12(1):23–30, Winter 1987.

Portnoy, S., Stromberg, R. E., and Newbold, P. A. *Acquiring and Enhancing Physicians' Practices.* Chicago: American Hospital Publishing, 1988.

Roberts, C. C., and Beck, E. C. *Marketing in Small and Rural Hospitals.* Chicago: American Hospital Publishing, 1989.

Schwartz, R. G., Oren, S. S., Dennis, C. A., and DeBusk, R. T. Measuring and Responding to Consumer Preferences for Medical Products and Services. AHA report no. AB08. Chicago: American Hospital Association, 1987.

Smith, R. J. Integrating the marketing function: a model for strategic management. *Health Marketing Quarterly* 3(2–3):13–17, Winter 1985–Spring 1986.

Van Doren, D. C., and others. Hospital marketing: strategy reassessment in a declining market. *Journal of Health Care Marketing* 9(1):15–24, Mar. 1989.

Wagle, J. S., and others. The role of the chief marketing executive in hospitals: a survey. *Health Care Strategic Management* 5(5):17–20, May 1987.

Williams, R. C. *Managing the Hospital Sales Team.* Chicago: American Hospital Publishing, 1988.

Winston, W. J. *How to Write a Marketing Plan for Health Care Organizations.* New York City: Haworth Press, 1985.

Materials Management Department

American Society for Hospital Materials Management. *Leadership and Diversification: Expanding the Role of Materials Management.* Annual conference proceedings, 1987.

American Society for Hospital Materials Management. *National Performance for Hospital Materials Management Operations.* Chicago: American Hospital Association, 1987.

American Society for Hospital Materials Management. *For Profit Ventures: Case Studies in Materials Management.* Chicago: American Hospital Association, 1988.

Coltey, R. W. Developing new measures of department productivity. *Hospital Materials Management* 13(8):13–14, Aug. 1988.

Giunipero, L. C. Inventory productivity practices of hospital material managers. *Hospital Materiel Management Quarterly* 10(3):15–22, Feb. 1989.

Kelliher, M. E., and Mannie, R. E. Coordinating Efforts Complementing Services and Progress: A Case Study. AHA report no. PU75. Chicago: American Hospital Association, 1986.

Roth, J. M., and Hagerty, D. Operational Audit of a Friesen Model Supply, Distribution and Processing Department. AHA report no. PU74. Chicago: American Hospital Association, 1986.

Sanderson, E. D. *Effective Hospital Materiel Management.* Rockville, MD: Aspen, 1985.

Scheyer, W. L. *Handbook of Health Care Material Management.* Rockville, MD: Aspen, 1985.

Simmons, P. A., and Schnitzer, M. E. Paired Comparison Constant Sum Methodology for Workload Determination in Purchasing. AHA report no. PU35. Chicago: American Hospital Association, 1986.

Medical Record Department

Beegle, S. C., and Wiesener, F. A. Developing a Straight Line Process in Medical Records Development: Streamlining Face Sheet and Chart Completion. AHA report no. MR36. Chicago: American Hospital Association, 1987.

Bettie, D. J., and Wooden, J. M. Automation of the Medical Records Department Yesterday, Today and Tomorrow. AHA report no. MR46. Chicago: American Hospital Association, 1987.

Bible, R. L. Back to Basics: Classic Management Engineering Techniques to Improve Medical Records Department Operations. AHA report no. MR59. Chicago: American Hospital Association, 1986.

Bruce, J. C. *Privacy and Confidentiality of Health Care Information,* 2nd ed. Chicago: American Hospital Publishing, 1988.

Cox, M. B. *Risk Management for the Department Head: Legal Aspects of Medical and Health Records.* El Cerrito, CA: Cox Publications, 1987.

Hansmann, J. Development of Computerized Productivity and Other Monitoring Systems for a Medical Records System. AHA report no. MR37. Chicago: American Hospital Association, 1987.

Jackovitz, D. S. Operational Audit Techniques: Problem Identification and Solution Development in a Medical Records Department. AHA report no. MR78. Chicago: American Hospital Association, 1986.

Joint Commission on Accreditation of Healthcare Organizations. *Medical Staff: Medical Record Function.* Chicago: JCAHO, 1988.

Keers, S. C., Kantutis, C. A., and Riehs, S. P. Implementing Quality and Productivity Measures through Japanese Management Techniques in Medical Records. AHA report no. MR35. Chicago: American Hospital Association, 1987.

Lethcoe, H. B., and Bowie, V. Work Processing Productivity for Medical Record Transcriptionists. AHA report no. MR38. Chicago: American Hospital Association, 1987.

McPhee, W. M. Records management efficiency. *New Zealand Hospital* 39(3):9, Apr. 1987.

Micheletti, J. A., and Schlala, T. J. Understanding the medical records department improves efficiency. *Healthcare Financial Management* 41(12):38, 40, 42 passim, Dec. 1987.

Page, J. A., and Pille, B. L. Successful Systems Analysis of the Medical Records Department: Enhancing Operational Effectiveness through Systems. AHA report no. MR32. Chicago: American Hospital Association, 1987.

Skurka, M. F. *Organization of Medical Record Departments in Hospitals,* 2nd ed. Chicago: American Hospital Publishing, 1988.

Medical Staff Office

American Medical Association. *Bylaws: A Guide for Hospital Medical Staffs.* Chicago: Department of Hospital Standards and Procedures, Division of Professional Relations, AMA, 1984.

American Medical Association. *Organization: A Guide for Hospital Medical Staffs.* Chicago: Department of Hospital Standards and Procedures, Division of Professional Relations, AMA, 1985.

American Medical Association. *Physician-Hospital Joint Ventures.* Chicago: AMA, 1986.

Bloom, H. *Corporatization of Health Care Delivery: The Hospital-Physician Relationship.* Chicago: American Hospital Publishing, 1986.

Boissoneau, R. The medical staff role: management in rural hospitals. *Hospital and Health Services Administration* 32(2):161–69, May 1987.

Eisele, C. W., Fifer, W. R., and Wilson, T. C. *The Medical Staff and the Modern Hospital.* Englewood, CO: Estes Park Institute, 1985.

Joint Commission on Accreditation of Healthcare Organizations. *Hospital Accreditation Program Scoring Guidelines: Medical Staff.* Chicago: JCAHO, 1988.

Joint Commission on Accreditation of Healthcare Organizations. *Medical Staff: Departmental Review.* Chicago: JCAHO, 1988.

Kernaghan, S. G. *Medical Staff Bylaws Handbook.* Edited by K. W. Porter. Chicago: American Hospital Publishing, 1987.

Matheson, G. W. Good management for good medicine: the role of the vice president for medical affairs. *Healthcare Executive* 3(5):30–33, Sept.–Oct. 1988.

McDermott, S. The new hospital challenge: organizing and managing physician organizations. *Health Care Management Review* 13(1):57–61, Winter 1988.

Shortell, S. M., and others. Economic regulation and hospital behavior: the effects on medical staff organization and hospital-physician relationships. *Health Services Research* 20(5):597–628, Dec. 1985.

Young, D. W., and Saltman, R. B. *The Hospital Power Equilibrium: Physician Behavior and Cost Control.* Baltimore, MD: Johns Hopkins University Press, 1985.

Zacks, D. M., and others. Organizing a medical staff. *Journal of the Medical Association of Georgia* 74(10):691–92, Oct. 1985.

Nursing Service

Blasak, R. E. Real Challenge: Changing Nurse's Roles to Implement Staffing Reductions. AHA report no. NR87. Chicago: American Hospital Association, 1987.

Coss, T. A. Nursing registries and economic efficiency. *Nursing Management* 20(1):50–51, Jan. 1989.

Curtin, L. L., and Zurlace, C. L. Nursing productivity: from data to definition. *Nursing Management* 17(6):32–34, 38–41, June 1986.

DeBlaise-Dietz, R., and Kachhal, S. K. Nursing Costs by DRG and Nursing Management. AHA report no. NR82. Chicago: American Hospital Association, 1986.

Douglass, L. M. *The Effective Nurse: Leader and Manager.* St. Louis: Mosby, 1988.

Douglass, L. M., and others. *Nursing Management and Leadership in Action.* St. Louis: Mosby, 1989.

Hanson, R. L. Core-Plus: Streamlined Patient Classification Tool Development. AHA report no. NR89. Chicago: American Hospital Association, 1987.

Health Care Education Associates Staff. *Models of Excellence for Nurse Managers.* St. Louis: Mosby, 1986.

Helmer, F. T., and Suver, J. D. Pictures of performance: the key to improved nursing productivity. *Health Care Management Review* 13(4):65–70, Fall 1988.

Helt, E. H., and Jelinek, R. C. In the wake of cost cutting, nursing productivity and quality improvement. *Nursing Management* 19(6):36–38, 42, 46–48, June 1988.

Henry, B., and others. *Dimensions of Nursing Administration.* Cambridge, MA: Blackwell Scientific Publications, 1988.

Hernandez, S. R., Kaluzny, A. D., Parker, B., Chae, Y. M., and Brewington, J. R. Enhancing nursing productivity: a social psychologic perspective. *Public Health Nursing* 5(1):52–63, Mar. 1988.

Jenkins, C. Automation improves nursing productivity. *Computers in Healthcare* 9(4):40–41, Apr. 1988.

Johnson, M., and McCloskey, J. *The Series on Nursing Administration.* Vol. 2. Reading, MA: Addison-Wesley, 1988.

Kahl, K., and Kuschel, A. Nursing Care Cost Identification and Productivity Management System. AHA report no. NR88. Chicago: American Hospital Association, 1987.

Kerfoot, K. M. Thinking administratively: a must for the effective nurse manager. *Nursing Economics* 6(3):139–40, May–June 1988.

Kirk, R., and Dunaye, T. M. Managing hospital nursing services for productivity. *Nursing Management* 17(3):29–32, Mar. 1986.

LaMonica, E. *Nursing Leadership and Management: An Experiential Approach.* Boston: Jones and Bartlett, 1986.

Meehan, M., and Price, C. Managing layoffs with minimum loss of productivity. *Nursing Administration Quarterly* 13(1):26–32, Fall 1988.

Minyard, K., Wall, J., and Turner, R. RNs may cost less than you think. *Journal of Nursing Administration* 16(5):28–34, May 1986.

Porter-O'Grady, T. *Creative Nursing Administration: Participative Management into the 21st Century.* Rockville, MD: Aspen, 1985.

Randall, A. The nursing shortage, the straight pin and productivity. *Healthcare Computing and Communications* 5(4):24–26, 28, Apr. 1988, and 5(5):41, May 1988.

Rantz, M., and Hauer J. D. Analyzing acute care nursing staff productivity. *Nursing Management* 18(4):33–4, 38–42, 44, Apr. 1987.

Rieder, K. A., and Lensing, S. B. Nursing productivity: evolution of a systems model. *Nursing Management* 18(8):33–35, 38–40, 44, Aug. 1987.

Rowland, H. S., and Rowland, B. L. *Nursing Administration Handbook,* 2nd ed. Rockville, MD: Aspen, 1985.

Seigel, H. Nurses improve hospital efficiency through a risk assessment model at admission. *Nursing Management* 19(10):38–47, Oct. 1988.

Silber, M. B., and others. *Dynamic Nurse Management: Competencies in a Changing Healthcare World.* San Diego: Cabashon Publishing, 1987.

Simms, L. M. *The Professional Practice of Nursing Administration.* New York City: John Wiley and Sons, 1985.

Smith, H. L., Mangelsdorf, K. L., Piland, N. F., and Garner, J. F. A retrospective on Japanese management in nursing. *Journal of Nursing Administration* 19(1):27–37, Jan. 1989.

Strasen, L. Redesigning patient care to empower nurses and increase productivity. *Nursing Economics* 7(1):32–35, Jan.–Feb. 1989.

Sullivan, E. J., and Decker, P. J. *Effective Management in Nursing.* Reading, MA: Addison-Wesley, 1985.

Weinstein, S. M. *Restructuring the Nursing Workload: Methods and Models to Address the Nursing Shortage.* Chicago: American Hospital Association, 1989.

Wenke, P. C. Nursing productivity: challenge for the '90s. *Nursing Management* 19(7):60, July 1988.

Williamson, W. J., Jr., and Johnston, J. Understanding, evaluating, and improving nursing productivity. *Nursing Management* 19(5):49–50, 52, 54, May 1988.

Yokl, R. T. Organizing support services can increase nursing efficiency. *Contemporary Longterm Care* 10(3):86, 88, Mar. 1987.

Young, L. C., and Hayne, A. N. *Nursing Administration: From Concepts to Practice.* Philadelphia: W. B. Saunders, 1988.

Pharmacy

Choich, R., Jr. Relationship of productivity analysis to departmental cost-accounting systems. *American Journal of Hospital Pharmacy* 45(5):1103–10, May 1988.

Covert, R. P. Management engineering in the hospital environment. *Topics in Hospital Pharmacy Management* 3(3):12–19, Nov. 1983.

Daniels, C. E., and others. The automation of information in pharmacy. *Topics in Hospital Pharmacy Management* 9(1):51–61, May 1989.

Day, D. L., Mason, M., and Reeme, P. D. Using a nursing-workload index to validate hospital pharmacy productivity. *American Journal of Hospital Pharmacy* 43(4):909–12, Apr. 1986.

DeBlaise-Dietz, R., and Kachhal, S. K. Improving Narcotics Control Using an Automated Bar Code Based Computer System. AHA report no. PH05. Chicago: American Hospital Association, 1987.

Fromberg, R., editor. *Monitoring and Evaluation: Pharmaceutical Services.* Chicago: Joint Commission on Accreditation of Healthcare Organizations, 1987.

Gouveia, W. A., and others. *Hospital Pharmacy Computer Systems.* Bethesda, MD: American Society of Hospital Pharmacists, 1987.

Loeb, A. J., and Kahl, K. Microcosting pharmacy services: a basic approach. *Topics in Hospital Pharmacy Management* 7(1):1–11, May 1987.

Lummus, R. A. Improving the Pharmacy Department through the Innovative Implementation of a Hospital Information System. AHA report no. PH49. Chicago: American Hospital Association, 1986.

Lyon, J. A. Personal computers: Rx for improving productivity. *Hospital Pharmacy* 22(11):1146, Nov. 1987.

Manness, L. J., and others. The development of a computerized hospital pharmacy workload measurement reporting system. *Canadian Journal of Hospital Pharmacy* 42(1):31–36, Feb. 1989.

Miller, L. R., and Darnell, S. R. Pharmacy Staffing Analysis through Implementation of a Workload and Productivity Reporting System. AHA report no. PH59. Chicago: American Hospital Association, 1986.

Siegel, J., and Geier, T. Workload monitoring systems for clinical pharmacy services. *Topics in Hospital Pharmacy Management* 7(1):33–47, May 1987.

Wilson, A. L. PHARMIS: a national pharmacy workload and productivity reporting system. *Topics in Hospital Pharmacy Management* 7(1):65–72, May 1987.

Zatkins, K. M., and Davis, N. M. A survey of hospitals with computerized incorporation of the pharmacy patient profile and medication administration record. *Hospital Pharmacy* 21(9):840, 845–46, 852–56, Sept. 1986.

Physical Therapy Department

American Physical Therapy Association. *The American Physical Therapy Association Public Relations Manual.* Alexandria, VA: APTA, 1986.

Andamo, E. M., editor. *Guide to Program Evaluation for Physical Therapy and Occupational Therapy Services.* New York City: Haworth Press, 1984.

Francis, K. *Computer Essentials in Physical Therapy.* Thorofare, NJ: Slack, 1987.

Ventrone, J. M., and others. Dressing for success: measuring productivity can ensure continuing success. *Healthcare Financial Management* 42(8):30–32, 34–38, 40, Aug. 1988.

Planning Department

Abendshien, J. *A Guide to the Board's Role in Strategic Business Planning.* Chicago: American Hospital Publishing, 1988.

Carpman, J. R., and others. *Design That Cares: Planning Health Facilities for Patients and Visitors.* Chicago: American Hospital Publishing, 1986.

Champagne, F., and others. Strategic planning for hospitals—a health-needs approach. *Long Range Planning* 20(3):77–83, June 1987.

Hardy, O. B., and Lammers, L. P. *Hospitals: The Planning and Design Process,* 2nd ed. Rockville, MD: Aspen, 1986.

Hospital Research and Educational Trust and Society for Healthcare Planning and Marketing of the American Hospital Association. *Environmental Assessment Workbook: Identifying the Hospital's Local Issues.* Chicago: American Hospital Publishing, 1989.

McMillan, N. H. *Planning for Survival: A Handbook for Hospital Trustees,* 2nd ed. Chicago: American Hospital Publishing, 1985.

Peters, J. P. *A Strategic Planning Process for Hospitals.* Chicago: American Hospital Publishing, 1985 [out of print].

Rice, J. A., and Creel, G. H. *Market-Based Demand Forecasting for Hospital Inpatient Services.* Chicago: American Hospital Publishing, 1985.

Stacey, S., and Leggat, S. Strategic planning: a practical guide. *Health Management Forum* 8(2):41–51, Summer 1987.

Public Relations

American Hospital Association. *A Basic Guide to Hospital Public Relations,* 2nd ed. Chicago: AHA, 1984.

Conwell, G. Public relations is related to the bottom line. *Texas Hospitals* 43(5):16–18, Oct. 1987.

Davis, B. How to start or improve your public relations program—without a large budget. *Hospital Topics* 64(3):10–13, 19, May–June 1986.

Gaudet, F., and others. Public relations: more than a good bedside manner. *Dimensions in Health Service* 62(3):14–15, Mar. 1985.

Ghiorse, P. W., and others. Preparing for the '90s. The integration of resource development, strategic planning, marketing, and public relations in the modern healthcare setting. *Journal of the National Association for Hospital Development,* Fall 1988, pp. 56–62.

Grant, J. Salesmanship for the hospital. *Journal of Hospital Marketing* 1(3–4):45–49, Spring–Summer 1987.

Klepper, M. Getting your message out: a new prescription. *Dimensions in Health Service* 62(3):20–21, Mar. 1985.

Norcross, D. R. Developing effective public relations activities. *Health Marketing Quarterly* 3(2–3):207–24, Winter 1985–Spring 1986.

Riggs, L. Staffing the hospital public relations function. *Healthmarketing* 4(5):4–6, Sept.–Oct. 1985.

Quality Assurance

Curtis, L. K. Measuring productivity in quality assurance. *Journal of Quality Assurance* 9(2):10–13, Spring 1987.

Donabedian, A. *Explorations in Quality Assessment and Monitoring.* Vol. III, *The Methods and Findings of Quality Assurance and Monitoring: An Illustrated Analysis.* Ann Arbor, MI: Health Administration Press, 1985.

Haley, R. W. *Managing Hospital Infection Control for Cost-Effectiveness.* Chicago: American Hospital Publishing, 1986.

Joint Commission for Accreditation of Healthcare Organizations. *Accreditation Manual for Hospitals.* Chicago: JCAHO, 1989.

Longo, D. R., Ciccone, K. R., and Lord, J. T. *Integrated Quality Assessment: A Model for Concurrent Review.* Chicago: American Hospital Publishing, 1989.

Orlikoff, J. E., and Vanagunas, A. M. *Malpractice Prevention and Liability Control for Hospitals,* 2nd ed. Chicago: American Hospital Publishing, 1988.

Spath, P. L., editor. *Innovations in Health Care Quality Measurement.* Chicago: American Hospital Publishing, 1989.

Radiation Therapy Department

Burns, M. *Trends in Nuclear Medicine.* Chicago: American Hospital Association, 1984.

Staples, M. Time and motion. Improving efficiency in radiation oncology. *Administrative Radiology* 7(9):35–36, 38–41, Sept. 1988.

Veale, F. H., III. Development of a Comprehensive Standard for a Radiation Oncology Department Located within a Major Teaching Hospital. AHA report no. RL02. Chicago: American Hospital Association, 1983.

Radiology Department

American College of Radiology. *Marketing for the Radiologist: An Introduction.* Reston, VA: ACR, 1988.

Bouchard, E. A. *Radiology Management: An Introduction.* Denver: Mosby, 1985.

Fedor, J., and Salvekar, A. Productivity monitoring of the non-technical staff. *Radiology Management* 9(1):32–34, Winter 1987.

Ganti, A. R., Rabushka, S., and Reiner, A. Individual Employee Productivity Monitoring to Determine Pay for Performance in Radiology. AHA report no. RL28. Chicago: American Hospital Association, 1986.

Happ, D., and Klee, B. Radiology Information System. AHA report no. RM16. Chicago: American Hospital Association, 1985.

Henschke, C. I., Balter, S., Whalen, J. P., and Colfelt, B. W. Diagnostic protocols for radiologic efficiency. *Administrative Radiology* 7(11):26–28, Nov. 1988.

Henschke, C. I., Balter, S., Whalen, J. P., Saint-Louis, L., Auh, Y., Cataldi, G., Goldman, A. B., Rosenblit, G., Sarkar, S., Winchester, P., and others. Organizing for radiologic efficiency in a DRG environment. *Investigative Radiology* 23(4):321–26, Apr. 1988.

McCue, P. Radiology information systems: looking to the future. *Applied Radiology* 16(11):49–50, Nov. 1987.

Melcher, C. Radiology information systems. A tool for improving efficiency and reducing cost. *Healthcare Computing and Communications* 3(10):67–68, Oct. 1986.

Rubenzer, B. F. Software for the personal computer: monthly productivity reporting. *Radiology Management* 8(1):41–43, Jan. 1986.

Suskin, S., and Gagnon, N. Grass roots productivity: productivity managed by the productive. *Radiology Management* 8(3):57–61, July 1986.

Renal Dialysis Department

Barbiano di Belgiojoso, G., and others. AIDS in dialysis centers: an emerging risk? *Contributions to Nephrology* 61:254–65, 1988.

Deber, R. B., and others. The multidisciplinary renal team: who makes the decisions? *Journal of the American Medical Record Association* 58(7):44–46, July 1987.

Sharrow, R. F. The renovation challenge: cost-effective appeal. *Michigan Hospitals* 24(5):33–35, May 1988.

Smith, D. G., and others. A comparison of charges for continuous ambulatory peritoneal dialysis and center hemodialysis. *Journal of Clinical Epidemiology* 41(9):817–24, 1988.

Stewart, W. K., and others. Patient load and medical staffing in adult dialysis units in the United Kingdom. *British Medical Journal [Clinical Research Ed.]* 293(6561):1545–48, Dec. 13, 1986.

Respiratory Care Department

Burgher, L. W. The qualified medical director of respiratory care: then and now. *Respiratory Management* 18(1):10–11, 14–18, Jan.–Feb. 1988.

Clark, R. A., and Landsborough, R. Comprehensive Productivity Monitoring for Respiratory Therapy. AHA report no. IT66. Chicago: American Hospital Association, 1984.

Fitch, B. Determining the Optimal Number of Respiratory Therapy Ventilators. AHA report no. IT39. Chicago: American Hospital Association, 1984.

Kim, M. K., and others. Applications of staffing, scheduling, and budgeting methodologies to hospital ancillary units. *Journal of Medical Systems* 13(1):37–47, Feb. 1989.

Packard, R. W., and Pettigrew, S. L. Respiratory Therapy System Space Study. AHA report no. IT71. Chicago: American Hospital Association, 1984.

Rohe, D. K., and Goodpasture, J. Automating Respiratory Therapy's Operational and Management Support Systems. AHA report no. IT38. Chicago: American Hospital Association, 1984.

Watson, D., and Strasen, L. The integration of respiratory therapy into nursing: reorganization for improved productivity. *Hospital and Health Services Administration* 32(3):369–77, Aug. 1987.

Wildman, G. Quality assurance information: developing actions and recommendations. *Journal of Quality Assurance* 10(4):21–24, Oct.–Nov. 1988.

Risk Management Department

Allen, P. *The Development of a Risk Management Program.* Ottawa, Ontario: Canadian Hospital Association, 1986.

Allen, P. Risk management program protects against financial loss. *Dimensions in Health Service* 63(5):24–25, June 1986.

Eubanks, P. Risk managers need clout. *Hospitals* 63(4):72, Feb. 1989.

Hathaway, G. E. Computerized documentation strengthens risk management. *Provider* 14(4):45, Apr. 1988.

Hospital Research and Educational Trust. *Managing Risks and Quality in Hospital-Sponsored Home Care.* Chicago: Institute on Quality of Care and Patterns of Practice, HRET, 1987.

Mason, B. C., and others. Risk management, quality assurance, and health care policy dilemmas. *Quality Assurance and Utilization Review* 4(2):49–55, May 1989.

McCue, P. Consultant services in quality assurance and risk management. *Applied Radiology* 17(11):23, 26, Nov. 1988.

McKerrow, W. The whys and hows of hospital risk management. *Health Law in Canada* 7(3):67–70, 91, 1987.

Micheletti, J., and others. Integrating risk management and quality assurance programs. *Contemporary Longterm Care* 11(11):79–83, Nov. 1988.

Orlikoff, J. E., and Vanagunas, A. M. *Malpractice Prevention and Liability Control for Hospitals,* 2nd ed. Chicago: American Hospital Publishing, 1988.

Penz, E. M. Integration of risk management and quality review. Part I: structure. *Journal of Quality Assurance* 10(3):14–15, Aug.–Sept. 1988.

Penz, E. M. Integration of risk management and quality review. Part II: outcomes. *Journal of Quality Assurance* 10(5):12–14, Dec. 1988–Jan. 1989.

Sanders, P. S. Risk management in practice. Maintaining defensible medical records. *Minnesota Medicine* 70(8):471, 473, Aug. 1987.

Shanahan, M. Confronting the software dilemma: specifications for a QA/RM information management system. *QRB: Quality Review Bulletin* 14(11):345–47, Nov. 1988.

Taravella, S. Active risk management. *Modern Healthcare* 19(20):32–34, 36–37, 42–44, May 19, 1989.

Social Services Department

American Hospital Association. *Proceedings of the Forum on Productivity Measurement in the Social Work Department.* Chicago: AHA, 1988.

Hubschman, L. *Hospital Social Work Practice.* New York City: Praeger, 1983.

Lurie, A., and Rosenberg, G., editors. *Social Work Administration in Health Care.* New York City: Haworth Press, 1984.

Thomas, A., and Domanski, M. Acuity-Based Productivity Monitoring System for a Hospital Social Work Department. AHA report no. MG20. Chicago: American Hospital Association, 1986.

Surgical Suite

Anonymous. Does optimal operating room utilization result in efficiency? *Osteopathic Hospital Leadership* 31(5):24, July–Aug. 1987.

Association of Operating Room Nurses. *AORN Operating Room Staffing Study.* Denver: AORN, 1985.

Association of Operating Room Nurses. *OR Management Anthology.* Denver: AORN, 1986.

Beitlek, K. Implementing Automation in the Operating Room: OR Bringing ORSOS™ on Line. AHA report no. OR24. Chicago: American Hospital Association, 1987.

Cowan, D. Improved productivity in the operating department—a challenge to management and designers alike. *Nursing RSA Verpleging* 2(10):14–19, 23, Oct. 1987.

Dreiser, K. J., Tamachunas, V. M., and McRobert, K. L. Variable Block Booking by Computer: A Demand-Based O.R. Case Scheduling Alternative. AHA report no. OR99. Chicago: American Hospital Association, 1987.

Ekbatani, S. F. Recovery Room Staffing Analysis Based on Patient Acuity. AHA report no. OR48. Chicago: American Hospital Association, 1986.

Falasco, P. R., and Eastaugh, N. A. Effective utilization of operating room services. *Health Matrix* 4(3):29–31, Fall 1986.

Karol, R. V., and Picard, N. Step by Step Structured Methodology for Productivity Improvement in the Operating Room. AHA report no. OR58. Chicago: American Hospital Association, 1986.

Little, M., editor. *Operating Room Risk Management, 1988.* Vols. 1 and 2. Plymouth Meeting, PA: ECRI, 1988.

Patterson, P. Mastering the fundamentals of OR productivity monitoring. *OR Manager* 2(2):1, 6–7, Feb. 1986.

Pitzer, M. E. Increasing productivity in the operating room with participative management. *Perioperative Nursing Quarterly* 3(2):19–21, June 1987.

Shevchik, P. S. F. Evaluation and Definition of the Surgery Department Personnel. AHA report no. OR57. Chicago: American Hospital Association, 1986.

Telecommunications Department

Chien, J., and Avila, M. E. *Assessing Your External Disaster Plan and Disaster Drills.* Los Angeles, CA: Hospital Council of Southern California, 1983.

Johnston, B. New "cures" for ailing communications. *Healthcare Computing and Communications* 5(7):43–44, July 1988.

Transportation Department

Bell, F. *Patient-Lifting Devices in Hospitals.* London: Croom Helm, 1984.

Schall, R. T. Increased productivity through a central transportation system. *Hospital Materiel Management Quarterly* 9(4):77–81, May 1988.